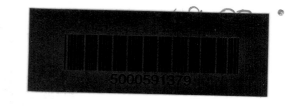

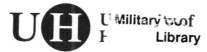

Magnetic Resonance Imaging
of Orthopedic Trauma

Magnetic Resonance Imaging of Orthopedic Trauma

Stephen J. Eustace, M.B., F.F.R. (R.C.S.I.)
Boston University School of Medicine
Boston Medical Center
Boston, Massachusetts

With 2 contributing authors

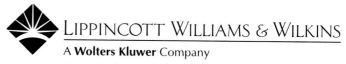

LIPPINCOTT WILLIAMS & WILKINS
A **Wolters Kluwer** Company
Philadelphia · Baltimore · New York · London
Buenos Aires · Hong Kong · Sydney · Tokyo

Acquisitions Editor: James Ryan
Developmental Editor: Delois Patterson
Manufacturing Manager: Tim Reynolds
Production Manager: Kathleen Bubbeo
Production Editor: Robin E. Cook
Cover Designer: Marsha Cohen
Indexer: Nancy Newman
Compositor: Maryland Composition
Printer: Courier Westford

Printed in the United States of America

9 8 7 6 5 4 3 2 1

Library of Congress Cataloging-in-Publication Data

Eustace, Stephen J.
    Magnetic resonance imaging of orthopedic trauma / Stephen J.
Eustace.
        p. cm.
    Includes bibliographical references and index.
    ISBN 0-412-15211-8
    1. Radiography in orthopedics.   2. Magnetic resonance imaging.
3. Musculoskeletal system—Wounds and injuries—Imaging.   4. Bones—
Wounds and injuries—Treatment.   I. Title.
    [DNLM: 1. Bone and Bones—injuries.   2. Bone and Bones—
radiography. WE 200E91m 1998]
RD734.5.R33E96 1998
616.7′ 107548—dc21
DNLM/DLC
for Library of Congress
                                                        98-27271
                                                            CIP

Muscoskeletal system - Radiography
                    "
diseases - Radiography

Care has been taken to confirm the accuracy of the information presented and to describe generally accepted practices. However, the authors, editors, and publisher are not responsible for errors or omissions or for any consequences from application of the information in this book and make no warranty, expressed or implied, with respect to the contents of the publication.

The authors, editors, and publisher have exerted every effort to ensure that drug selection and dosage set forth in this text are in accordance with current recommendations and practice at the time of publication. However, in view of ongoing research, changes in government regulations, and the constant flow of information relating to drug therapy and drug reactions, the reader is urged to check the package insert for each drug for any change in indications and dosage and for added warnings and precautions. This is particularly important when the recommended agent is a new or infrequently employed drug.

Some drugs and medical devices presented in this publication have Food and Drug Administration (FDA) clearance for limited use in restricted research settings. It is the responsibility of the health care provider to ascertain the FDA status of each drug or device planned for use in their clinical practice.

To my mother and father, to my daughters Sarah and Emma,
but above all, to Nicola, a million thanks. This is for you!

Contents

Contributors

Stephen J. Eustace, M.B., F.F.R. (R.C.S.I.) *Associate Professor of Radiology, Section Head of Musculoskeletal Radiology, Boston University School of Medicine and Boston Medical Center, 88 East Newton Street, Boston, Massachusetts 02118*

Hernan H. Jara, Ph.D. *Associate Professor of Radiology, Section Head of Radiologic Physics, Boston University School of Medicine and Boston Medical Center, 88 East Newton Street, Boston, Massachusetts 02118*

Elias R. Melhem, M.D. *Assistant Professor of Radiology, Section Head of Neuroradiology, Boston University School of Medicine and Boston Medical Center, 88 East Newton Street, Boston, Massachusetts 02118*

Illustrations:

Matthew DiMasi, M.D. *Radiology Resident, Boston University School of Medicine and Boston Medical Center, 88 East Newton Street, Boston, Massachusetts 02118*

Proofreader:

Adel Assaf, M.D., F.R.C.P. *Assistant Professor of Radiology, Department of Musculoskeletal Radiology, McGill University Health Centres, 1650 Cedar Avenue, Montreal, Quebec H3G 1A4, Canada*

Foreword

Magnetic resonance imaging (MRI) in the musculoskeletal system was first applied as a replacement for less satisfactory examinations, such as polytomography and arthrography. It demonstrated similar ranges of disease with better accuracy for the physician and greater comfort for the patient. Newer applications of this maturing technology are being developed to study diseases for which there has been no previous role for diagnostic imaging. In the musculoskeletal system, the cutting edge has become acute trauma. Although other modalities are sufficient to demonstrate fractures and dislocations, MRI is without peer in demonstrating the soft tissue and the less dramatic bone and joint components of trauma. The diagnosis and treatment of these elements of musculoskeletal injury may prove to be as important in restoring health and function as fixing fractures and reducing dislocations. As the medical, social, and economic advantages of precise and timely diagnosis in the setting of acute trauma become more apparent, the use of MRI in this setting can be expected to increase rapidly. This book is a pragmatic and comprehensive guide to this new territory.

The book begins with a description of the basic principles of MRI and how it differs from conventional radiography and computed tomography. This is followed by two chapters describing more advanced techniques for generating MR images and the pragmatic application of these techniques to the musculoskeletal system in clinical settings using standard equipment. The final introductory chapter explains the basis of musculoskeletal MR image interpretation, with correlation to clinical setting, anatomy, and physiology, biomechanics of injury mechanisms, and physiological responses to injury. The remaining eight chapters are organized by region and include the foot and ankle, the knee, the pelvis and hip, the cervical spine, the thoracolumbar spine, the shoulder, the elbow, and the wrist and hand. Each chapter has an overview of special considerations of patient positioning and imaging protocols unique to the region, including detailed, suggested protocols for addressing specific clinical concerns. The clinical aspects of trauma that are unique to the anatomic region are described and specific types of injuries to bones, joints, and soft tissues are discussed and illustrated. Correlation and comparison to other modalities of imaging are frequent, placing the current and potential role of MRI in context.

I have known Stephen Eustace for a number of years. He has become one of our specialty's acknowledged experts on this timely topic. This book is a complete work, reflecting the author's vision, energy, and diligence. The book is a scholarly exposition on the state of the art of MRI in musculoskeletal trauma, presented in the guise of a practical clinical guide, enhancing one's conceptual understanding while helping one obtain diagnostic images. The book is not only useful for practicing radiologists, but also for emergency room physicians and orthopedic trauma surgeons. It is a masterful effort for which I congratulate the author.

Felix S. Chew M.D.
Professor of Radiology
Wake Forest University School of Medicine
Winston-Salem, North Carolina

Foreword

Magnetic resonance imaging (MRI) has changed the practice of medicine perhaps more than any other medical technology developed over the past quarter of a century. Not only are physicians now able to view images of the body and distinguish organs and tissues based on their chemical makeup, but the field has evolved to the point where MRI can be used to facilitate real-time interventional medicine. The physician can watch what he or she is doing with the kind of visual image never before possible.

When first introduced, MRI was embraced by the medical community, and no one hesitated to use it even before they understood its scientific basis or its true diagnostic potential. In large measure, this is still true today. However, armed with educational materials such as this volume, these issues should be brought into clearer view, at least for the orthopedic trauma surgeon. In this handsome, well-illustrated text, Stephen Eustace and colleagues have assembled a series of chapters that provide an exceptionally clear and well-organized approach to the subject. The book begins with a thorough and understandable presentation of the physics of MRI and then applies this fundamental information to all of the important musculoskeletal tissues, including bone, cartilage, synovium, and marrow. The images are exceptionally clear and the text includes important tips on how radiologists or radiology technicians can enhance the clarity of their own images, such as in the evaluation of postoperative patients who have had hardware implanted to stabilize their fractures.

The chapters are ordered to present, in sequence, the events that the clinician experiences when caring for the orthopedic trauma patient. This begins with a discussion of patient positioning and imaging protocols and then describes the images of soft tissues even before osseous structures are reviewed. This unique approach makes a lot of sense, as this is the way these injured tissues should be approached from a clinical perspective.

The book also contains valuable discussions of topics in MRI that have never before been so clearly presented. These include the use of advanced techniques such as fast imaging, MR-based arthrography, and angiography. The organization of the chapters around anatomical structures or regions helps the reader to understand how this new information and these new technologies are differentially effective in aiding the clinician with diagnostic challenges and preoperative planning strategies. The use of black and white images and line drawings, including fracture classifications, is a particularly effective way of presenting the information. The material is easy to understand and remember.

The contributors to this book deserve both our congratulations and thanks. With this new knowledge and information it should be possible for us to render more rapid and effective orthopedic care to those who have sustained musculoskeletal injuries. Equally as important, it will enhance the preparation of a future generation of clinicians who will be caring for orthopedic trauma patients.

Thomas A. Einhorn, M.D.
Chairman, Department of Orthopedics
Boston University School of Medicine
Boston Medical Center
Boston, Massachusetts

Preface

Irishmen Colles and Smith are credited with the early clinical descriptions of distal radial fractures in the late eighteenth and early nineteenth centuries. Although these descriptions are founded on clinical examination alone, they have endured the test of time; despite advanced imaging, they are still widely employed in clinical practice. Such descriptions emphasize osseous injury alone, however, and overlook the potential impact of concomitant injury to adjacent soft tissues. Therefore, traditional orthopedic repair of distal radial fractures, similar to fractures at other sites, has been confined to repair of osseous injury alone, and persistent morbidity in many patients has remained unexplained.

Although magnetic resonance imaging (MRI) has revolutionized both radiology and orthopedics, allowing noninvasive evaluation of both bone and soft tissues, its use in patients following orthopedic trauma has been limited by cost, availability, and the constraints of time. Decreased imaging cost incurred by current rapid imaging, paralleled by wider availability of hardware now being deployed adjacent to emergency or trauma rooms, threatens to alter current practices, despite the stranglehold of insurers. Anticipating such changes, this volume outlines both accepted and evolving uses of MRI in trauma. This book reviews basic physics principles of MRI, emphasizing a clinical rather than an academic understanding; reviews newly developed fast-imaging techniques; and describes practical applications, protocols, and diagnostic appearances encountered following acute trauma.

Stephen J. Eustace

Acknowledgments

I offer particular thanks to J. T. Ferrucci, chairman of the Department of Radiology at Boston University School of Medicine and Boston Medical Center, a continual source of inspiration and guidance. He is the ultimate mentor. I thank all my colleagues, including Kent Yucel, Oliver Pomeroy, Matt Barish, Victor DeCarvalho, Sid Pollack, Dan O'Connor, Ewa Kuligowska, Peter Clarke, Richard Tello, and Helen Fenlon, for support.

Special thanks are offered to Bill Buff, Dan Williamson, Esterbrook Longmaid, and all the radiologists and radiographers in the Mater Misericordiae Hospital, Dublin, Ireland, where my career began.

Thanks are offered to all the technologists and staff in MRI at Boston Medical Center, including Teresa, Bethann, Peter, Rafael, Todd, Lisa, Rick, Julie, Soren, and Cruz; to Ginette, PeeWee, and David in photography.

Last, but not least, thanks are extended to my coauthors Hernan Jara and Elias Melhem for their efforts, to Matt Dimasi for beautiful illustrations, to Steve Valentine and Art Newberg for images, to Adel Assaf who proofread and advised on all chapters, to William Conn at Lunar, to Deane Witney at Phillips, and finally to the editorial and publishing staff at Lippincott Williams & Wilkins.

CHAPTER 1

Basic Principles of Magnetic Resonance Imaging

Hernan H. Jara and Stephen J. Eustace

Magnetic resonance imaging (MRI) is a technique in which images are computer generated from data obtained from two separate methods: the nuclear magnetic resonance (NMR) induction method and the spatial encoding method. These combined NMR induction–spatial encoding methods are known generically as MRI pulse sequences. The great majority of MRI pulse sequences used in clinical practice are designed to probe the most abundant form of nuclear magnetization found in biological tissues, that of the hydrogen nuclei (protons) present in the organs of a patient who is immersed in a strong magnetic field. Because the magnitude of this particular form of nuclear magnetism is proportional to the local density of protons, the fundamental delineation of organs in clinical MRI reflects the relative concentrations of protons among the tissues in the imaging section.

In practice, the application of an MRI pulse sequence is a cyclic process during which the sample is exposed to a semirepetitive series of brief bursts of resonant radiowave energy (radiofrequency or RF pulses) and of brief magnetic

field perturbations (position-tagging gradient pulses). The duration of each pulse sequence cycle is known as the repetition time and is universally denoted by TR. Every cycle of the pulse sequence begins with an RF pulse the purpose of which is to initiate the NMR signal; this is referred to as the excitation pulse. The measurement of the NMR signal is performed a certain time after the excitation pulse, at an operator-adjustable time that is referred to as the echo time (TE). The position-tagging pulses are accommodated between the time of excitation and TE.

The MRI pulse sequences may be viewed as streams of RF pulses, magnetic field gradient pulses, and time spacings between these pulses. The pulses, which are transmitted in four channels—one RF signal generation channel and three spatial encoding channels—are arranged in time according to rules compatible with NMR physics, spatial encoding physics, and the desired scan properties (contrast weighting, spatial resolution, anatomic coverage, image orientation, artifact reduction techniques). The RF and gradient pulses may be used in innumerable combinations, thus leading to a confusingly large number of possible MRI pulse sequences. The three most important criteria useful in the categorization of MRI pulse sequences are: (a) the type(s) of NMR signal acquired, (b) the combination of spatial encoding methods used, and (c) whether one or several differently encoded

---

H. H. Jara: Department of Radiology, Section of Radiologic Physics, Boston University School of Medicine and Boston Medical Center, Boston, Massachusetts 02118.

S. J. Eustace: Department of Radiology, Section of Musculoskeletal Radiology, Boston University School of Medicine and Boston Medical Center, Boston, Massachusetts 02118.

signals are acquired per sequence cycle: i.e., conventional versus hybrid pulse sequences.

PRINCIPLES OF MAGNETIC RESONANCE IMAGING

Magnetic resonance images are made of picture elements (pixels), each of which is assigned a brightness that is proportional to the amount of magnetization present at that location in the patient, at the time of measurement. Pixels are displayed adjacent to each other to form a two-dimensional gray-scale shaded map of the spatial distribution of proton magnetization in the selected imaging slice. Each pixel represents a small volume of tissue(s) known as the imaging voxel, or simply voxel. The size, the shape, the location, and the image intensity of the voxels are determined during the application of the pulse sequence from several patient-emitted NMR signals with different spatial encodings (Fig. 1).

Nuclear Magnetic Resonance Induction Method

Because soft tissues contain very large numbers of protons per unit volume, it is customary to describe their magnetic properties at a macroscopic level. To this end, the (macro-

scopic) magnetization is defined the vector sum of all the magnetic moments contained in a unit volume. It represents the magnetic polarization inside a material when it is immersed in a magnetic field. In the absence of external stimuli, the magnetization generated in the organs of a patient by a homogeneous magnetic field is referred to as equilibrium longitudinal magnetization because it does not change in time and is parallel to, and in the same direction as the parent magnetic field. The equilibrium longitudinal magnetization is a vector that has a magnitude and a direction, and although the direction is constant throughout the patient, the magnitude may change from location to location because tissues may differ in their proton content, thus leading to the concept of volumetric distribution of equilibrium longitudinal magnetization inside a magnetized patient (Figs. 2 and 3).

In the NMR induction method, the longitudinal magnetization, which is not directly detectable, is transformed into detectable transverse magnetization by absorption of a burst of radiowaves at the resonance (Larmor) frequency, the value of which is proportional to magnetic field strength. The burst of resonant radiowaves is known as the RF excitation pulse, and its net effect is to rotate the longitudinal magnetization, thus removing it from the equilibrium value (Fig. 4). The angle by which the longitudinal magnetization

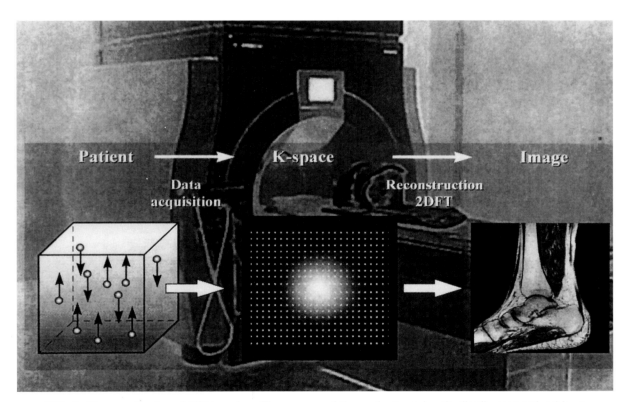

FIG. 1. The mechanics of MR imaging. The organs of the patient are longitudinally magnetized by a very strong and homogeneous magnetic field. An imaging pulse sequence is applied, thus generating detectable transverse magnetization. The generated NMR signals are spatially encoded before measurement and stored in computer memory. The resulting raw data are not visually interpretable because they are scrambled during the application of the MRI pulse sequence by the spatial encoding pulses. The raw data, which are referred to as k-space data, are computer reconstructed, thus generating the anatomic image.

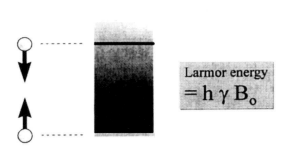

Larmor energy

$$= h \gamma B_o$$

B_0

FIG. 2. Magnetic resonance Larmor energy equation. The Larmor equation states that the energy of a magnetic moment that is aligned antiparallel to the magnetic field is higher than the energy of a magnetic moment aligned parallel to the magnetic field. It further states that the energy difference is proportional to the product of the strength of the magnetic field, the gyromagnetic ratio, and Planck's constant. This energy is important in MRI for two reasons: (a) it is the resonant energy for the excitation RF pulse, and (b) it is proportional to the frequency of precession of the magnetic moments after excitation. Hence, the frequency of precession and therefore the signal are proportional to the magnetic field, a property used to encode the signal by means of magnetic field gradients.

is rotated, known as the flip angle, is proportional to the energy of the RF excitation pulse and therefore can be easily controlled by adjustment of the RF power delivered to the transmit coil. In general, an RF pulse with arbitrary flip angle is possible, thus transforming pure longitudinal magnetization into a combination of longitudinal and transverse magnetization components. Following the application of the excitatory pulse, both the transverse and longitudinal components return to the equilibrium state in a process generating

an MR signal (Fig. 5). The motion induced by recovery may be described as a gyration on the surface of a cone that collapses rapidly onto the longitudinal axis, followed by a slower one-dimensional recovery about the longitudinal axis toward the positive equilibrium value. The gyrational portion of this motion is known as Larmor precession and is characterized by a relaxation time T2*. The one-dimensional portion is known as recovery of longitudinal magnetization and is characterized by a recovery time T1 (Fig. 6).

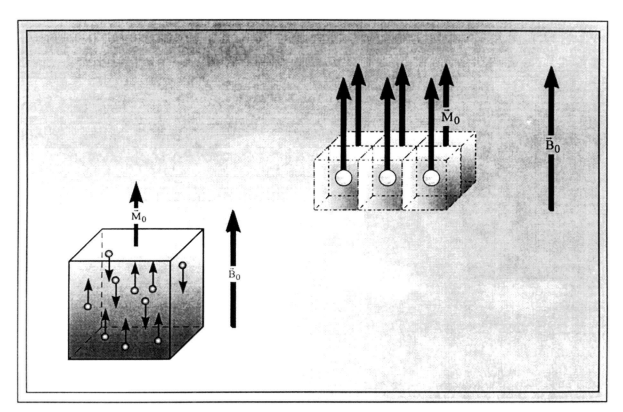

FIG. 3. Equilibrium longitudinal magnetization. The equilibrium longitudinal magnetization *M* represents the response of a tissue to an external magnetic field B_0 at a macroscopic level. Specifically, it is defined as the sum of individual magnetic moments contained in a unit volume. Because the sum includes the parallel as well as the antiparallel magnetic moments, which cancel each other, the equilibrium longitudinal magnetization of a tissue at room temperature is small. For this reason, MRI is viewed as a low-sensitivity imaging modality.

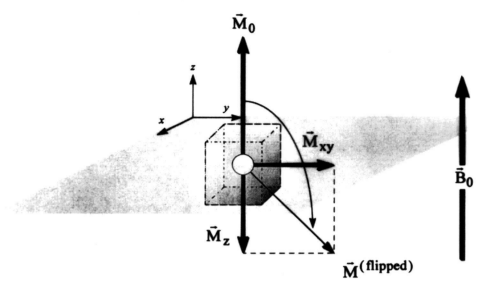

FIG. 4. Separation of flipped magnetization into transverse and longitudinal components. Magnetization that has been flipped away from the positive longitudinal equilibrium value M_0 can be decomposed into two orthogonal components termed the transverse magnetization (M_{xy}) and the longitudinal component (M_z). The angle by which an RF pulse flips the equilibrium magnetization is proportional to the energy contained in the excitation. In principle, any flip angle is possible; the effect of a 145° pulse is used in this hypothetical example because it generates transverse and longitudinal components of equal magnitudes.

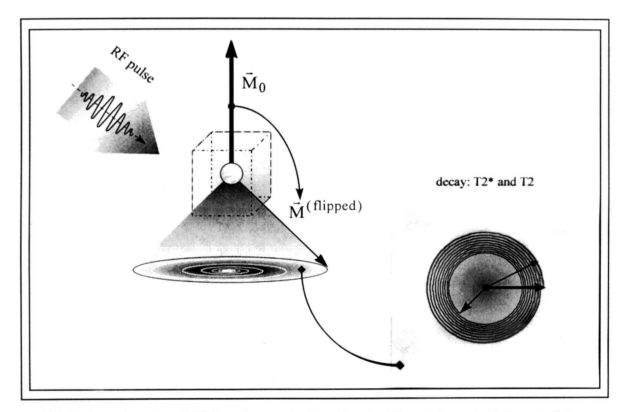

FIG. 5. Dynamic motion of RF-flipped magnetization. After the RF excitation pulse is turned off, the flipped magnetization moves on the surface of a cone that collapses toward the longitudinal axis. The speed at which the cone collapses is inversely proportional to the T2* (FID) or T2 (spin-echo) of the tissue. Viewed from below, the tip of the transverse magnetization describes a spiral curve. Signal is generated for as long as the transverse magnetization is nonzero or, equivalently, for as long as the cone remains open.

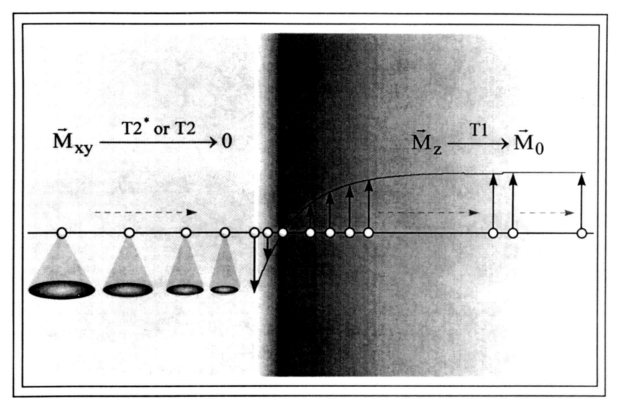

FIG. 6. Flipped magnetization returns to equilibrium, T2 decay and T1 recovery. For most tissues, the transverse magnetization component returns to its null equilibrium value much faster than the longitudinal component returns to the positive M_0 value. Because of the large disparity between the short T2 and the longer T1 values observed in most tissues, MRI signals are available for measurement for only a small fraction of the time during which the pulse sequence is applied. For this reason, conventional MRI pulse sequences are inherently slow.

In general, any transverse magnetization component generated during a pulse sequence rotates freely in the transverse plane and simultaneously decreases in amplitude at a rate that is tissue dependent, a phenomenon known generically as T2* decay. Because of the rotational motion, the angle or phase between the transverse magnetization vector and a fixed reference direction increases continually in time. Most important to MRI, the rate at which the phase changes, namely the Larmor frequency of precession, is a linear function of the "instantaneous" magnetic field value at the specific position of the transverse magnetization. If for any reason the local value of the magnetic field changes, the Larmor frequency of precession changes proportionally and instantly. It is this magnetic field-tracking property of the Larmor frequency of precession that is used to encode spatially the transverse magnetization distribution inside the patient in three spatial dimensions. Spatial encoding is accomplished in MRI with pulsed magnetic field gradients that alter the magnetic field distribution inside the patient in known linear patterns for brief periods of time.

Nuclear Magnetic Resonance Signals

An NMR signal is a voltage induced in a receiver coil by the transverse magnetization sum corresponding to all the tissues excited by the RF pulses. The signal-contributing tissues are typically contained in a thin slice (two-dimensional imaging) or thicker slab (three-dimensional imaging) of the patient. The time dynamics of NMR signals and that of the transverse magnetization distributions they represent are closely related. Because the time dynamics of transverse magnetization is that of a free precession in two dimensions that is accompanied by a comparatively fast amplitude reduction rapidly approaching zero (generically known as T2* decay), NMR signals simultaneously oscillate and decay in time. The principal mechanism by which NMR signals decay in time is loss of phase synchronicity or phase coherence among the individual contributors to the signal, which are known as transverse magnetization isochromats or simply isochromats. Two isochromats at positions differing in magnetic field value will gyrate at different frequencies, thus losing phase coherence. In other words, T2* signal decay is predominantly caused by the magnetic field inhomogeneities inside the patient, a phenomenon secondary to the magnetic field-tracking property of the Larmor frequency. Furthermore, the rate of signal decay (1/T2*) is a function of the homogeneity of the magnetic field in the patient: the more inhomogeneous, the faster the decay rate, or, equivalently, the shorter the T2* value. The different contributions to the final inhomogeneity of the magnetic field distribution inside a patient are (a) imperfections in the main magnetic field, (b) macroscopic field variations caused by differences in the magnetic response (susceptibility) of organs and cavities in the body, and (c) microscopic field fluctuations caused at any given site by the neighboring atoms and molecules. Of these, the former two contributions are constant in time and may therefore be alleviated by an applied 180° pulse inherent in the spin-echo pulse sequence. In the standard terminology, the relaxation time associated with the so-called free induction decay signal (FID) is T2*, and the comparatively longer relaxation time associated with spin echoes that are RF-rephased is referred to as T2.

In summary, the number of pulses in the RF channel determines the type of NMR signal generated. The simplest pulse sequence uses only one RF pulse per TR cycle and generates an FID signal that decays rapidly in time. Next, the spin-echo pulse sequence uses two RF pulses, a 90° excitation followed by a 180° refocusing pulse, to generate spin-echo signals in which the dephasing effects of static magnetic field inhomogeneities have been compensated. Furthermore, when spatial encoding is incorporated into NMR pulse sequences, MRI pulse sequences are obtained. Those MRI pulse sequences using one RF pulse per TR cycle are referred to as fast field-echo (FFE) or gradient echo (GE) pulse sequences, designations that are manufacturer specific. Those MRI pulse sequences based on the SE principle are referred to as conventional spin-echo (CSE), a designation adopted by all major manufacturers.

Spatial Encoding Methods

Magnetic field gradients are spatially inhomogeneous magnetic fields, the strength of which increases at a constant rate in a given direction in space. The rate of change of magnetic field gradients is commonly expressed in milli-Teslas per meter (mT/m), and MRI scanners are equipped with three gradient coils, which are connected to gradient amplifiers that supply electric power. Collectively, such an imaging subsystem is capable of generating magnetic field gradients along each of the three main orthogonal directions by energizing one gradient coil at a time or any oblique direction by energizing two or more gradient coils simultaneously.

Three different spatial encoding methods based on magnetic field gradient pulses can be used to partition the volumetric magnetization field existing inside the patient in any desired direction. These methods, known as slice selection (SS), phase-encoding (PE) signal preparation, and frequency-encoding (FE) signal measurement, are used in one combination or another in all MRI pulse sequences to partition the volumetric magnetization field in three orthogonal directions. In the most common combination of these three methods, known as two-dimensional (2D) Fourier-transform imaging, (a) a slice is selected with the SS method, (b) the slice is phase-encoded (PE) along one of the two in-plane directions, and finally, (c) it is frequency-encoded (FE) in the remaining orthogonal in-plane direction. Although phase-encoding preparation is performed before the measurement of the NMR signal, frequency encoding is performed as the signal is acquired and digitized. This three-stage process is repeated sequentially, varying only the degree of phase encoding in every cycle, for a total number of cycles equal to the desired number of pixels in the PE direction (Fig. 7).

Although the SS, PE, and FE methods rely on the magnetic field-tracking property of the Larmor frequency, they are conceptually and practically different from each other. With the SS method, the volumetric magnetization field is partitioned in one direction at the time of excitation. The SS method uses two pulses that are applied simultaneously: a gradient pulse that alters linearly the Larmor resonance condition in one direction and an RF pulse with a limited frequency content (bandwidth). The net effect of this combination of pulses, when applied simultaneously, is to selectively excite only those tissues contained inside a thin slice oriented orthogonal to the direction of the gradient where the resonance condition is satisfied. The SS approach is a direct imaging method because the data generated can be viewed directly and do not need computer reconstruction. On the other hand, PE and FE are indirect spatial encoding methods in which the isochromats are made spatially distinguishable by phase and frequency, respectively, and are made identifiable by inverse Fourier transformation. With the PE method, a linear phase spread in one direction of the field of view (FOV) is imprinted on the magnetization field by applying a gradient pulse some time between RF excitation and signal measurement. With the FE method, a linear frequency spread

FIG. 7. **(A)** Gradient-echo pulse sequence diagram. A free-induction decay signal is formed following the application of the 90° excitation pulse. The diagram includes the radiofrequency (RF), the slice-select (SS), the phase-encode signal preparation (PE), and the frequency-encode (FE) signal measurement channels. To simulate the T2* decay, a *bar* with gray-scale shading has been included at the bottom. **(B)** Spin-echo pulse sequence diagram. A free-induction decay signal is formed following the application of the 90° excitation pulse. Because of the dephasing effects of magnetic field inhomogeneities, the FID decays comparatively fast in time. The signal is partially recovered following the application of a refocusing 180° RF pulse, which generates a Hahn spin-echo signal, which is used for imaging. The diagram includes the radiofrequency (RF), the slice-select (SS), the phase-encode (PE) signal preparation, and the frequency-encode signal measurement (FE) channels. The gray-scale *shaded bar* included at the bottom illustrates the time evolution of the FID and the spin-echo signals.

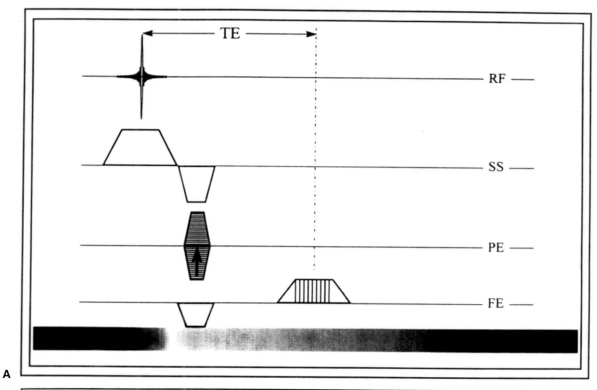

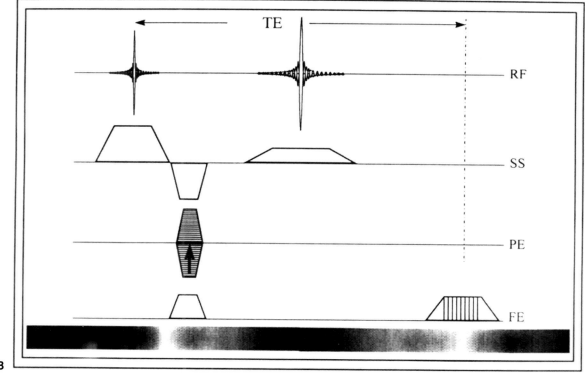

is imprinted on the magnetization field along the remaining orthogonal direction of the FOV. In practice, this is accomplished by applying a gradient pulse with constant amplitude in that direction during the measurement of the spatially encoded signal. The PE and FE methods are most commonly implemented as Fourier methods that generate Fourier-transformed raw data, which in turn require a one-dimensional inverse Fourier transformation in each direction to produce the anatomic image. With Fourier encoding methods, the dimension of the voxel along each direction is inversely proportional to the area under the waveform of the gradient pulse. A gradient waveform is a plot of the gradient strength (mT/m) as a function of time. For a given pulse duration and maximum gradient strength, the maximum-area waveform is rectangular in shape. Because the maximum gradient strength that any scanner can produce is limited, the rectangular gradient waveform is the theoretic ideal shape for efficient use of the gradient capability of the system.

In summary, to generate an MR image—that is, a spatially resolved map of the tissue magnetizations in a two-dimensional section of the body—the transverse magnetization field must first be position-tagged or, equivalently, spatially encoded in three orthogonal directions. Additionally, a tagging reversal technique for determining the local values of the transverse magnetization (spatial decoding) is necessary. Whereas spatial encoding is accomplished with a combination of the SS, PE, and FE encoding methods described above, spatial decoding results from computer postprocessing of the raw spatially encoded data, a process known as image reconstruction. The raw data generated by most pulse sequences used in clinical practice are encoded in such a manner that if displayed in image format, they are not directly interpretable. This is because the raw data have been separated into frequency and phase components by a mathematical procedure called Fourier transformation during the application of the pulse sequence. As a consequence, in order to generate an anatomic image, the raw data must be inverse-Fourier transformed. The raw data and the anatomic image are two representations of the transverse magnetization field in different spaces: the geometric image space and the frequency–phase raw data space. In the standard physics terminology, the Fourier codomain of the image space is referred to as k-space.

Contrast Weighting and Magnetization Dynamics in Tissues (T1, T2*, and T2)

Although the longitudinal and the transverse magnetizations are two components of the same physical property, namely the vector sum of all the magnetic moments contained in a unit volume of tissue, the two vector components change very differently in time when removed from their respective equilibrium values: positive for the longitudinal component and zero for the transverse component. Although the time dynamics of longitudinal magnetization is that of a relatively slow one-dimensional recovery toward the posi-

TABLE 1. *Nuclear magnetic resonance relaxation times of human tissues*

Tissue	T1 @ 4.1 T(*) (msec)	T1 @ 1.5 T (msec)	T1 @ 0.5 T (msec)	T2 (msec)
Adipose		260	215	84
Liver		490	323	43
Kidney		650	449	58
Spleen		780	554	62
White matter	833.9 ± 23.7	790	539	92
Muscle		870	600	47
Gray matter	1,281.7 ± 42.6	920	656	101
Blood		1,000		600
CSF	3,285.6 ± 331.8	4,000	4,000	2,000

tive equilibrium value (T1 recovery), the time dynamics of transverse magnetization is that of a free precession in two dimensions that is accompanied by a comparatively fast amplitude reduction rapidly approaching the zero value (generically known as T2* decay). Furthermore, except in the case of simple bodily fluids such as CSF and bile, for which the longitudinal and transverse time scales of return to equilibrium are comparable, for most soft tissues the return to equilibrium of the longitudinal component is approximately tenfold faster than the return of the transverse component to its null equilibrium value. Most important to diagnostic imaging is the fact that the characteristic rates at which the longitudinal magnetization recovers and the transverse magnetization amplitude decays in time are functions of the microscopic spatial distribution of the magnetic field inside the tissues, and consequently, these characteristic rates depend on the molecular structure of the tissues. The NMR relaxation times of selected human tissues are outlined in Table 1.

THE ARCHITECTURE OF THE MRI SCANNER

The architecture of an MRI scanner may be described in terms of the functions it must perform. The basic functions and the associated components are (a) to magnetize the patient (the magnet), (b) to generate and to apply pulses (pulse sequence software/hardware, amplifiers, and coils), (c) to collect the raw data (coils and receivers), (d) to Fourier-reconstruct the images (array processor), and (e) to display and to archive the images (host computer) (Fig. 8).

Magnetic Field Generation

Before imaging can be performed, the patient must be magnetized, ideally with a very strong, very stable, and extremely homogeneous magnetic field. The strength of a magnetic field is measured in Tesla (T) in the metric International System (SI) of units. The most common whole-body magnets found in clinical practice generate magnetic fields with the following strengths: 1.5 T, 1.0 T, and 0.5 T, but fields of up to 4.0 T have been demonstrated. In comparison, the

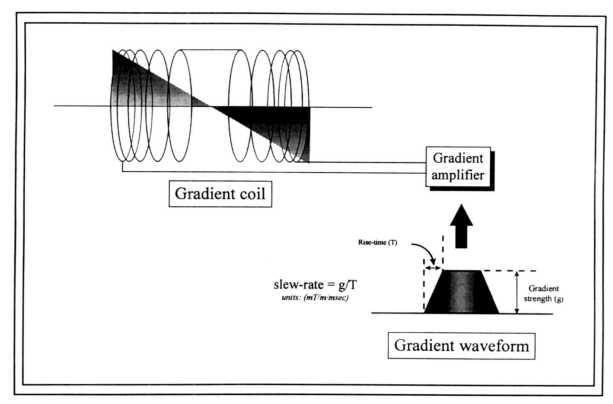

FIG. 8. Generation of magnetic field gradients. The figure shows schematically the wiring of a coil that generates a magnetic field that increases linearly in one direction in space. This linear magnetic field is known as a gradient. The MRI scanners are equipped with three coils that generate magnetic field gradients along the three orthogonal directions in space. Gradients are applied to the patient for finite periods of time, which are generally very short; hence the concept of gradient pulses. The most efficient and therefore the most common way to apply magnetic field gradients in time is with time waveforms that are of trapezoidal shape. The area underneath the gradient waveforms of the PE and FE pulses is inversely proportional to the corresponding voxel dimension. All the gradient waveforms in a pulse sequence are computer generated and transmitted to the digital inputs of the corresponding gradient amplifier, which in turn energizes the gradient coil for the duration of the pulse.

Earth's magnetic field (approximately 50 μT) is 10,000 to 80,000 times weaker. High-field magnets use a large and powerful superconducting coil that is immersed in a bath of liquid helium to keep the wire of the coil at a very low temperature (approximately 4.2°K). At this temperature the wire is in the so-called superconducting state in which there are no resistive electric losses, and consequently, the magnet remains energized permanently. The superconducting coils are close solenoids that are positioned horizontally, thus generating a horizontally oriented magnetic field (Fig. 9). The patient is inserted inside the bore of the magnet, which is the cylindrical hollow cavity of the superconducting coil, where the magnetic field is most intense and homogeneous (typically, magnetic variations are less than 10 parts per million). Other magnet designs include permanent magnets and resistive electromagnets. Permanent magnets consist of two plates of highly magnetized material and opposed polarity. In these magnets, which do not consume electric power, the magnetic field is vertical, and the maximum strength is limited to about 0.3 T. Magnetic resonance imaging scanners

based on resistive electromagnet designs are rare. These use water-cooled resistive coils made with copper or aluminum wire and consume between 50 and 100 kW of electric power. The maximum magnetic field strength resistive magnet designs can generate is limited by heat generation to approximately 0.5 T.

To further improve the homogeneity of the main magnetic field, MRI scanners are equipped with a shim system, which in general consists of a set of iron sheets and special shim coils wound on the surface of the bore tube. Shim systems are energized by a separate set of power supplies and may be active or passive.

Pulse Sequence Generation and Delivery

As described above, MRI pulse sequences consist of four separate streams of pulses or pulse sequence channels. These streams of pulses are electrically transmitted during the scan, from the pulse sequence controller to the RF and gradient coils, via appropriate amplifiers, which supply the necessary

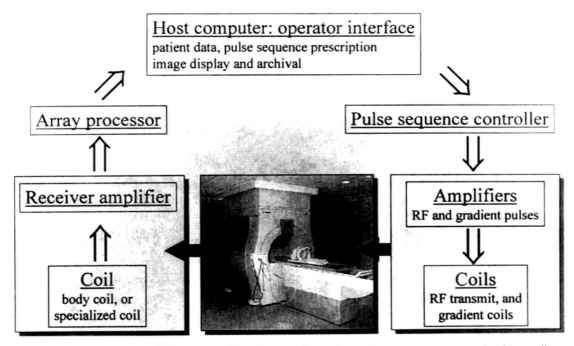

FIG. 9. Architecture of an MRI scanner. The diagram shows the main components, organized according to function. Also shown is the pathway followed by operator commands, pulse sequences, and image data. The imaging subsystem **(right)** consists of amplifiers (RF and gradients), the excitation RF coil, and the gradient coils used to encode the signals. The detection subsystem **(left)** consists of the receiver coil and the hardware involved in the signal amplification pathway.

electrical energy. Special purpose coils are positioned in the bore of the magnet around the patient: RF coils to generate and to detect the NMR signals and a set of three separate gradient coils to generate the pulsed magnetic field gradients used for three-dimensional spatial encoding.

Radiofrequency coils are specialized antennas that can convert an electric current into electromagnetic radiowaves when used in transmit mode or, conversely, convert electromagnetic waves into electric currents when used in receive mode. The pulse sequence stream of RF pulses is delivered to the patient by transmit coils, which produce a very homogeneous and precise radiowave field in the patient, thus generating NMR signals from all the organs excited. The emerging NMR signals are detected collectively with the so-called receive coil. The RF coils vary in size and shape. Most scanners are equipped with a large, nonremovable coil known as the body coil. In principle the same coil may be used for the transmit and the receive functions. However, in high-spatial-resolution applications, the receive function is handled by a smaller receive coil that may be positioned closer to the imaged organs, thus affording images with improved signal-to-noise ratio.

Gradient coils consist of wires wound on the surface of a cylinder that is positioned parallel to and inside the bore of the magnet. The geometry of the wire windings is such that when the coil is electrically energized, a magnetic field that increases linearly in one direction (gradient magnetic

field) is generated. A simplified diagram of a coil that generates a magnetic field gradient parallel to the main axis of the magnet is shown in Fig. 9. The overall imaging flexibility afforded by a modern MRI scanner in terms of achievable spatial resolution and imaging speed is mostly limited by the gradient capabilities of the imaging subsystem. The gradient capabilities are commonly quantified by two figures of merit, namely, the maximum gradient strength and the slew rate. As the name implies, the maximum gradient strength is the strongest gradient the subsystem can generate. The slew rate is a measure of both the rise time to maximum (rise time) and the gradient strength of the system, which is measured in milli-Teslas per meter per millisecond. In the last few years, the figures of merit for the typical clinical MRI scanner have improved from gradients of 10 mT/m with a slew rate of 20 mT/m per msec to 25 mT/m with a slew rate of 100 mT/m per msec.

Data Acquisition and Reconstruction

The electric signals generated in the receiver coil during the scan are amplified, digitized, and stored in computer memory. The digital data are then sent to the array processor, which is a computer designed to perform digital Fourier transformations at the highest speed. The fastest array processors currently available can reconstruct 20 images per second, each with 256 × 256 matrix size. This figure is likely to improve as computer technology evolves continually.

IMAGE PROPERTIES

In the end, the utility of any medical image should be assessed in terms of the diagnostic power afforded by the information it contains. Although the concept of diagnostic power is observer dependent and therefore to some extent subjective, image quality may be judged on more quantitative grounds. In this regard, one must consider image spatial resolution, contrast resolution, signal to noise, and, finally, the practical issue of acquisition time.

Spatial Resolution

The spatial resolution of an MR image refers to the fineness with which the volumetric distribution of transverse magnetization is partitioned by the pulse sequence. It is a measure of the technique's (resolving) power to separate spatially the small structures and the fine detail features present in the imaged object. Spatial resolution is inversely related to voxel size and therefore spatial resolution improvements result from reductions in either the slice thickness (SS direction) or in any of the in-plane voxel dimensions along the PE or FE directions (Fig. 10).

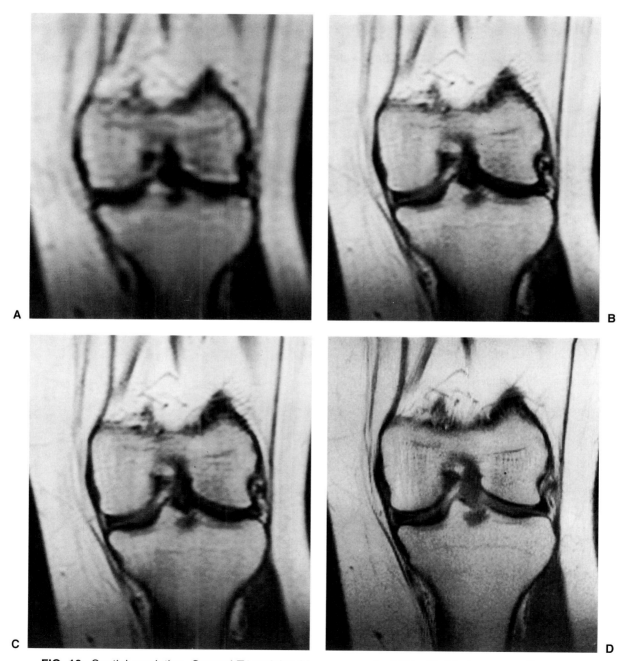

FIG. 10. Spatial resolution. Coronal T1-weighted images acquired **(A)** with 64 phase-encoding steps, **(B, C)** with 128 phase-encoding steps, and **(D)** with 256 phase-encoding steps.

Most 2D pulse sequences produce voxels in which the SS dimension is several times longer than the PE and FE dimensions. When voxels with more isotropic dimensions are desired, this is better achieved with three dimensional (3D) pulse sequences, which use phase encoding along two directions and frequency encoding in the remaining third, i.e., make use of a (PE, PE, FE) combination.

Each of the in-plane voxel dimensions is directly calculated as the ratio of the field of view and the matrix size in the corresponding direction. For instance, the voxel size in the frequency-encoding direction is a function of the image field of view and of the number of frequency-encoding steps, with an otherwise identical equation applicable for the phase-encoding directions.

Two different methods may be used to decrease an in-plane voxel dimension: (a) to decrease the FOV while maintaining fixed matrix size, referred to as the "zoom" technique in analogy with the photography terminology, or (b) to increase matrix size while maintaining a fixed FOV. Assuming that no other pulse sequence parameter is changed, the zoom technique leads to higher spatial resolution at the expense of coverage, whereas scanning at a higher matrix size leads to higher spatial resolution at the expense of scan time. In general, independently of the method used, higher spatial resolution is always obtained at the expense of overall signal-to-noise ratio.

Spatial Resolution

Slice thickness
Field of view
Number of phase and frequency encoding steps

Signal-to-Noise Ratio

Signal-to-noise ratio refers to the sensitivity of an MRI technique to a particular tissue. It is defined as the image intensity of the tissue divided by the standard deviation of the noise level present in the image in any homogeneous region in the image; that is, signal to noise is a function of the ratio of signal in tissue and signal in background noise.

In practice, signal to noise can be measured from the image by means of region-of-interest (ROI) measurements of tissue and background noise.

Four factors determine the signal-to-noise ratio of any given tissue: (a) the signal sensitivity factor, (b) the measurement statistics factor, (c) the number of protons contained in the imaging voxel, and (d) a pulse sequence-weighting factor that expresses the level of T1 recovery and of T2 decay that the tissue experiences with the application of the pulse sequence.

The signal sensitivity factor is a measure of the sensitivity of the experimental setup to the tissue of interest. This factor represents the imaging qualities of the receiver electronics–receiver coil combination. This factor is of practical interest to the MRI user to the extent that it is greatly influenced by the coil geometry and by the positioning of the coil relative to the organ of interest. In general, maximum sensitivity is achieved by positioning the receiver coil as close as physically possible to the desired imaging volume. Also important is the selection of a coil with a coverage exceeding only slightly the desired imaging volume (Fig. 11).

The measurement statistics factor is equal to the square root of the total measurement time per image during which NMR signals are being sampled, i.e., the square root of the sum of NSA × NPE × T sampling. It describes the effects of the measurement statistics as well as the noise generated during the imaging experiment. This factor is of interest to MRI users to the extent that it outlines possible avenues to improve tissue signal by increasing any of the three factors under the square-root sign. These avenues are always available but have trade-offs: longer scan times result from increasing either NSA or NPE, and more severe chemical shift artifact results from increasing T sampling. The chemical shift phenomenon, which is reviewed later in this chapter, consists of a spatial shift along the FE direction of the image, which may be experienced by tissues containing protons in chemical species other than water. In practice, improving signal by increasing either NSA or NPE or both is scan-time inefficient because of the square root dependence. Because

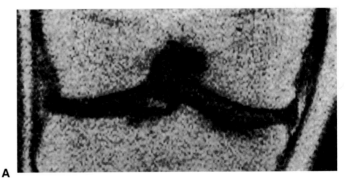

A

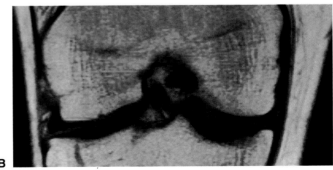

B

FIG. 11. Signal to noise. Coronal T1-weighted image of knee acquired **(A)** with body coil with poor signal relative to noise and **(B)** with a dedicated quadrature knee coil with optimum signal to noise.

the scan time is proportional to these variables, increasing scan time by a factor of two results only in approximately 40% improvement in image signal.

The number of protons contained in the imaging voxel is the product of the average longitudinal magnetization density at a given location and the voxel volume as defined by the pulse sequence. This factor is a measure of the number of proton magnetic moments contributing to the image intensity associated to an individual pixel. The practical implication of this term is that higher spatial resolution (i.e., smaller voxel) comes inevitably at the expense of poorer signal, all other parameters being equal.

The pulse sequence weighting factor depends on both the pulse sequence and the tissue. It represents the influence of the type of pulse sequence (FFE, CSE, etc.), the pulse parameters (TR, TE, flip angle [FA], etc.), and the tissue NMR properties (T1, T2*, T2,...) on the resulting image appearance of that tissue.

The existence of the pulse sequence weighting factor, which is tissue dependent, sets MRI apart from all known medical imaging modalities in terms of contrast flexibility, because such a large number of different pulse sequences is possible.

Factors Affecting Image Signal-to-Noise Ratio

Excitatory pulse sequence
Magnetic field strength
Receiver coil
Slice thickness
Field of view
Matrix dimensions—number of phase and frequency encoding steps
Number of signal averages (NSA)

Contrast Resolution

Pulse Sequence Weighting

Contrast between two tissues, A and B, is commonly expressed in relation to the noise level present throughout the image by the so-called contrast-to-noise ratio, which is the difference of the individual signal-to-noise ratios; i.e., contrast-to-noise ratio equals the difference in signal-to-noise ratio at point A relative to the signal-to-noise ratio at point B.

Intrinsic Image Contrast

Before excitation, atoms with unpaired protons, possessing charge and hence angular momentum, align or rotate around the z axis of a magnetic field (the parent field) generated by the imaging magnet. Such alignment results in a net magnetization vector in the z axis described as longitudinal magnetization. Random rotation around the z axis (out of

phase) results in neutralization of magnetization in the xy plane or absence of transverse magnetization.

Following excitation, spins are deflected to the xy plane. Deflected spins now rotate in phase or as a single vector in the xy plane, which results in the presence of transverse magnetization. Magnetic vectors, now oriented in the xy plane, lack longitudinal magnetization.

Following excitation and removal of the excitatory pulse, spins or in-phase magnetic vectors in the xy plane begin to dephase, leading to a loss of transverse magnetization. As protons dephase in the transverse plane, they reorient to the parent field and regain longitudinal magnetization.

Recovery of longitudinal magnetization, which generates the T1 signal, occurs more slowly than loss of transverse magnetization, which generates the T2 signal. If excitatory pulses are repeatedly applied to tissue, movement of induced magnetic vectors becomes negligible, which is described as a steady state. If the excitatory pulse is applied repeatedly immediately following recovery of longitudinal magnetization, before complete loss of transverse magnetization, sequential pulses induce steady-state transverse magnetization, and therefore, yielded signal is from recovery of longitudinal magnetization (T1 weighted). In contrast, if sequential excitatory pulses are applied after a delay that allows not only recovery of longitudinal magnetization but also complete loss of transverse magnetization, tissue weighting in the yielded image is a function of the time at which signal is sampled (the echo time or TE). If signal is sampled early, it will contain both T1- and T2-weighted information (a function of the tissue proton density); if signal is sampled late, it will contain predominantly T2-weighted information.

Intrinsic image contrast, although manipulated by both repetition time and echo time, is primarily a function of the tissue type. Tissues with complex macromolecules (facilitating rapid transfer of energy), such as fat, recover longitudinal magnetization and lose transverse magnetization rapidly following excitation; tissues with unpaired protons not influenced by complex macromolecules, such as free water, recover longitudinal magnetization and lose transverse magnetization slowly following excitation (Fig. 12).

Extrinsic Image Contrast

Although intrinsic factors predominantly dictate contrast, manipulation of methods of exciting and sampling signal contribute to contrast observed in the generated image.

Spin-echo pulse sequences generate signal by applying a 90° excitatory pulse and then a refocusing 180° pulse before sampling the generated echo. Observed tissue contrast in this setting is a function of both how frequently tissue is reexcited (TR) and the time at which generated signal is sampled (TE).

Fast field-echo (gradient-echo) pulse sequences use an excitatory pulse sequence of sufficient power to only partially deflect protons. Generated signal is sampled only following refocusing by the application of reversed gradients (faster than the 180° refocusing pulse inherent in the spin-

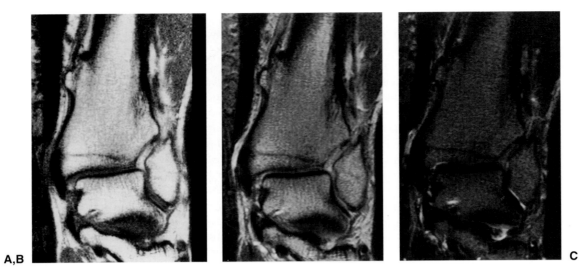

FIG. 12. Contrast resolution. Coronal image of the ankle showing effect of both echo and repetition time on image contrast: **(A)** TE 15 msec, TR 500 msec; **(B)** TE 15 msec, TR 2,000 msec; **(C)** TE 80 msec, TR 2,000 msec. Improved contrast between cortex and marrow yielded on T1-weighted scan. Incidental note is made of sessile osteochondroma.

echo sequence). With fast field-echo techniques, observed contrast reflects the magnitude by which protons are deflected (the flip angle, small flip angles enhancing T2 contrast and high flip angles enhancing T1 contrast) and both the TR and TE.

Fat-suppressed imaging, suppressing signal generated by fatty yellow marrow, forms the foundation of most musculoskeletal imaging protocols; the abundance of signal-rich yellow marrow throughout both the axial and appendicular skeleton, if unsuppressed, may lead to obscuration of sites of abnormality. Fat-suppressed imaging may be achieved by either inversion-recovery or spectral presaturation techniques.

Inversion-recovery sequences achieve suppression by applying a 180° inversion pulse immediately before a typical spin-echo pulse sequence. Tissues begin to reorient and regain longitudinal magnetization immediately following an inversion pulse. After 160 msec (at 1.5 T) (two-thirds the T1 value of fat), recovering magnetic vectors from fat align both with and against the main magnetic field in equal amounts (the null point), resulting in effective cancellation of magnetization from vectors induced by fat. If tissue is excited by a spin-echo sequence applied, just as fat is, at the null point (160 msec at 1.5 T), signal is generated by all tissues but fat (Fig. 13). By lengthening the inversion time, the same technique may be used to suppress different tissues, including water (FLAIR, fluid attenuated inversion recovery, inversion time TI 2,400 msec). Because inversion recovery relies on tissue T1 values (predominantly reflecting intrinsic tissue components), suppression is little affected by variations in field homogeneity.

In contrast, spectral presaturation of fat requires absolute field homogeneity. Because precession frequencies are intimately related to local field strength, any variation in magnetic field homogeneity will affect precession frequencies. In the presence of inhomogeneity, the precession frequency of fat in one voxel may differ from its precession frequency in another voxel. An applied saturation pulse at a particular frequency may therefore suppress fat at one point in an image and not at another. Such field inhomogeneities are most marked at the extremity of the coil systems and thus impact on the imaging of joints. Developments in coil technology have dramatically improved field homogeneity and now allow routine improved uniform frequency-selective saturation and suppression of signal from fat.

Artifacts

Artifacts refer to unwanted image features without correlation in the imaged object. These features, which arise from imperfections in the imaging technique and/or hardware limitations, may appear in an image as artificial intensity patterns, geometric distortions, or spurious ghosting. In practice, the most common artifacts encountered with modern MRI scanners in proper working conditions originate from one of the following: (a) magnetic field inaccuracies (susceptibility artifacts), (b) tissue motion, (c) existence of multiple resonant frequencies (chemical shift artifacts), (d) inadequate spatial resolution (truncation artifacts), and (e) tissues extending beyond the imaging volume along the PE direction (aliasing or wraparound artifacts). The typical image appearance of these artifacts, their causes, and the measures commonly used to alleviate their adverse effects are reviewed in the following.

Susceptibility Artifacts

These artifacts result from deviations in the value of the magnetic field inside the patient during the application of

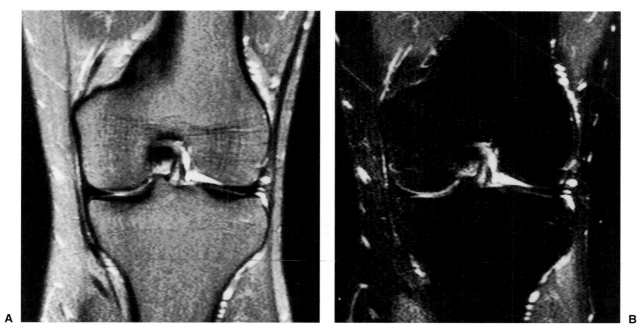

FIG. 13. Inversion time. Coronal inversion recovery image (TE 20 msec, TR 2,000 msec) of the knee acquired with **(A)** an inversion time of 100 msec with poor fat suppression and **(B)** with an inversion time of 160 msec with optimum fat suppression.

the pulse sequence. Because modern scanners generate very homogeneous parent magnetic fields and highly linear magnetic field gradients, inaccuracies in the values of these are caused mainly by magnetic susceptibility variations within the patient. When present, these magnetic susceptibility variations distort the parent magnetic field as well as the magnetic field gradients used for spatial encoding. Because

the function of the parent magnetic field is very different from that of the magnetic field gradients, the resulting artifacts may be categorized accordingly. For example, first, inaccuracies of the main magnetic field cause a faster decay rate (i.e., shorter $T2^*$) of the NMR signals in fast-field or gradient-echo pulse sequences. In regions of large magnetic field variations, the shortening of $T2^*$ may lead to complete

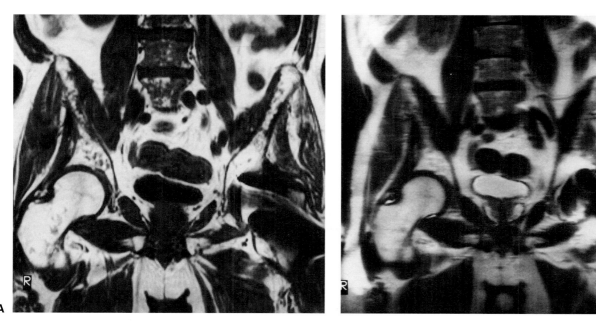

FIG. 14. Susceptibility artifact. **(A)** Coronal T1-weighted image shows distortion and signal loss adjacent to left hip fixation screws. **(B)** Coronal turbo spin-echo image shows marked reduction in artifact adjacent to the hardware component, allowing visualization of the adjacent soft tissues.

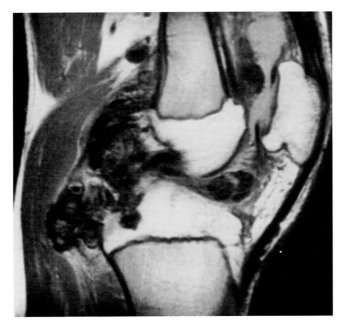

FIG. 15. Susceptibility artifact. Sagittal T1-weighted (TE 15 msec, TR 500 msec) image shows a lobular synovial mass with diffuse signal hypointensity secondary to hemosiderin-induced susceptibility artifact typical of pigmented villonodular synovitis.

signal loss even at the shortest TE possible, as determined by the capabilities of the imaging subsystem. These so-called susceptibility artifacts are substantially alleviated in spin-echo pulse sequences as a consequence of the rephasing effect of the 180° refocusing pulse (Figs. 14–16). Second, inaccuracies in the magnetic field gradients deteriorate the quality of the spatial encoding process, thus potentially lead-

ing to a number of spatial encoding artifacts, including geometric deformation, spatial misregistration, and partial signal loss from incomplete gradient balance. These artifacts are most noticeable when the susceptibility gradient magnitude is a significant fraction of the imaging gradient. Susceptibility gradients are strongest near the interface between two materials with different magnetic susceptibilities (Fig. 17). Susceptibility artifacts are therefore more prominent near anatomic interfaces separating two magnetically dissimilar materials. Important examples of such areas include soft tissue–air interfaces near the nasal cavities, bone marrow–calcified bone, and soft tissue–metal in the case of patients with metallic orthopedic hardware.

Artifacts Caused by Tissue Motion

Movement of tissues during imaging interferes with the spatial encoding processes used in the pulse sequence. Because the time interval between successive measurements in the FE direction is several orders of magnitude shorter than that in the PE direction, motion artifacts are almost exclusively observed along the phase-encoding direction. Depending on the properties of flow and on the pulse sequence parameters, motion-related artifacts may appear as image intensity smearing or as well-organized fainter replicas of the moving organs, which are referred to as ghosts. Vessel ghosting by flowing blood is also a common occurrence. Sources of motion artifacts active during the time scale of conventional MRI include (from slowest to fastest) involuntary patient motion, respiration, peristalsis, vascular flow, and cardiac pulsations (Fig. 18).

A number of methods have been used with varying degrees of success to counteract the adverse effects of motion

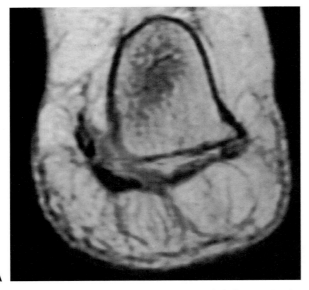

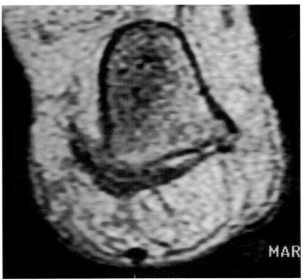

A   B

FIG. 16. Susceptibility artifact. **(A)** Coronal spin-echo T1-weighted image of the hindfoot in a patient with suspected soft tissue foreign body. **(B)** Coronal fast field-echo image (lacking refocusing 180° pulse) of the same patient shows susceptibility blooming at the site of the soft tissue foreign body.

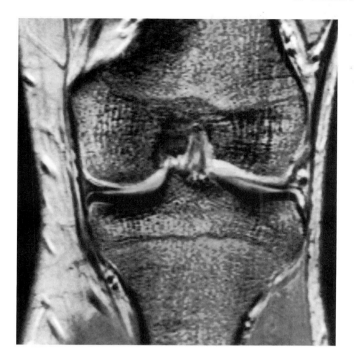

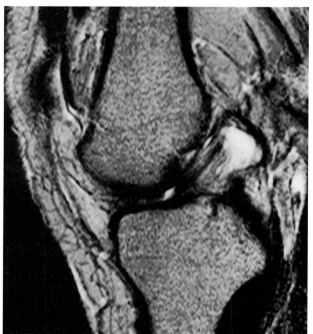

FIG. 17. Susceptibility artifact. Coronal T2-weighted fast field-echo image (flip angle 30°, TE 15 msec, TR 500 msec) of the knee showing prominence of trabeculae within metaphyseal cancellous bone. Conspicuity of trabeculae is enhanced (actually distorted) by susceptibility artifact resulting from the different magnetic susceptibility of cellular marrow and acellular bony trabecular seams.

in MRI. Some of these methods, including increased NSA, fat suppression, presaturation pulses, ordered phase encoding, and gradient moment nulling, may be referred to as indirect methods because they do not counteract directly the main cause of the problem, which is the acquisition of imaging information with the organs in different positions at different times. Instead, indirect methods are used to reduce the severity of motion artifacts by either averaging (increasing NSA), eliminating the signals and consequently the ghosts of moving tissues, which are not relevant for diagnosis (fat suppression and presaturation pulses), or by (partially) correcting the erroneous phases caused by motion (ordered

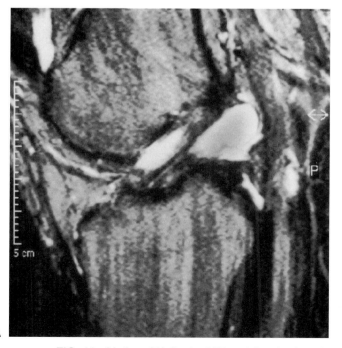

A

B

FIG. 18. Motion. (A) Sagittal T2-weighted spin-echo image of the knee shows pulsation artifact in the phase-encoding direction obscuring visualization of anterior cruciate ligament ganglion cyst. (B) Sagittal T2-weighted image in the same patient with phase-encoding in the superoinferior orientation without associated pulsation artifact.

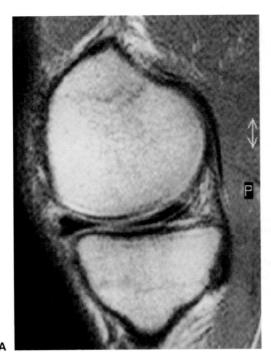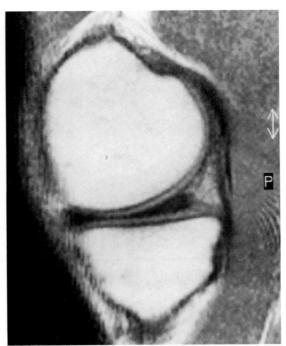

A   B

FIG. 19. Motion. **(A)** Sagittal T1-weighted spin-echo image of the knee showing a pseudotear of the posterior horn of the medial meniscus secondary to subtle motion-induced ghosting artifact. **(B)** Sagittal T1-weighted turbo spin-echo image of the same patient acquired in 1 min minimizes motion artifact and shows a normal posterior horn of the medial meniscus.

phase-encoding and gradient-moment nulling). Alternatively, direct motion artifact reduction techniques, which include rapid image acquisition (Fig. 19), respiratory triggering, cardiac triggering, and breath holding, attempt to acquire the imaging data with all tissues in the same location at all times. These techniques will be reviewed in more detail in the context of rapid imaging pulse sequences.

Chemical Shift Artifacts

The Larmor frequency of protons varies depending on the structure of the hydrogen-containing molecules. This phenomenon, which is known generically as chemical shift, is a direct consequence of the magnetic field-tracking property of the Larmor frequency. In the case of different chemical species, the local magnetic fields differ because the surrounding electron clouds modify differently the magnetic field at the site of the proton. In biological tissues, the two proton-containing chemical species of interest are water and lipids. The Larmor frequency difference between protons in water and protons in lipids is a very small fraction of the parent magnetic field, approximately 3.5 parts per million (ppm). In a 1.5-T magnetic field, this translates to a 220-Hz frequency difference, approximately. As a consequence, the chemical shift artifact, which is also referred to as a chemical shift spatial offset, consists of an apparent spatial offset of the lipid-containing voxels relative to the water-containing voxels in the frequency-encoding direction. The magnitude of this spatial offset is inversely proportional to the amplitude of the frequency-encoding gradient applied during signal readout. Specifically, the amount of chemical shift is a function of the frequency difference between fat and water and of the readout bandwidth (Figs. 20 and 21).

Truncation Artifacts

These artifacts, which manifest in an image as ripples that occur near a sharp tissue interface in a parallel linear pattern, result from undersampling of the tissue interface in the Fourier domain. Consequently, their severity decreases with decreasing voxel size.

Aliasing Artifacts

An anatomic region of the patient that extends beyond a border of the field of view appears on the opposite border, superimposed on the desired image (Fig. 22). Aliasing artifacts are a consequence of the limitations of the phase-encoding and the frequency-encoding methods, whereby tissues extending beyond the borders of the field of view are tagged with integer multiples of the phases and of the frequencies associated with the tissues within the field of view and are indistinguishable to the scanner. In practice, only aliasing artifacts in the phase-encoding direction are of concern to

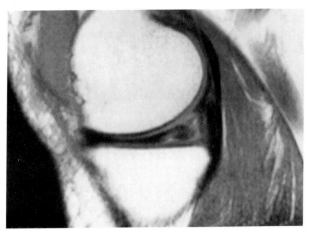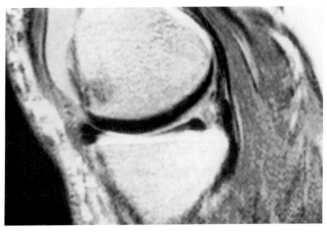

A

B

FIG. 20. Chemical shift artifact. **(A)** Sagittal turbo spin-echo image shows an oblique tear of the posterior horn of the medial meniscus. **(B)** Sagittal spin-echo, echo planar image shows obscuration of meniscal tear as a result of chemical shift misregistration artifact. Note apparent absence of cortex in tibial plateau, accompanied by apparent thickening of cortex over the femoral condyle.

the user because the extra frequency content in the MRI signals is eliminated electronically at a hardware level by means of filtering. Unfortunately, no such filtering means are available to selectively eliminate the extra phase content of the MRI signals, and consequently, alternative measures are implemented to counteract the adverse effects of aliasing

artifacts in the phase-encoding direction. These include (a) the foldover suppression method, whereby the field of view is doubled in size during the scan and only the tissues contained in the desired field of view are displayed; (b) the use of receiver coils with sensitivity extending only slightly over the desired field of view; and (c) spatial presaturation pulses,

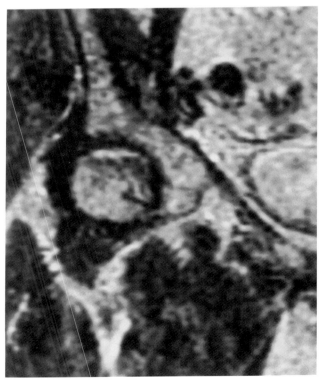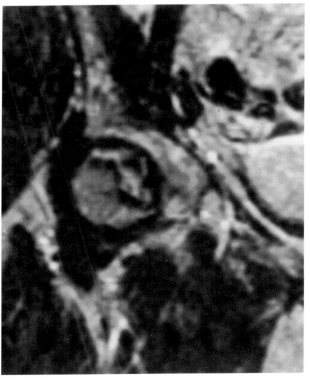

A

B

FIG. 21. Chemical shift artifact. **(A)** Coronal T2-weighted spin-echo image shows double-line sign at the site of femoral head avascular necrosis (readout bandwidth 16 kHz). **(B)** Coronal T2-weighted spin-echo image shows more marked double-line sign in the same patient in an image acquired with a narrowed readout bandwidth (2 kHz) enhancing chemical shift artifact.

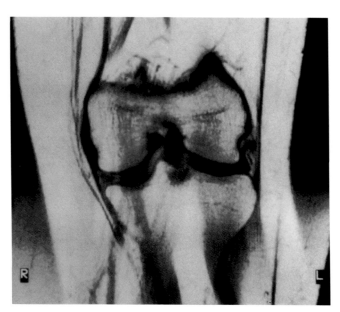

FIG. 22. Aliasing: phase wraparound. Coronal T1-weighted spin-echo image shows image of the thigh superimposed on the knee as a result of wrap-around artifact.

which reduce the MRI signals stemming from tissues beyond the desired field of view.

CONVENTIONAL MRI PULSE SEQUENCES

The physical principles and the mechanics of MR imaging were delineated in the preceding sections of this chapter. These lead to the concept of magnetization mapping by means of an MRI pulse sequence with which the volumetric distribution of magnetization inside a patient is effectively partitioned into voxels, potentially weighted by any of a number of variables (proton density, T1, T2*, T2, etc.), and measured, thus generating an MR image with a given spatial resolution and contrast. Because the vast majority of pulse sequences used clinically acquire the imaging data in the Fourier codomain or k-space, the rationales used in, and the technical issues associated with, pulse sequence design are easier to understand when expressed in k-space terminology. For this reason, the structure of k-space and the mechanics of pulse sequence scanning in k-space are studied in the following sections.

Fourier Codomain: Structure of k-Space

k-Space is the (digital) depository of the discrete measurements performed by a Fourier-transform MRI pulse sequence. The array of k-space data has the same number of elements as the reconstructed MR image; in other words, k-space and image space (x-space) have identical matrix size. These two spaces contain equivalent imaging information in terms of spatial resolution and contrast and therefore are referred to as imaging codomains. The information is, how-

ever, stored in very different forms: whereas data points in x-space are organized according to spatial position coordinates within the field of view, in k-space data points are organized according to the phase and frequency imprinted on them by the spatial encoding process (Fig. 23). A deeper understanding of k-space may be gained from studying its structural features as they relate to the most important image properties, namely spatial resolution, signal to noise, and contrast weighting. First, with respect to spatial resolution, the separation between data points in k-space in each scanning direction is inversely proportional to the product of the number of points sampled in each direction and the desired voxel dimension in each direction.

Equivalently, the scanning step in k-space in each direction is inversely proportional to the desired field of view in that direction.

Second, with respect to signal to noise, because the data points near the center of k-space are the least dephased by the spatial encoding gradients, these contain the strongest signal elements. Consequently the majority of the signal-to-noise information and therefore the overall contrast to noise (see preceding section) of the image are contained in the central portion of k-space. On the other hand, the information contained in data points located at increasing distance from the center of k-space contains weaker elements of the signals that have been dephased to a greater extent by the spatial encoding gradients to reproduce the finer details in the image.

In summary, in Fourier transform MRI, the voxel dimensions are determined by the spacing of the data points in k-space, and the relative image intensities associated to these voxels are determined by the relative signal content between the central and the outer regions of k-space. The MRI pulse sequences scan in k-space, acquiring spatially encoded data points in a successive pattern until the acquisition of the full data set consisting in NPE × NFE is completed.

Pulse Sequence Trajectories in k-Space

During a scan, Fourier transform MRI pulse sequences acquire the NPE × NFE k-space data points successively. The mechanics of these pulse sequences is such that after a phase-encoding pulse is applied, a series of NFE frequency-encoding steps and measurements follows very rapidly. For this reason, Fourier-transform MRI pulse sequences are said to scan on a k-line by k-line basis. Each k-line is parallel to the frequency-encoding direction and contains NFE data points that correspond to the same phase-encoding cycle. Equivalently, each k-line contains the signal generated during a single phase-encoding step. In this context, the scanning process may be represented by a path in k-space, which is commonly referred to as the k-space trajectory of the pulse sequence. In the case of conventional pulse sequences (FFE and CSE), the trajectory starts at the bottom of k-space and proceeds upward following a zigzag pattern until all NPE k-lines are acquired.

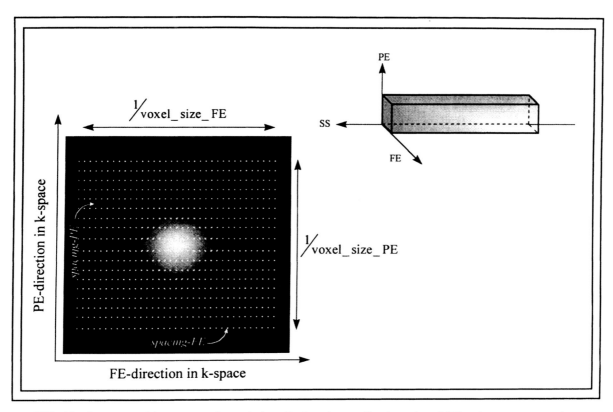

FIG. 23. Structure of *k*-space and voxel size. During the application of an MRI pulse sequence, the raw data are stored in computer memory in a format known as *k*-space, which is not anatomically interpretable. However, the structure of *k*-space has properties with very simple geometric interpretation: (a) the spacing of data points in each direction is equal to the inverse of the field of view in that direction, (b) the size of *k*-space is equal to the inverse of the voxel size in that direction, (c) application of a pulse sequence can be described as a trajectory in *k*-space, (d) the strongest signal data points, which contain primarily the SNR and contrast information, are stored in the central section of *k*-space, and (e) weaker signal data points containing mostly the geometric detail information of the image are stored in the periphery of *k*-space.

Scan Time

Magnetic resonance image acquisition involves tissue excitation by an applied excitatory pulse, localization of induced signal by the application of three orthogonal gradients, and signal acquisition by receiver coils (the equivalent of radio antennas).

To create an image, which is essentially composed of multiple signal samples (dictated by the image matrix or the number of phase- and frequency-encoding steps), the process must be repeated until signal is sampled from all points in the image. Sampled signal is oriented within *k*-space, with the highest amplitude signal responsible for contrast filling the center of *k*-space, and the signal with the least amplitude acquired by the highest-order phase-encoding gradients filling the periphery of *k*-space responsible for edge enhancement. The Fourier transform of signal within *k*-space converts signal from the frequency domain to a digital form. In the digital form, signal is assigned to individual pixels within the image matrix and subsequently assigned a gray scale.

In such a way, an excitatory pulse is applied, gradients are switched, and an echo is sampled (at a time TE) and is encoded in *k*-space. After a period of time to allow recovery or loss of tissue magnetization following the initial applied excitatory pulse (TR dictated by whether T1 or T2 tissue weighting is required), an excitatory pulse is reapplied, gradients are switched again, and another echo is sampled. To fill a matrix, samples would have to be taken from each voxel; in other words, gradients would have to be switched 256 × 256 times, with resultant impact on acquisition time. This is overcome by sampling signal in lines, localizing signal within each line on the basis of changes in phase induced by phase-encoding gradients and frequency imposed by frequency-encoding gradients. Therefore, the time to acquire a single image is a function of the time that must be waited between the application of each radiofrequency pulse (TR) and the number of phase-encoding lines in the image. To improve image signal, the process may be completely repeated a second time, improving image signal 1.4 times, and so on (image signal is proportional to the square root of the number of excitations). Total acquisition time for a single slice is therefore:

acquisition time = TR (repetition time, a function of required image contrast resolution) × NPE (number of phase-encoding acquisitions, a function of required image spatial resolution) × NSA (number of signal averages, a function of required image signal to noise)

In practice, while we are waiting for tissue within a slice to recover following the application of a radiofrequency pulse, several contiguous slices are excited, their number dictated primarily by the time that must elapse before the initial slice can be reexcited (TR) and how early excited tissue is sampled (TE) (approximately 15 slices for TE 20 msec, TR 500 msec). In effect, although it may take 5 min to acquire one slice, up to 15 slices may be aquired at the same time without any impact on overall acquisition time. If additional slices are required to allow complete coverage of a region of interest, this can be achieved simply by increasing the repetition time, allowing more time to excite additional slices; for example, increasing TR from 500 msec to 600 msec will increase the number of slices acquired from 15 to 18 without great impact on either acquisition time or contrast.

REFERENCES AND SUGGESTED READING

1. Hashemi RH, Bradley WG. *MRI The Basics.* Baltimore: Williams & Wilkins, 1997.
2. Stark DD, Bradley WG, eds. *Magnetic Resonance Imaging, 2nd ed, vols 1 and 2.* Chicago: Mosby, 1992.
3. Horowitz AL. *MRI Physics for Radiologists—A Visual Approach, 2nd ed.* New York: Springer-Verlag, 1992.
4. Lufkin RB. *The MRI Manual.* Chicago: Mosby, 1990.
5. Hennig J, Nauerth A, Friedburg H. RARE imaging: a fast imaging method for clinical MR. *Magn Res Med* 1986;3:823–833.
6. Elster AD. *Questions and Answers in Magnetic Resonance Imaging.* Chicago: Mosby, 1994.

CHAPTER 2

Advanced Magnetic Resonance Imaging

Hernan H. Jara and Stephen J. Eustace

INTRODUCTION

Many approaches to pulse sequence design, geared to counteract the intrinsic slowness of conventional MRI, have been investigated. The most fruitful approaches stem from the following four general scan acceleration principles:

1. Multislice two-dimensional scanning.
2. Rapid imaging with conventional pulse sequences: reduction of TR.
3. Rapid imaging with hybrid pulse sequences: effective reduction of NPE.
4. Reduced k-space acquisitions: reduction of NSA.

Multislice Two-Dimensional Scanning

To scan sequentially a clinically useful number of slices would require a very long scan time. For example the sequential acquisition of 20 slices (NSA 1, NPE 256, TR 2 sec) would require almost 3 hr. The MRI is slow mainly because each TR cycle consists of a very short active time, which is approximately equal to TE, and a comparatively much longer inactive time, approximately equal to the difference TR − TE, used solely for the purpose of T1 recovery. Multislice two-dimensional (2D) scanning is a ''parallel'' or multiplexing acquisition technique whereby the TR − TE inactive time is used to interrogate unexcited slices at

H. H. Jara: Department of Radiology, Section of Radiologic Physics, Boston University School of Medicine and Boston Medical Center, Boston, Massachusetts 02118.

S. J. Eustace: Department of Radiology, Section of Musculoskeletal Radiology, Boston University School of Medicine and Boston Medical Center, Boston, Massachusetts 02118.

other locations. If the number of slices does not exceed a certain maximum number, dictated by the amount of inactive time available (TR), the multislice 2D scan time of a group of slices and the sequential scan time of one slice are approximately equal (Fig. 1).

For example, for TR = 2 sec, TE = 100 msec, NSA = 1, and NPE = 256, approximately 20 slices can be scanned for the time of one (i.e., 8.5 min).

Although multislice 2D imaging brings the scan efficiency of MR imaging to a level compatible with routine clinical operation, the minimum scan times of many pulse sequences affording adequate coverage and modest spatial resolution are still on the order of 10 min.

Short-TR Rapid Conventional Imaging

Acceleration methods based on shortening TR can easily be used to drastically reduce the scan time of conventional pulse sequences. In this respect, TR is a convenient scan time control variable that may be adjusted continuously over a very wide range of values extending several orders of magnitude. Furthermore, whereas the upper limit for this range can be tens of seconds, or even infinity for single-shot techniques, the lower limit approaches TE, i.e., only a few milliseconds. Therefore, for extremely short TRs, the potential scan time reductions are dramatic; for example, for TR = 6 msec, TE = 3 msec, NSA = 1, and NPE = 256, the scan time for two slices is approximately 1.54 sec. Note that although this scan time is very short and approaches the acquisition times in CT, because TR is only twice TE in this example, the package contains only two slices.

There are, however, difficulties associated with short-TR

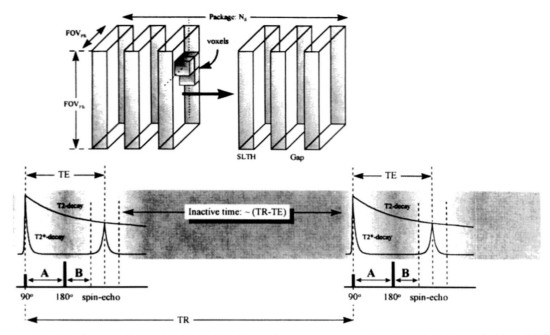

FIG. 1. Multislice two-dimensional imaging. The pulse sequence acceleration principle applied to a CSE pulse sequence. The inactive time (TR − TE) that is needed for recovery of longitudinal magnetization in slice 1 is used to interrogate other slices. This principle allows interrogation of a package of slices in approximately the same time required to scan one slice. The number of slices contained in a package is TR and TE dependent; specifically, N = TR/TE.

scanning, particularly signal-to-noise penalties and less contrast flexibility. In clinical practice, short-TR pulse sequences are mostly used for T1-weighted imaging, which may be either FFE (GE)-based or CSE-based. However, because the minimum TRs and TEs achievable with FFE (GE) sequences are shorter than with CSE sequences, the highest scan time reductions are obtained with the former. Also, short-TR pulse sequences are used to image flow, leading to MR angiography. A drawback associated with short-TR scanning is signal-to-noise degradation from magnetization saturation effects, a phenomenon that increases as a function of decreasing TR (Fig. 2). For a given TR and T1 combination, the extent of signal loss from saturation effects may be reduced by lowering the flip angle to maintain a larger "reserve pool" of unsaturated positive longitudinal magnetization available for each TR cycle. Accordingly, flip angle can be used to manipulate the contrast weighting of short-TR pulse sequences: strongest T1 tissue differentiation among tissues is achieved with large flip angles, in the range from 70° to 90°.

Perhaps the most important limitation encountered with short-TR scanning is the lack of a rapid and reliable pulse sequence affording T2-weighting comparable to the CSE pulse sequence. In the short-TR regime, the mechanism for achieving T2 weighting is very different and more delicate than that with long-TR/TE CSE sequences because it relies on preservation of transverse magnetization coherence in the steady state, a phenomenon that is very flow/motion sensitive. The acceleration method of choice to produce reliable

and rapid T2-weighted scans is by means of hybrid RARE (Rapid Acquisition with Relaxation Enhancement) pulse sequences.

Hybrid Pulse Sequences

If, instead of reducing TR, several differently encoded *k*-lines are acquired following one RF excitation, a very different pulse sequence acceleration method results. The pulse sequences using this method are termed hybrid because, for each excitation, the signal is read using a phase and frequency encoding mixture by the so-called hybrid readout, also known as the echo train. Hybrid pulse sequences are grouped in families that are defined according to the type of signals (field echoes versus spin echoes) acquired during the hybrid readout: only field echoes in echo-planar imaging (EPI), only spin echoes in hybrid RARE, and a combination of field and spin echoes in GraSE.

Hybrid RARE is the generic denomination for a family of hybrid spin-echo pulse sequences that includes the original single-shot RARE sequence as well as the more modern variants termed fast spin echo (FSE) and turbo spin echo (TSE). The defining architecture of these pulse sequences (Fig. 3) is the use of one 90° excitation radiofrequency pulse followed by the so-called hybrid RARE readout, which generates and acquires multiple spin-echo signals with different phase encodings. Accordingly, the hybrid RARE readout can be viewed schematically as a succession of pulse sequence element modules of equal duration that acquire differently

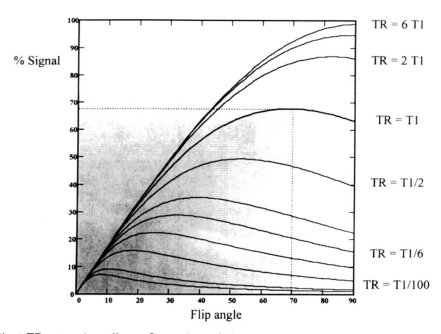

FIG. 2. Short-TR saturation effects. Saturation refers to the signal loss of a tissue that results from exciting the tissue at a faster rate than it will recover according to its T1 value. The graph shows that when TR is shorter than T1, maximum SNR is obtained at a lower flip angle. It also shows the drastic overall SNR penalties that can result from operating pulse sequences at TRs much shorter than the tissue T1s.

phase-encoded spin-echo k-lines. Technically, hybrid RARE pulse sequences are accelerated versions of the CSE pulse sequences. The pulse sequence variables associated with the hybrid RARE readout are: (a) the number of k-lines acquired by the hybrid RARE readout, which is known as echo-train length (ETL) or turbo factor, depending on the manufacturer; (b) the time interval elapsed between consecutive spin-echo signals, known as echo spacing (ES); and (c) the effective echo time (TE_{eff}), which determines the extent of T2

weighting in a form analogous to the variable TE in CSE sequences. TE_{eff} is defined as the time of acquisition of the k-line(s) with zero or near-zero phase encoding that are positioned centrally in k-space. Hybrid RARE sequences are faster because they acquire imaging data at times during which their CSE counterparts are inactive. For hybrid sequences, the scan time of the package is reduced to: scan time = NSA × NPE × TR/turbo factor or ETL.

For this reason, the scan time reduction obtained with

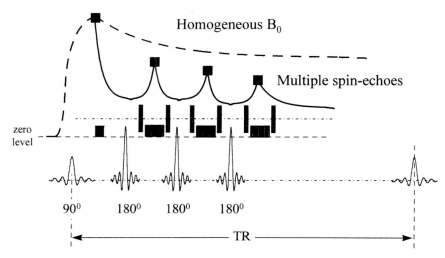

FIG. 3. Rapid acquisition with relaxation enhancement (RARE) platform. Unlike conventional spin echo, multiple 180° refocusing pulses are applied following each 90° excitatory pulse, yielding multiple echoes as part of the RARE (fast spin-echo or turbo spin-echo sequence).

hybrid pulse sequences may be thought of as an effective reduction in the number of k-lines acquired. Note, however, that the effective scan time acceleration is not as high as the equation seems to imply because the number of slices in a package is also reduced: number of slices = TR/(ETL × ES). Therefore, the real scan time reduction depends on both the ETL used and the minimum echo spacing achievable by the gradient subsystem. In practice, even with maximum gradient strengths as low as 10 mT/m, for the same coverage, the scan time of a T2-weighted hybrid RARE pulse sequence with ETL = 8 is approximately four times shorter than that of its CSE counterpart.

Fast or Turbo Spin-Echo Imaging: Practical Considerations

Coverage Versus Acquisition Time
Repetition Time
Echo Time
Echo Train Length: Acquisition Time Versus Blur
Echo Spacing: Acquisition Time Versus Signal to Noise
Echo to View Mapping Profile: Linear Versus Low-High Versus Half-Scan

Fast or Turbo Spin-Echo Advantages and Disadvantages

Rapid Image Acquisition
Decreased Magnetic Susceptibility: Decreased Metal Artifact
Magnetization Transfer Effects: Decreased Conspicuousness of Cuff Tears
Image Blur: Impaired Detection of Meniscal Tears
J Coupling: Bright Fat Impairs Differentiation of Fat from Subacromial Fluid
Decreased Acquisition Time at the Expense of Decreased Coverage

---

T1 versus T2 Contrast Using RARE-Based Sequences

With RARE-based sequences, image contrast, like conventional spin-echo sequences, is a function of both the time at which signal is sampled and the repetition time. Unlike conventional spin-echo sequences, where each echo is sampled at the same time following excitation, using fast or turbo spin-echo sequences, multiple sequential echoes are acquired for each excitatory pulse at progressively longer times following excitation and, therefore, at a progressively longer TE. The echo time ascribed to the image (that determines image contrast) is therefore the effective TE and is dictated by the time of echoes filling the center of k-space. If the center of k-space is filled initially and additional echoes are used to fill the periphery of k-space, the effective TE is short, affording T1 contrast. Such a mapping scheme is termed low-high or centric. If, in contrast, acquired echoes initially fill the periphery of k-space, it is the echoes in the middle of the acquired train that fill the center of k-space

and determine the effective TE. Such a mapping scheme is termed linear (Fig. 4).

With linear mapping, the periphery of k-space, responsible for edge enhancement, is filled with signal-rich echoes, and images are sharp. In contrast, with low-high (centric) mapping, the periphery of k-space is filled with signal-poor echoes, and sharpness is lost. By using a short echo train or turbo factor (short turbo factor allows the use of a short TR-enhancing T1 contrast), even the echoes at the end of the train are signal-rich, and so edge enhancement is not lost.

In such a way, T1-weighted turbo spin-echo images are yielded with an effective TE of 15 msec using low-high mapping, with a short repetition time of 500 msec, by using a short echo train. In contrast, T2-weighted images are

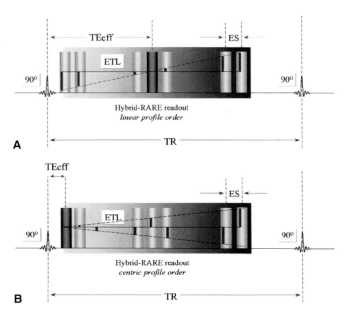

FIG. 4. (A) Hybrid RARE pulse sequence diagram, linear profile order. Simplified hybrid RARE (rapid acquisition with relaxation enhancement) pulse sequence diagram shows the linear profile order that is most useful for T2-weighted applications. Except for the phase-encoding pulses, all other pulses of the hybrid RARE readout are not shown. Note that TE$_{eff}$ (the time at which the $k = 0$ k-line is acquired) divides hybrid RARE readout into two parts of equal duration. Strength of the phase-encoding gradient pulses increases linearly from beginning to end in a symmetric form. To simulate uneven T2 weighting of the acquired profiles, this hybrid RARE readout has superimposed gray-scale shading. **(B)** Hybrid RARE pulse sequence diagram, centric profile order. Simplified hybrid RARE (rapid acquisition with relaxation enhancement) pulse sequence diagram shows the centric profile order that is most useful for proton-density-weighted and T1-weighted applications. Except for the phase-encoding pulses, all other pulses of the hybrid RARE readout are not shown. Note that TE$_{eff}$ is shortest because the $k = 0$ k-line is acquired at the beginning of the hybrid RARE readout. Strength of the phase-encoding gradient pulses increases at later times in an alternate form. To simulate uneven T2 weighting of the acquired profiles, this hybrid RARE readout has superimposed gray-scale shading.

yielded by an effective TE of 80 msec, a repetition time of 2,000 msec, an average echo train of 6, and linear echo to view mapping (Fig. 5).

Specific Issues

Improved In-Plane Spatial Resolution

With RARE-based sequences, a series of echoes are acquired within the same slice for each applied excitatory pulse before excitation of the neighboring slice. In contrast, with conventional sequences, only one echo in the slice is acquired before the apparatus moves to and excites a neighboring slice. Acquiring several echoes in the slice before moving to another slice theoretically improves the in-plane resolution, although this is not clinically evident.

Fat Bright

With RARE-based sequences, induced J coupling effects result in preservation of signal by fat even on heavily T2-weighted scans. Such retained signal may impair the ability to differentiate fat from fluid, particularly in the subacromial bursa, where identification of fluid is used as a marker of a full-thickness cuff tear. This potential difficulty is overcome by the use of frequency-selective presaturation of fat on T2-weighted turbo or fast spin-echo sequences.

Image Blur

Although extended echo trains facilitate rapid image acquisition, acquisition time = NPE × TR × NSA/turbo factor or echo train length. Longer echo trains are associated with greater image blur. Signal in extended echoes is less, and so the periphery of k-space is filled with signal-poor echoes. Similarly, sampling times are accelerated in order to accommodate extended echo trains, reducing yielded signal in sampled echoes.

Reduced Susceptibility

Ferromagnetic components become magnetized when placed in a superconducting magnet and, in so doing, generate their own magnetic field. Spins immediately adjacent to the induced magnetic field in the piece of metal hardware, under its influence, dephase rapidly following excitation, resulting in signal loss. The application of serial refocusing pulses as part of a RARE type sequence reduces dephasing and therefore reduces induced loss of signal.

Magnetization Transfer Effects

RARE-based sequences sample a train of neighboring echoes for each excitatory pulse. Movement of saturated spins between successive refocusing pulses may result in some saturation of signal in extended echoes. Such saturation may lead to some loss of T2 signal hyperintensity, potentially decreasing conspicuity of pathology. Magnetization transfer signal saturation has received particular attention in

relation to the diagnosis of rotator cuff tears, where identification of persistent signal on the T2-weighted image is used to differentiate tendinitis from cuff tear.

Coverage Versus Acquisition Time

The terms fast or turbo spin echo are somewhat misleading. Although RARE-based sequences allow rapid imaging, because a series of echoes is acquired for a given excitatory pulse, more time is spent within the excited slice than with a conventional spin-echo sequence. In such a way, there is less time to excite additional neighboring slices before the initial slice is reexcited at the given TR. Fast acquisition is therefore at the expense of coverage. The greater the echo train length, the faster the image acquisition, the less the amount of coverage.

HASTE, GraSE, and Echo Planar Imaging

Half Fourier Acquisition Turbo Spin Echo (HASTE)

For applications requiring even shorter scan times, conventional and hybrid pulse sequences may be combined with partial Fourier imaging to generate scans that are substantially shorter for the same spatial resolution and anatomic coverage because they acquire only a portion of the data. Partial Fourier scan reductions are possible because up to 75% of the k-space data are redundant with the standard Fourier acquisition methods (because each half of k-space is a mirror of the other, conjugate synthesis). In practice, the so called half-Fourier scans acquired approximately 60% of the k-lines and therefore result in a 40% scan time reduction. Because only a fraction of the k-space data are acquired for every slice, this method is often described as a fractional excitation, i.e., fractional NSA or fractional NEX (number of excitations). Single-shot half-Fourier scans are particularly useful for abdominal applications and also to scan uncooperative patients.

GraSE

GraSE, or gradient-echo spin-echo hybrid, is a further hybrid of the RARE platform. In an attempt to facilitate more rapid image generation, gradient reversals are interspersed between each refocusing 180° pulse such that images have both gradient-echo and spin-echo information (Fig. 6). Image quality is therefore dictated by the number of refocusing pulses (echo train length or turbo factor), the number of interspersed gradient reversals (echo planar factor), the echo spacing, and the echo to view mapping order. In effect, GraSE images present information enhanced by susceptibility, improving detection of meniscal tears, yet without significant distortion of bone as a result of the spin-echo component (Fig. 7).

acquisition time = TR × NPE × NSA/ETL × EPI factor

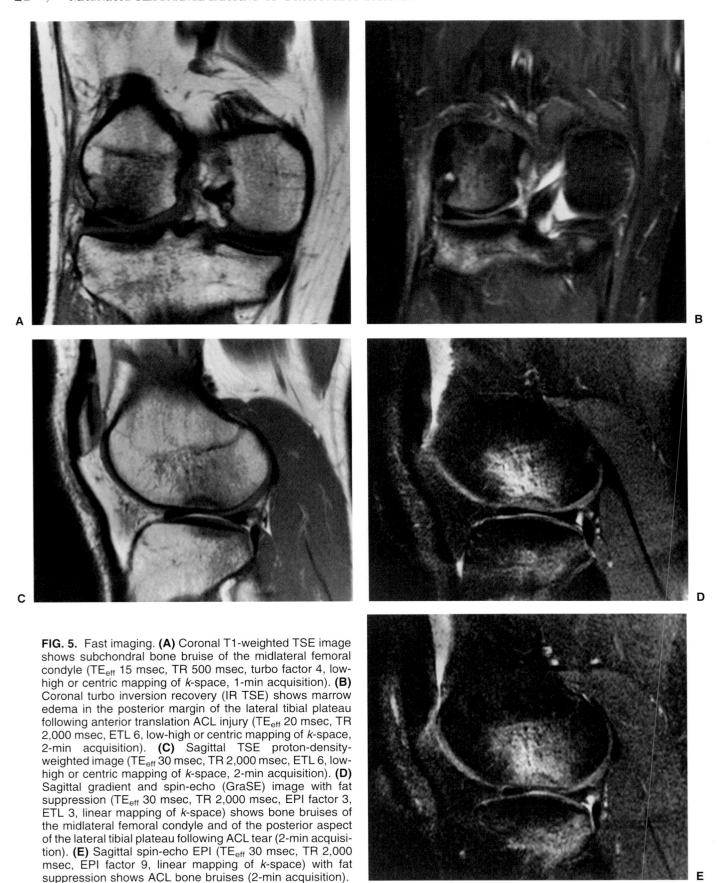

FIG. 5. Fast imaging. **(A)** Coronal T1-weighted TSE image shows subchondral bone bruise of the midlateral femoral condyle (TE$_{eff}$ 15 msec, TR 500 msec, turbo factor 4, low-high or centric mapping of *k*-space, 1-min acquisition). **(B)** Coronal turbo inversion recovery (IR TSE) shows marrow edema in the posterior margin of the lateral tibial plateau following anterior translation ACL injury (TE$_{eff}$ 20 msec, TR 2,000 msec, ETL 6, low-high or centric mapping of *k*-space, 2-min acquisition). **(C)** Sagittal TSE proton-density-weighted image (TE$_{eff}$ 30 msec, TR 2,000 msec, ETL 6, low-high or centric mapping of *k*-space, 2-min acquisition). **(D)** Sagittal gradient and spin-echo (GraSE) image with fat suppression (TE$_{eff}$ 30 msec, TR 2,000 msec, EPI factor 3, ETL 3, linear mapping of *k*-space) shows bone bruises of the midlateral femoral condyle and of the posterior aspect of the lateral tibial plateau following ACL tear (2-min acquisition). **(E)** Sagittal spin-echo EPI (TE$_{eff}$ 30 msec, TR 2,000 msec, EPI factor 9, linear mapping of *k*-space) with fat suppression shows ACL bone bruises (2-min acquisition).

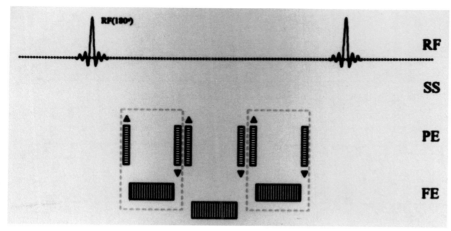

EPI factor = 3 *(in this example)*
ADCS improvement product (TF x EPI) factors

FIG. 6. GraSE. Diagram shows three gradient reversals interposed between refocusing 180° pulses, representing the building module for the GraSE sequence.

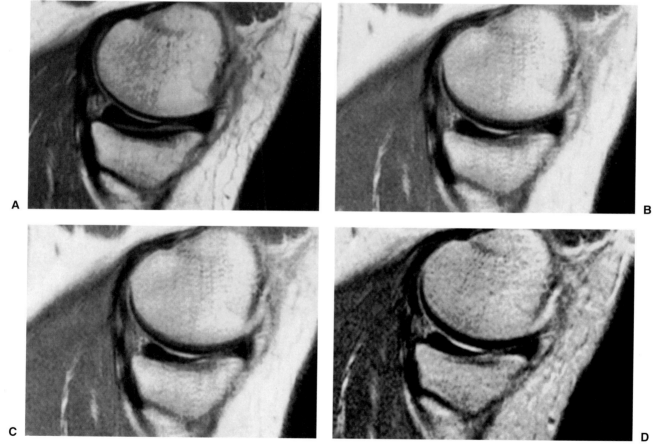

FIG. 7. Fast imaging. **(A)** Sagittal turbo spin-echo image (low-high or centric profile order, ETL) shows a wrinkled medial meniscus without tear. **(B)** Sagittal gradient-echo spin-echo hybrid (GraSE) image acquired with low-high or centric mapping of *k*-space (EPI factor 3, ETL 3) shows loss of edge enhancement as periphery of *k*-space filled with low-amplitude echoes. **(C)** Sagittal gradient-echo spin-echo hybrid (GraSE) image acquired with low-high or centric mapping of *k*-space (EPI factor 3, ETL 3) shows loss of edge enhancement as periphery of *k*-space filled with low-amplitude echoes. **(D)** Sagittal gradient-echo spin-echo hybrid (GraSE) image with same parameters as in image **C** but now with linear mapping of *k*-space (EPI factor 3, ETL 3) shows restoration of edge enhancement but in so doing generates more T2 weighting.

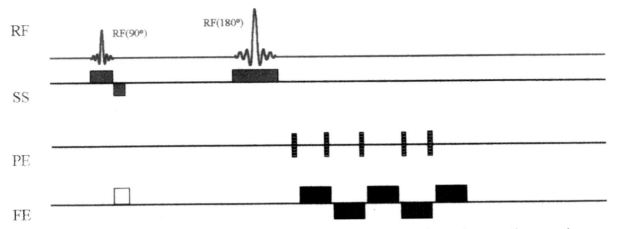

FIG. 8. Echo planar imaging. Diagram shows multiple gradient reversals, each generating an echo following an initial spin-echo 90°, 180° excitatory pulse. Such a sequence is termed spin-echo, echo planar imaging.

Echo Planar Imaging

Echo planar imaging (EPI), although it is gradient-echo based, also mirrors RARE imaging. Following an excitatory pulse, a train of echoes is acquired generated by a train of gradient reversals (Fig. 8). With such a technique, the entire *k*-space can be filled in one excitation or shot. Reflecting long echo trains, extended echoes have minimal amplitude, and therefore, acquired images have little signal relative to noise. To improve image signal-to-noise ratio, images may be acquired in multiple shots or with shorter echo trains at the expense of time.

Echo planar sequences may follow either a partial flip excitation (gradient echo) or a conventional spin-echo excitation (spin-echo EPI).

Both GraSE and EPI images are markedly distorted by both magnetic susceptibility and multidirectional chemical shift artifact (see Fig. 7). Chemical shift artifact increases as echo train length is increased, resulting in marked image distortion of single-shot images. Diagnostic images are therefore obtained with a multishot technique, particularly when supplemented by frequency-selective fat saturation (see Fig. 5).

Image Artifacts Distorting MR Imaging of Bone

Magnetic Susceptibility

Magnetic susceptibility describes the potential of elements to become magnetized. Contrast on MR images reflects the tendency of different elements to become magnetized and therefore reflects magnetic susceptibility. Bone includes cortical compact bone with poor susceptibility, which surrounds medulla containing loosely packed marrow with interdigitating trabeculae. At the interfaces of elements where susceptibilities differ, signal loss may distort image detail. Susceptibility differences are enhanced on gradient-echo images including GraSE and EPI and decreased on spin-echo-based sequences (particularly turbo spin echo and HASTE). Marrow-based susceptibility differences may lead to obscuring of subtle fractures on gradient-echo-based sequences.

Chemical Shift

Signal is localized in space at MR imaging on the basis of phase and frequency. Such a method is effective if tissues are uniform. However, because two tissue types predominate, fat and water, and fat spins at a frequency 220 Hz slower than free water, any signal being localized according to an induced gradation in frequencies undergoes a shift at fat–water interfaces leading to misregistration in space. Chemical shift effects or misregistration of signal distorts images, particularly in the frequency axis. Chemical shift distorting fine detail is particularly obvious using both EPI and GraSE sequences in which the artifact is multidirectional. The artifact is increased by increasing EPI factor. In such a way, a multishot technique with reduced EPI factor decreases chemical shift artifact. Such artifact reduction is at the expense of increased acquisition time. If frequency-selective fat saturation is used, fat–water interfaces are eliminated, and the artifact is removed. Frequency-selective fat saturation may be applied to single-shot EPI images in such a way that image acquisition time is unaffected.

RAPID MRI: SPECIALIZED HARDWARE

Scan-time reductions can be obtained either by reducing the total amount of data acquired by the pulse sequence or by using very busy pulse sequences in which the inactive times are at an absolute minimum. This latter approach, which is preferable for most applications, includes short-

TR conventional pulse sequences as well as hybrid pulse sequences. These sequences can be very demanding on the scanner's hardware because RF and gradient pulses must be amplified and delivered accurately to the patient in a very rapid succession. Furthermore, in the pursuit of faster scans affording higher spatial resolution and larger anatomic coverage, the spatial encoding gradient pulses must have increasingly higher amplitudes, and these must be switched on and off in very short times. Consequently, newer imaging subsystems should handle increasing levels of electric and magnetic powers and also must be capable of switching these powers very rapidly, ideally in a small fraction of a millisecond. Furthermore, these imaging subsystems should be very stable and accurate to minimize image artifacts. Taken together, these performance requirements translate into difficult engineering problems relating to the design and the construction of high-power-gradient amplifiers and large-bore-gradient coils.

Advanced Imaging Subsystems

Although very powerful imaging subsystems (maximum gradient amplitude > 50 mT/m and slew rate > 100 mT/m per msec) suited for small-bore research scanners have been available for a number of years, scaling up these designs to fit large-bore clinical MRI scanners has been difficult and consequently much slower. The main difficulty originates from the steep increase in the electrical power required to energize larger-bore gradient coils: the electric power increases as the fourth or fifth power of the coil radius. Consequently, the size and cost of the gradient amplifiers increase substantially. More problematic, however, is the amount of heat and the loud audible noise generated by the gradient coils. Typically, gradient coils designed to operate above 15 mT/m are fluid cooled. As a consequence, their design is more complicated, and scanners equipped with powerful imaging subsystems require additional hardware components to circulate the cooling fluid. Despite careful structural designs, noise generation by large-bore gradient coils is still a persistent problem that requires patients to wear ear protection. Currently, the specifications for an advanced imaging subsystem are approximately 25 mT/m maximum gradient strength with a slew rate of 100 mT/m per msec. These performance figures are likely to be improved in the coming years as manufacturers continue seeking solutions to the technological problems associated with the generation of strong magnetic field gradients (Fig. 9).

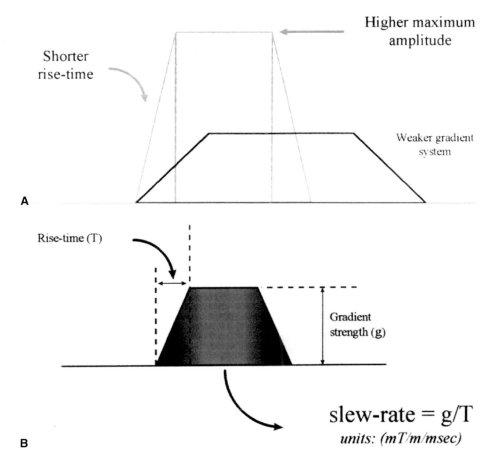

FIG. 9. Improvements in magnetic field gradient power. **(A)** Strong and fast gradients. Figure illustrates the improvements in maximum gradient strength and slew rate of the gradient waveforms obtainable with more powerful imaging subsystems (gradient coils and gradient amplifiers). **(B)** Magnetic field gradients: strength and switching speed. Diagram showing effect of rise time and gradient amplitude on slew rate.

Sensitivity Improvements

The additional gradient power afforded by high-performance gradient subsystems may be utilized in different ways. Clinically, the most desirable "investments" of additional gradient power are geared to either shorten scan times, increase spatial resolution, increase anatomic coverage, or produce shorter minimum echo times. Accordingly, to take full advantage of all the capabilities afforded by improvements in magnetic field gradient performance, MRI scanners should ideally be equipped with more advanced signal detection subsystems. Of particular interest is the development of detection subsystems with improved signal detection sensitivity and with larger anatomic coverage. The so-called phased-array coils offer the high signal sensitivity of small surface coils in combination with the large anatomic coverage of lower SNR typical of larger receiver coils. Phased-array coils consist of a number of surface coils, typically four to six, which are individually connected to separate independent signal amplification channels. The individual coil elements may be arranged in a linear pattern to increase anatomic coverage or in a wrap-around configuration to further improve the SNR. Linear phased arrays are most useful for spine and lower extremity imaging, and wrap-around phased arrays are ideal for abdominal and brain applications. The main drawbacks of phased-array systems are the greater expense of the coil plus the additional receiver channels and severalfold increase in reconstruction times.

DEDICATED EXTREMITY LOW-FIELD MRI SYSTEMS

To overcome the impact of patient claustrophobia and to reduce cost, there has been extensive interest in the development of open-design low-field MRI systems dedicated for extremity imaging (Lunar Artoscan, Genoa, Italy; Magna SL, Magnalab, New York, NY). These systems, which use a permanent magnet, generate comparatively weaker magnetic fields, the strengths of which currently range between 0.2 and 0.35 T.

Low-field systems need considerably less shielding and therefore can be deployed in small rooms with much reduced risk of deleting either computer disks or credit cards, unless these are placed directly within the bore of the magnet. Besides these practical advantages, low-field systems also benefit from much reduced artifacts from chemical shift misregistration, susceptibility variations and secondary to metallic orthopedic hardware. In particular, the magnetic field distortion induced by orthopedic components is significantly reduced, thus allowing diagnostic visualization of soft tissues adjacent to the metal components (discussed in Chapter 3).

The main limitations of low-field systems include limited

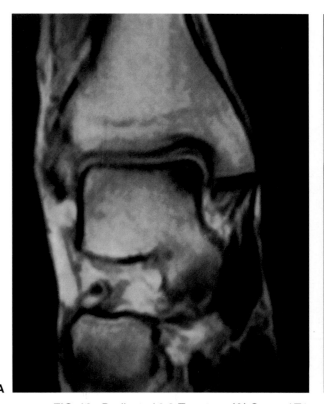

A

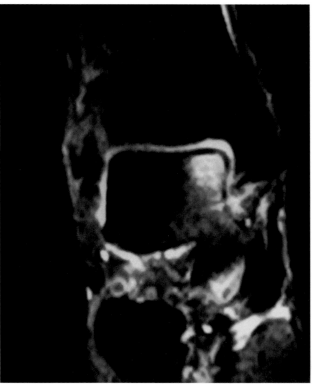

B

FIG. 10. Dedicated 0.3-T system. **(A)** Coronal T1-weighted spin-echo and **(B)** inversion recovery images show a posttraumatic osteochondral lesion of the talar dome. (Courtesy of Lunar Artoscan, Madison, WI.)

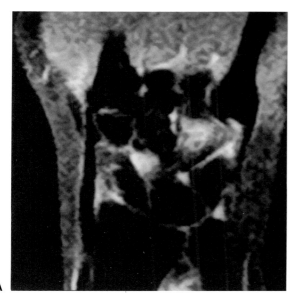
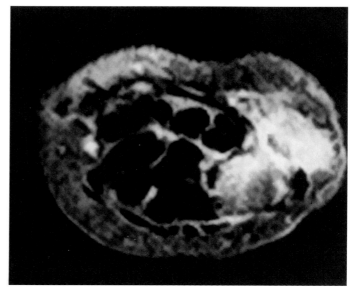

A

B

FIG. 11. Dedicated 0.3-T system. **(A)** Coronal and **(B)** axial inversion recovery images show extensive edema throughout the body **(A)** and the hook of hamate at the site of an occult fracture. (Courtesy of Lunar Artoscan, Madison, WI.)

field of view (approximately 11 cm), limited tissue coverage, and, most important, reduced overall signal-to-noise ratio (Table 1). Furthermore, unlike high-field systems, where water and fat peaks can be distinguished spectrally, the two peaks have considerable overlap at low field strengths. For this reason, frequency-selective fat suppression is technically challenging, and inversion recovery fat suppression technique has been the alternative of choice. Although all T1 values are shorter at low field strength, the T1 relative differences among tissues are approximately maintained: the inversion recovery time is reduced from about 140 msec at 1.5 T to about 80 msec at 0.3 T. Inversion recovery techniques are T1-selective and not chemically selective; therefore, the signal stemming from gadolinium-enhanced tis-

sues with short T1 values close to that of fat may be suppressed.

Approximation of fat and water peaks on low-field-strength systems almost eliminates both magnetic susceptibility and chemical shift misregistration artifacts, improving image quality. Similarly, although compatible fat saturation and contrast enhancement techniques are not available on low-field systems, when employed, the shortened T1 values of tissue at low field enhance the potency of gadolinium (reducing the required imaging dose) (Figs. 10–12).

TABLE 1. *Differences between permanent and superconducting MR systems*

Low field: 0.3-T systems	Superconducting systems: 0.5–1.5 T
Low signal to noise	High signal to noise
Improved signal with multiple NEX	
Increased acquisition times	Decreased acquisition times
Decreased maximum tissue coverage (11 cm)	
IR fat suppression	IR and frequency-selective fat suppression
Extremely sensitive to gadolinium	
T2* approximates T2	
Gradient echo equivalent to spin echo	Routine use of fast spin echo
Improved imaging of post op patients	Hardware artifacts

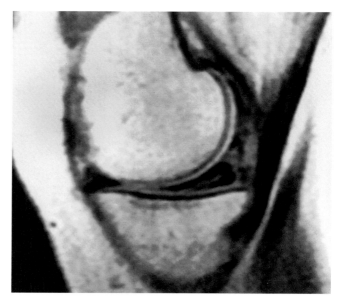

FIG. 12. Dedicated 0.3-T system. Sagittal proton-density-weighted image shows an oblique tear through the posterior horn of the medial meniscus extending to the inferior surface. (Courtesy of Lunar Artoscan, Madison, WI.)

APPENDIX: MANUFACTURER-DEPENDENT VARIATIONS IN PULSE SEQUENCE TERMINOLOGY (GENERAL ELECTRIC AND SIEMENS VERSUS PHILIPS)

Inversion recovery (IR)

Gradient echo (GE) (General Electric and Siemens Medical Systems) is the same as *fast field echo* (FFE) (Philips Medical Systems)

Conventional spin echo (CSE) (all manufacturers)

RARE fast spin echo (FSE) (General Electric) is the same as *turbo spin echo* (TSE) (Philips Medical Systems)

Fast inversion recovery is the same as *inversion recovery turbo spin echo* (IR TSE) (Philips Medical Systems)

REFERENCES AND SUGGESTED READING

1. Edelman RR, Hesselink JR, Zlattkin MB, eds. *Clinical Magnetic Resonance Imaging, 2nd ed, vol 1.* Philadelphia: WB Saunders, 1996.
2. Stark DD, Bradley WG, eds. *Magnetic Resonance Imaging, 2nd ed, vols 1 and 2.* Chicago: Mosby, 1992.
3. Horowitz AL. *MRI Physics For Radiologists—A Visual Approach, 2nd ed.* New York: Springer-Verlag, 1992.
4. Lufkin RB. *The MRI Manual.* Chicago: Mosby, 1990.
5. Hennig J, Nauerth A, Friedburg H. RARE imaging: a fast imaging method for clinical MR. *Magn Res Med* 1986;3:823–833.
6. Elster AD. *Questions and Answers in Magnetic Resonance Imaging.* Chicago: Mosby, 1994.
7. Hashemi RH, Bradley WG. *MRI—The Basics.* Baltimore: Williams & Wilkins, 1997.
8. Edelman RR, Wielopolski P, Schmitt F, et al. Echoplanar MR imaging. *Radiology* 1994;192:600–612.
9. Peterfy CG, Roberts T, Genant HK. Dedicated extremity MR imaging: An emerging technology. *Radiol Clin North Am* 1997;35:1–20.

CHAPTER 3

Applied Magnetic Resonance Imaging Techniques

Stephen J. Eustace

This chapter reviews basic MR techniques employed to allow successful imaging of articular cartilage, synovium, marrow, para-articular vascular structures, and finally postoperative patients with metal hardware *in situ* (Fig. 1).

IMAGING CARTILAGE

The histology of cartilage shows five organized layers, predominantly composed of water. Chondrocyte size and mineralization increase in deeper layers, in contrast to water content (1,2). In such a way, at magnetic resonance, images of articular cartilage show three layers: a surface hypointense (submillimeter) layer (corresponding to the lamina splendens at histology), a dominant hyperintense proton-rich parenchymal midzone (corresponding to the tangential, transverse, and radial zones at histology), and a third deep hypointense zone of mineralized cartilage that merges with underlying cortex (corresponding to the calcified zone deep to the tidemark at histology) (3) (Fig. 2).

Because of its abundance of water, cartilage is readily imaged using magnetic resonance. Despite innumerable descriptions of techniques employed to improve its visibility, existing techniques may be simply divided into either T1 or T2 categories.

On T1- and proton-density-weighted sequences, cartilage generates more signal than synovial fluid; on T2-weighted (both true T2- and T2*-weighted) sequences, cartilage generates less signal than synovial fluid.

On T1- and proton-density-weighted images, cartilage may be enhanced by the application of a frequency-selective fat saturation pulse, irrespective of whether images are derived from spin-echo or gradient-echo pulse sequences. On fat-suppressed images, cartilage becomes dramatically hyperintense relative to suppressed yellow marrow and synovial fluid as a result of signal rescaling (4) (Figs. 3 and 4). The use of partial flip angle techniques allowed the acquisition of three-dimensional (3D) fat-suppressed T1-weighted images without significant impact on time, enhancing spatial resolution.

Successful T2*-weighted cartilage imaging may be achieved using partial flip angle gradient or fast field-echo techniques. With such techniques, contrast between synovial fluid and cartilage may be enhanced by the application of an off-resonance pulse, 1,500 Hz off the resonant frequency of free water (Figs. 5–8). Protons or water molecules, par-

S. J. Eustace: Department of Radiology, Section of Musculoskeletal Radiology, Boston University School of Medicine and Boston Medical Center, Boston, Massachusetts 02118.

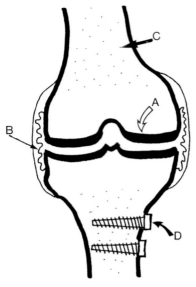

FIG. 1. Coronal representation of knee joint demonstrating articular components: A, cartilage; B, synovium; C, marrow; D, hardware.

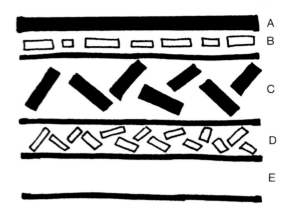

FIG. 2. Diagrammatic representation of structure and configuration of articular cartilage. Layer A, lamina splendens; layer B, tangential zone; layer C, transverse zone; layer D, radial zone; layer E, calcified zone. The size of collagen fibers increases in deeper layers, whereas the water content and organization decrease in deeper layers.

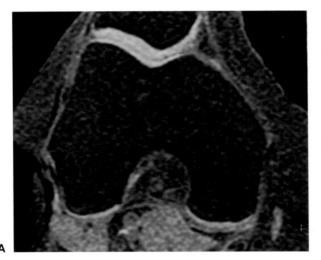

A

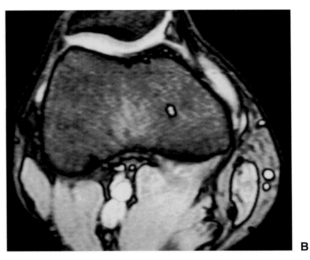

B

FIG. 3. (A) T1-weighted fast field-echo axial image (flip angle 70°) with fat suppression shows dramatic signal hyperintensity within patellofemoral cartilage as a result of signal rescaling. (B) T2-weighted fast field-echo image (flip angle 30°, TR 500 msec, TE 15 msec) shows signal hypointensity within articular cartilage relative to adjacent synovial fluid.

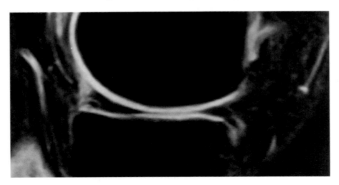

FIG. 4. Sagittal T1-weighted fast field-echo image of the knee with fat suppression shows dramatic signal hyperintensity within articular cartilage. Incidental note is made of oblique tear to inferior surface of the posterior horn of the medial meniscus.

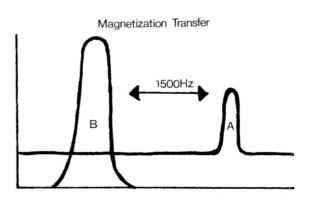

FIG. 5. Diagram showing resonant peak of free water (A) and saturation pulse 1,500 Hz off resonance.

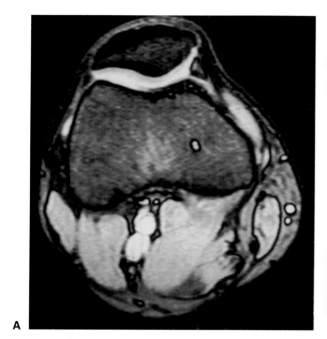 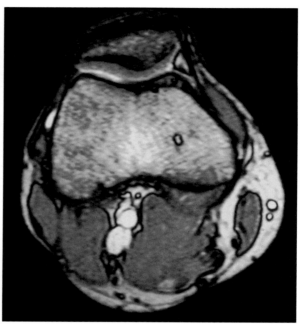

FIG. 6. Axial T2-weighted fast field-echo images without **(A)** and with **(B)** off-resonance saturation pulse.

tially bound are influenced by large macromolecules within cartilage, precessing up to 1,500 Hz slower than free water become saturated by the applied pulse, enhancing contrast between it and free hyperintense synovial fluid. This tech-

nique is termed gradient or fast field echo with off-resonance magnetization transfer (5). Such a technique may be used to image both articular cartilage and the unossified pediatric growth plate, particularly at the elbow (6) (Fig. 9).

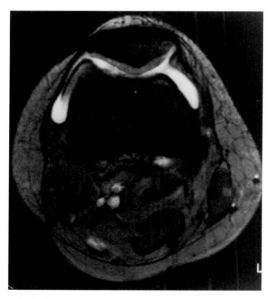

FIG. 7. Axial T2-weighted fast field-echo image with off-resonance magnetization transfer saturation pulse shows heterogeneous signal hyperintensity within cartilage of the lateral patellar facet at a site corresponding to fibrillation or grade 1 chondromalacia.

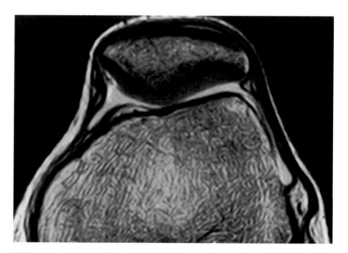

FIG. 8. Axial T2-weighted three-dimensional FFE-echo planar image of patellofemoral cartilage acquired on a Powertrack 3000 system (Philips Medical Systems) with a TR of 30, TE of 14, flip angle of 35°, 14-cm field of view, 3-mm slice thickness, 512 phase encodes, four excitations, with off-resonance magnetization transfer saturation, in 2 min 34 sec. (Courtesy of Philips Medical Systems, Shelton, CT.)

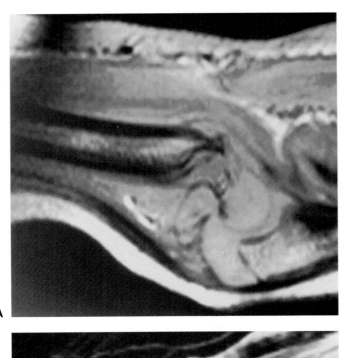

A

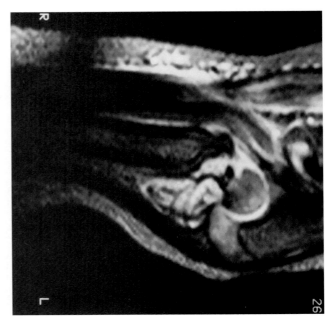

B

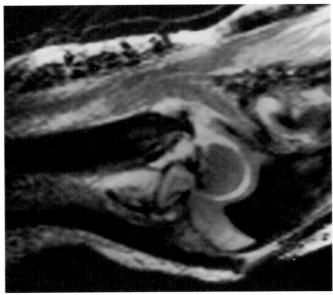

C

FIG. 9. (A) Sagittal T1-weighted image (TR 500 msec, TE 15 msec) of a transphyseal fracture of the distal humerus. (B) Sagittal T2-weighted fast field-echo image of the same patient. (C) Sagittal T2-weighted fast field-echo image with off-resonance magnetization transfer saturation shows enhanced contrast between unossified cartilage and free synovial fluid.

T2-turbo or fast spin-echo sequences with spectral fat saturation facilitate the acquisition of images with similar contrast between cartilage and joint fluid. With a short echo train of six and linear *k*-space mapping, images with a TR of 2,000 and an effective TE of 80 msec are rapidly acquired. Retained signal within fat as a result of the J coupling effect may be negated by a frequency-selective fat saturation pulse. Magnetization transfer effects theoretically result in signal loss within articular cartilage and enhance observed contrast between it and synovial fluid (7).

Although the diffusion imaging technique (to be discussed later in the chapter) allows the detection of subtle foci of cartilaginous degeneration, its use in evaluating posttraumatic cartilage injury has not, to date, been exploited.

Techniques to Image Cartilage

T1- or Proton-Density-Weighted Imaging
T1- or Proton-Density-Weighted Imaging with Fat Suppression
T2*-Weighted Technique
T2*-Weighted Technique with Off-Resonance Magnetization Transfer (Flip 30, TR 500 msec, TE 15, 512 × 512 matrix (50% scan percentage), Off-Res MT, NSA 2)
T2-Weighted Turbo or Fast Spin-Echo Imaging with Fat Saturation
Diffusion Imaging

IMAGING SYNOVIUM

Although synovial inflammation may follow articular trauma, interest in quantification and imaging has been most marked in patients with synovitis complicating inflammatory arthritis (8). Synovium contains abundant partially bound fluid or protons as a result of associated hypervascularity. Quantities of free water decrease in patients with chronic disease or following treatment, as inflamed synovium becomes replaced by fibrous tissue (9) (Fig. 10).

The presence of abundant water within synovial matrix results in the generation of signal characteristics similar to those of free water or synovial fluid on T1- and T2-weighted scans, limiting its routine visualization and detection. Visibility may be improved by using either gadolinium enhancement or a delayed-echo heavily T2-weighted technique.

Following intravenous administration of gadolinium (20 cc gadopentate dimeglumine), synovium enhances diffusely, improving its visibility relative to adjacent unenhanced structures. Within minutes of enhancement, synovium begins to secrete small amounts of gadolinium into synovial fluid, dramatically increasing the extent of observed enhancement and potentially leading to inadvertent overestimation of total synovial volume (10).

Recognizing the potential to overestimate synovial volume using the dynamic gadolinium technique, many now advocate the use of heavily T2-weighted, unenhanced scans similar to those used to characterize hepatic hemangiomas. In effect, synovium, isointense to free synovial fluid at an echo time of 80 msec, generally becomes hypointense to free synovial fluid at an echo time of 160 msec. Partially bound protons or fluid in synovium retain T2 signal at 80 msec but, under the influence of synovial macromolecules, dephase and lose T2 signal before protons in free water (11) (Fig. 11).

An alternate technique employs a saturation off-resonance pulse to improve contrast between hyperintense synovium and adjacent free synovial fluid. Exploiting the effect of macromolecules within synovium, an applied off-resonance pulse saturates partially bound protons, reducing the observed synovial T2 signal. Such a technique enhances con-

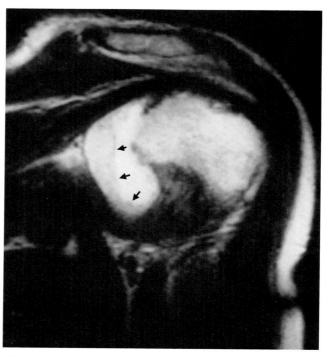

FIG. 11. Coronal oblique heavily T2-weighted turbo spin-echo image of the anterior margin of the shoulder shows a rind of inflamed synovium marginating the axillary recess *(arrows)* (TR 3,000, TE$_{eff}$ 140, turbo factor 6) in a patient with acute inflammatory synovitis.

trast between synovium and free synovial fluid (similar to the cartilage technique) (12) (Fig. 12).

The use of both diffusion imaging and of a combined fluid attenuated inversion recovery (FLAIR) technique with fat

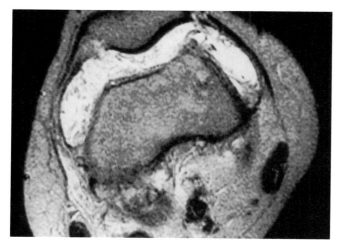

FIG. 10. Axial T2-weighted spin-echo image of the knee shows feathery filling defects within a large suprapatellar joint effusion secondary to chronic synovitis in a patient with rheumatoid arthritis.

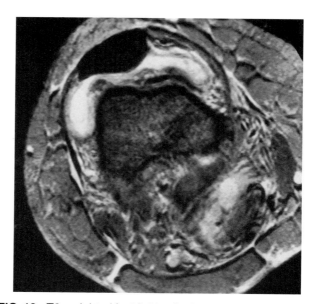

FIG. 12. T2-weighted fast field-echo image of the patellofemoral articulation in a patient with acute inflammatory synovitis. Contrast between a smooth rind of synovium and synovial fluid is enhanced by an off-resonance magnetization transfer saturation pulse.

saturation to characterize synovitis is currently under review (discussed later in this chapter).

Techniques to Image Synovium

T1-Weighted Technique After Gadolinium Enhancement
T2-Weighted Technique
T2-Weighted Technique with Off-Resonance Magnetization Transfer
T2-Weighted Technique with Delayed Echo (TE, 160 msec)
FLAIR with Frequency-Selective Fat Saturation
Diffusion Imaging

MARROW IMAGING: IN-PHASE/OUT-OF-PHASE TECHNIQUE

In adolescence, red marrow is converted to yellow marrow in the extremities, in part as a result of temperature differences in the axial and appendicular skeleton (13). Diaphyseal red-to-yellow marrow conversion precedes metaphyseal conversion, and distal conversion precedes proximal conversion. In such a way, marrow conversion typically occurs in the diaphyses of long bones and then in the metaphyses and occurs in distal long bones (tibia, radius, and ulna) before proximal (femur, humerus). Varying quantities of red marrow remain within the pelvis, the spine, and calvarium through adulthood, resulting in observed signal heterogeneity at these sites (14) (Figs. 13 and 14).

In response to oxygen demands of athletics and chronic lung disease, some individuals reconvert yellow to red marrow in the metaphyses and even in the diaphyses of long bones in adulthood. It is common to see metaphyseal red marrow in joggers, cigarette smokers, and for an unexplained reason in overweight middle-aged women (15). The presence of epiphyseal red marrow is pathologic, except that subarticular red marrow persists in the humeral head (16), a feature most commonly seen in patients with red cell packing disorders such as sickle cell disease and more recently in patients with chronic renal failure on erythropoietin supplements (Fig. 15).

Yellow marrow, as the name implies, is essentially fat (90% fat, 10% water), and as a result, reflecting rapid dissipation of energy to complex macromolecules recovers longitudinal magnetization (short T1) and loses transverse magnetization rapidly (short T2). Red marrow, in contrast, is cellular (20%) and contains significant quantities of water (40%), which has delayed recovery of longitudinal magnetization and loss of transverse magnetization following excitation (17).

In such a way, yellow marrow is hyperintense on T1- and hypointense on T2-weighted scans and suppresses on both inversion recovery and spectral presaturation scans, whereas red marrow is isointense to muscle on T1, T2, and fat-suppressed (inversion recovery and spectral presaturation techniques) images.

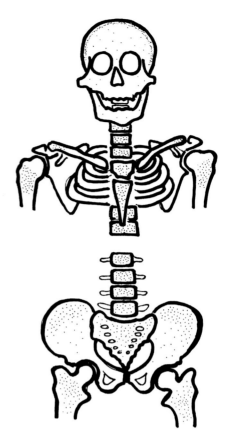

FIG. 13. Diagrammatic representation of the distribution of red marrow *(speckled areas)* within the axial and appendicular skeleton in adulthood.

Sites of marrow heterogeneity, occurring either as a result of primary yellow marrow conversion in the spine or as a result of red marrow reconversion in the extremities, often create diagnostic confusion in patients with known malignancies. In this setting, the chemical shift Dixon technique

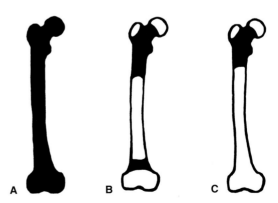

FIG. 14. Diagrammatic representation of red–yellow marrow conversion in the appendicular skeleton (the right femur) with aging. **(A)** Dark area indicating extensive red marrow in infancy. **(B)** Residual red marrow within proximal and distal metaphyses in second decade. **(C)** Residual proximal metaphyseal red marrow in adulthood.

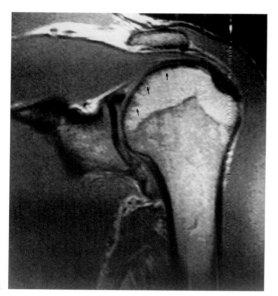
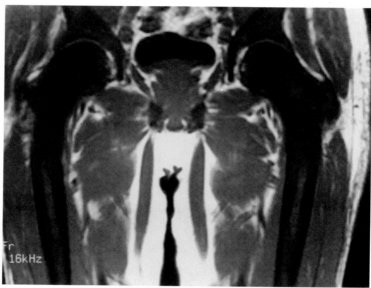

A   B

FIG. 15. (A) Coronal oblique T1-weighted spin-echo image of the shoulder shows extensive metaphyseal red marrow with subarticular red marrow rests *(arrows)*. (B) Coronal T1-weighted spin-echo image of the proximal femora shows replacement of normal fatty marrow by hypointense marrow infiltrate secondary to mastocytosis.

(in-phase/out-of-phase imaging) (previously used to characterize adrenal masses, fatty infiltration of the liver, and to enhance background tissue suppression at MRA) may be employed to differentiate benign red marrow from malignant tumor infiltration (17).

The in-phase/out-of-phase technique utilizes the fact that red marrow has approximately equal quantities of fat (40%) and water (40%) in contrast to tumor deposits, which are predominantly water or proton-rich (90%).

At rest, magnetic vectors from fat and water within a voxel align with the main magnetic field in the z axis, the sum of the two vectors accounting for a strong magnetic vector in

the direction of the main field (the z axis). Following excitation by an applied radiofrequency pulse at the Larmor frequency, water molecules or free protons uninfluenced by an adjacent macromolecule precess or spin at a slightly faster rate than protons bound to fat (Fig. 16). At 1.5 T, water precesses at 220 Hz faster than fat. Because the induced magnetic vector from water rotates faster than the vector created by fat, after each cycle the vectors move apart such that at a certain point the vectors are diametrically opposed. At the time when vectors are opposed, the sum of the two vectors results in a net loss of magnetization and therefore a relative loss of signal. If there are equal quantities of fat and water, as occurs in red marrow, there will be a marked reduction in signal on opposed-phase images and summation of signal on in-phase images (Fig. 17). If a voxel contains either predominant fat or water (as in metastasis, 90% water), there will be little signal cancellation on out-of-phase images, and observed signal will remain unchanged on opposed images (17) (Fig. 18).

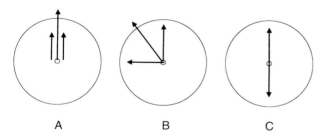

A   B   C

FIG. 16. In phase out phase chemical shift imaging. Diagram showing fat and water vectors in phase, resulting in a large net magnetic vector immediately following excitation **(A)**, with gradual loss of phase in time because water precesses faster than fat **(B)** until a point when magnetization vectors from fat and water are diametrically opposed **(C)**. In the presence of equal quantities of fat and water, summed vectors result in cancellation of magnetization.

To Calculate Sampling Times for In and Out of Phase (at 1.5 T in This Case) Using Gradient Echo

$-\frac{1}{2} \times 1/(220 \text{ Hz}) = 2.3$ msec: out of phase if signal is sampled 2.3 msec following excitation; TE = 2.3

$-1 \times 1/(220 \text{ Hz}) = 4.6$ msec: in phase if signal is sampled 4.6 msec following excitation; TE = 4.6

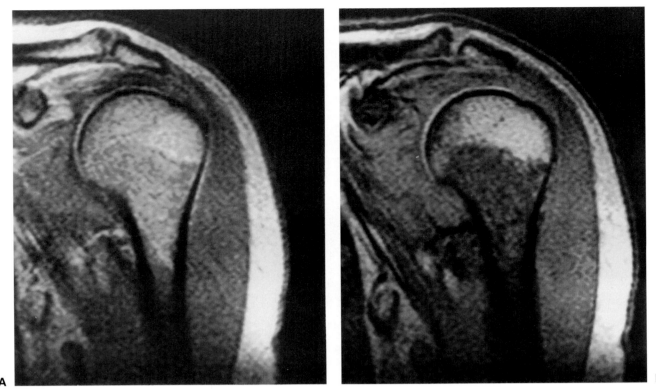

FIG. 17. Coronal oblique T1-weighted fast field-echo images of the shoulder acquired **(A)** at 1.5 T, at a TE of 4.6 msec (in phase), show summation of magnetization with relative red marrow hyperintensity, and **(B)** at a TE of 6.9 msec (out of phase) with relative red marrow hypointensity.

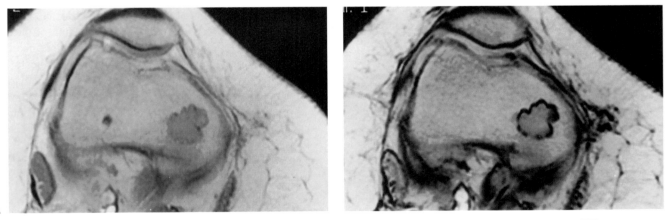

FIG. 18. Axial images of marrow deposit at the level of the patellofemoral articulation. **(A)** In phase (TE 4.6 msec), showing matrix signal similar to articular cartilage. **(B)** Out of phase (TE 6.9 msec), showing preservation of matrix signal and confirming that the deposit is not a residual red marrow rest (biopsy-revealed enchondroma).

WHOLE-BODY IMAGING TECHNIQUES

Although primarily employed as a marrow-imaging tool in patients with known malignancies, whole-body imaging techniques are also occasionally employed in patients with pathologic fractures to localize the site of a suspected pri-

mary tumor, to identify additional metastatic deposits, or as an alternative to skeletal survey in children referred with suspected child abuse to localize occult fractures.

With a RARE platform, fast gradients (rise time less than 200 μsec), and a moving table top, rapid imaging may be performed using turbo or fast spin-echo, HASTE, GraSE, or EPI sequences (see Chapter 2).

With a turbo inversion recovery sequence and a maximum field of view (45 cm), whole-body imaging may be achieved by four contiguous, slightly overlapping, coronal acquisitions (18) (Fig. 19).

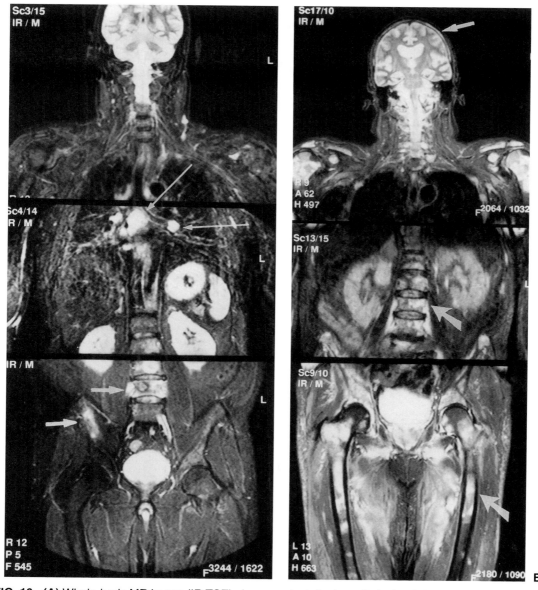

FIG. 19. (A) Whole-body MR image (IR TSE) shows metastatic deposits in the right ilium *(white arrow)*, L4 vertebral body *(white arrow)* in association with subcarinal adenopathy *(long arrow)* in a patient with metastatic prostate carcinoma. **(B)** Whole-body MR image shows diffuse marrow infiltration (hyperintense foci; *arrows*) in a patient with multifocal skeletal lymphoma.

Turbo STIR Whole-Body Imaging Protocol

Coronal Acquisition
Maximum Field of View
Inversion Time 160 msec
TE 20–40 msec
TR 2–4,000 msec
Slice Thickness 8 mm

MAGNETIC RESONANCE ARTHROGRAPHY: DIRECT AND INDIRECT TECHNIQUES

There has been extensive recent interest in the use of MRI to evaluate internal joint structures following administration of intra-articular contrast. Although the technique is often used to evaluate patients with chronic joint pain, arthrography is also frequently used to evaluate patients with suspected labral tears, chondral injury, or loose bodies following dislocation or direct joint trauma.

Contrast may be introduced to the joint either by direct needle puncture or indirectly following intravenous contrast injection (19).

Following intravenous contrast administration, contrast is gradually secreted to the joint space by enhancing synovium. Although the amount of secreted contrast is minimal (intra-articular gadolinium is not detectable at fluoroscopy or computed tomography 30 min following intravenous injection), the dramatic changes in magnetization induced by small amounts of intra-articular gadolinium as it diffuses through joint fluid result in a dramatic arthrographic effect. (It is not gadolinium contrast but the response it induces in the adjacent fluid that is being imaged) (20).

Elements with unpaired orbital electrons (paramagnetic substances) become magnetized in a magnetic field and orient in the direction of the parent field. As such, they locally enhance or strengthen the effects of the parent field and will enhance recovery of longitudinal magnetization in adjacent spins following excitation. The element in the periodic table with the greatest number of unpaired electrons is gadolinium, with seven (deoxyhemoglobin has four unpaired outer electrons; methemoglobin has five). Thus, small amounts of gadolinium induce strong local enhancement of the parent field manifest by extensive changes in longitudinal recovery in adjacent spins. At arthrography, gadolinium enhances longitudinal recovery within joint fluid (20).

Indirect MR Arthrography

Indirect gadolinium arthrography requires secretion of contrast from synovium into the joint space, most marked in patients with active synovitis. In such a way, the technique is unlikely to be successful if performed on patients in the absence of a preexisting joint effusion (reflecting synovitis). When employed, exercise is used to enhance vascular flow to synovium and deliver contrast (0.1 mmol/kg Gd-DTPA) to the joint. Imaging is undertaken 15 to 30 min following intravenous injection (21).

Direct Arthrography

Direct arthrography describes direct injection of contrast to the joint space before MR imaging. Although early interest in this technique was based on the use of intra-articular gadolinium injection and fat-suppressed T1-weighted imaging (22), there has been recent interest in the use of iodinated contrast and T2-weighted imaging or a hybrid technique in which gadolinium and iodinated contrast are mixed, allowing a conventional fluoroscopic arthrogram before gadolinium-enhanced T1-weighted MR imaging (23).

Gadolinium-enhanced T1-weighted images are signal-rich, overcoming limitations imposed by poor surface coils. When available, dedicated surface coils facilitate excellent signal-rich T2-weighted image acquisition without the requirement for intra-articular gadolinium (Figs. 20–23).

The primary advantage of the gadolinium technique versus the T2 technique is that unless a formal contrast arthrogram is performed in conjunction with the T2 technique, it may be unclear whether fluid identified in the subacromial bursa at the time of MRI preexisted the arthrogram (reflecting subacromial bursitis) or whether it entered the bursa at arthrography secondary to a cuff tear. In contrast, if gadolinium is identified in the subacromial bursa, it is definitive evidence of rotator cuff tear with communication between the injected shoulder joint and the subacromial space. The described hybrid technique in which gadolinium is mixed with iodinated water-soluble contrast allows acquisition of both a formal radiographic arthrogram and a fat-saturated T1-weighted MR arthrogram (23).

Because of the sensitivity of gadolinium, only 0.1 ml of gadolinium is added to 20 ml of normal saline (0.1 ml Gd DTPA is added to 20 ml of bacteriostatic saline) for routine

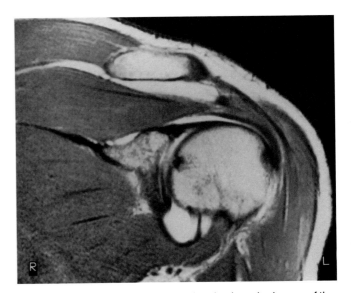

FIG. 20. Coronal oblique T1-weighted spin-echo image of the shoulder following direct gadolinium (1 in 200) arthrography showing an intact supraspinatus tendon and a type 2 bicipito-labral complex.

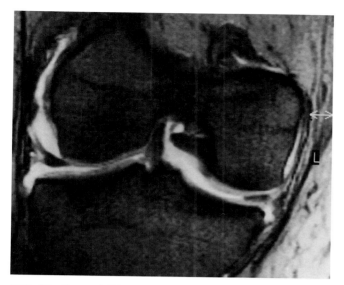

FIG. 21. Coronal T2-weighted fast field-echo image of the knee following direct intra-articular injection of normal saline with enhanced contrast between joint fluid and cartilage by an additional off-resonance magnetization transfer saturation pulse. Patient has undergone a previous partial medial meniscectomy.

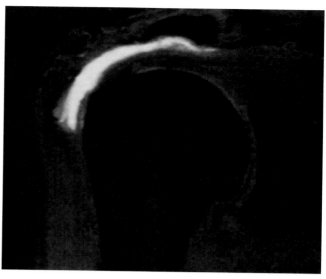

FIG. 23. Coronal oblique T1-weighted image of the shoulder with fat suppression following direct injection of contrast to the subacromial bursa; MR bursography was employed in the search for a superior surface tear.

gadolinium MR arthrography, 0.1 ml gadolinium is added to 15 ml iodinated contrast and 5 ml 1% lidocaine when undertaking the hybrid technique (lidocaine reduces discomfort induced by joint distension).

In addition to conventional positioning, additional imaging in the ABER (abducted, external rotation) hand behind the head position with imaging in the coronal oblique plane is occasionally employed at shoulder arthrography to allow detection of undisplaced anteroinferior labral abnormalities (Bankart, Perthe, ALPSA, and HAGL injuries discussed in Chapter 10) (24).

Injection of air bubbles, extravasation of contrast, and injection of excessive amounts of gadolinium are potential pitfalls in the technique.

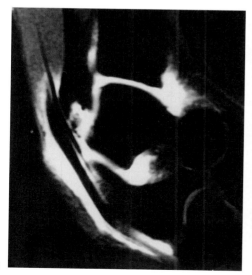
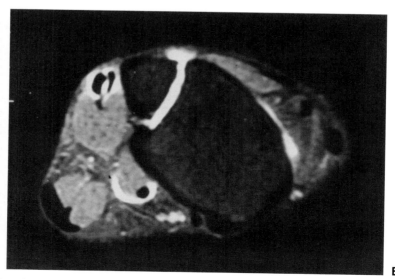

A

B

FIG. 22. Coronal **(A)** and axial **(B)** T1-weighted images with frequency-selective fat saturation of the ankle following direct injection of gadolinium (1 in 200). Coronal image shows extravasation of contrast to the peroneal tendon sheath following disruption of the calcaneofibular ligament. Axial image shows additional disruption of the anterior tibiofibular ligament. Courtesy of M. Barish, M.D., Boston Medical Center, Boston, MA.

Magnetic Resonance Arthrography Techniques

Indirect: 0.1 mmol/kg dose Gd-DTPA 15 to 30 min after exercise
Direct: 0.1 ml gadolinium in 20 ml normal saline
Direct Hybrid: 0.1 ml gadolinium in 15 ml iodinated contrast and 5 ml 1% lidocaine
Conventional Spin-Echo T1-Weighted Images with Fat Suppression in Coronal Oblique, Sagittal, and Axial Planes.

MAGNETIC RESONANCE ANGIOGRAPHY

Traditional evaluation of fractures has concentrated on osseous evaluation, overlooking associated soft tissue injury, frequently the cause of long-term morbidity. Detection of associated injury to vessels has traditionally required formal contrast angiography, and therefore, it has only been identified if specifically sought. Routine use of noninvasive MR venography in patients following pelvic fractures has led to frequent identification of deep pelvic vein thrombosis in this patient group (25). Similar use of MR angiography in fractures at other sites, particularly around the knee, allows earlier and more frequent detection of posttraumatic arterial injury.

Four methods of acquiring MR angiograms are currently employed: "time of flight," dynamic gadolinium-enhanced "time of flight," phase-contrast, and black blood angiography.

"Time-of-Flight" Partial Flip-Angle MR Angiography

"Time-of-flight" MR angiograms are generated by addition of information obtained on serial contiguous axial images (source data) using a maximum-intensity projection algorithm (MIP reconstruction).

Source images are generated using a T1-weighted partial flip angle sequence (images are based on the recovery of longitudinal magnetization); i.e., a flip angle of 50° to 80° generates T1 weighting (Fig. 24).

Signal in background tissue is suppressed by the repeated rapid application of excitatory pulses, which induce background steady state or saturation. A short repetition time (short TR) therefore improves background suppression.

In contrast, optimum signal is yielded by spins within a vessel entering the slice only if the excited spins move out of the slice before they can be reexcited and saturated by the reapplied excitatory pulse (short TR). Moving out of the slice and avoiding a reapplied pulse forestalls steady state or saturation. Spins within the vessel recovering longitudinal magnetization generate signal.

To achieve improved background suppression, signal is sampled at a time when fat and water are out of phase: signal in background tissue, containing opposed fat and water components, decreases, whereas signal in vessels containing water alone is retained (out-of-phase TE = 2.3 msec at 1.5 T).

The more spins are deflected by an applied excitatory

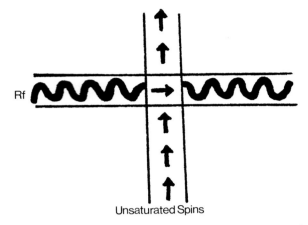

FIG. 24. Diagram demonstrating radiofrequency pulse repeatedly applied to a slice resulting in tissue saturation. Blood flowing perpendicular to the axis of the RF pulse brings unsaturated spins, which are excited and generate signal as they move out of the slice (before becoming reexcited and eventually saturated).

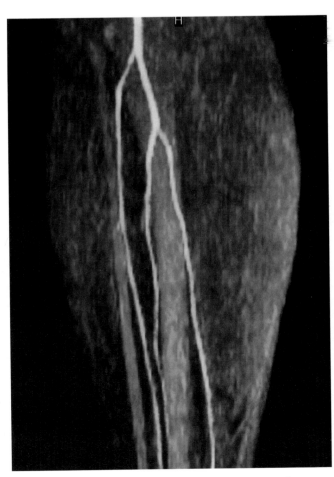

FIG. 25. Maximum intensity projection (MIP) coronal reconstruction of the popliteal trifurcation generated from multiple axial source images (TR 30 msec, TE 6.9 msec, flip angle 50°).

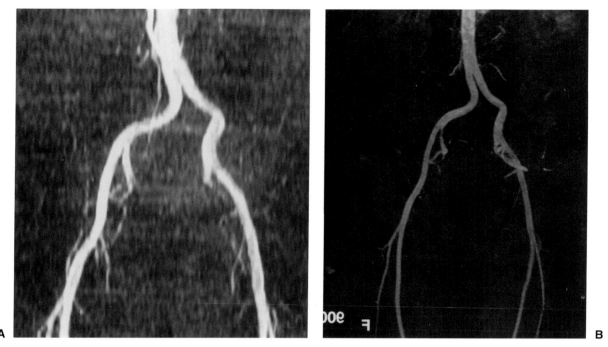

FIG. 26. Coronal MIP reconstruction of pelvic arteries generated from **(A)** axially acquired two-dimensional time-of-flight source data and **(B)** from coronally acquired source data (in the same patient) following a 40-mg gadolinium bolus.

pulse (higher flip angle), the greater the T1 weighting, and hence a larger signal is generated. Nevertheless, the more the spins are deflected, the greater the amount of time required to recover longitudinal magnetization, increasing the likelihood of reexcitation of spins within the vessel before complete recovery of magnetization and therefore increasing the potential for saturation. If flow is slow, and if repetition time is not altered, it is therefore necessary to lower the flip angle, allowing quicker recovery of magnetization, to avoid vessel saturation (Figs. 25 and 26).

Thus, time-of-flight angiography involves trade-offs among repetition time (TR), flip angle, and flow rate or practical trade-offs between background tissue saturation and generation of signal within vessels (26).

Dynamic Gadolinium

Gadolinium, enhancing the local parent field, induces rapid recovery of longitudinal magnetization by spins within an enhanced vessel. Rapid recovery facilitates more frequent reapplication of excitatory pulses, without inducing saturation of spins within the vessel. Shorter repetition time facilitates faster image acquisition (acquisition time = TR × NPE × NSA). Similarly, faster recovery of longitudinal magnetization allows use of higher flip angles (without saturation) and hence the generation of more signal within excited vessels.

Obliquely oriented vessels in the pelvis or tortuous peripheral vessels are vulnerable to in-plane saturation effects using unenhanced technique. Unenhanced spins or protons within

iliac vessels, staying in plane, become reexcited by the reapplied excitatory pulse before complete recovery of magnetization and become partially saturated. Saturated spins are manifest as signal loss, which is occasionally misinterpreted as indicating vascular stenosis. Gadolinium-enhanced spins recover magnetization rapidly before reexcitation and therefore do not become saturated. Gadolinium-enhanced imaging is therefore routinely employed to evaluate both pelvic and tortuous peripheral vessels (27) (Figs. 27–29).

Phase-Contrast Angiography

This technique involves application of equal and opposite excitatory gradients. The effect of an initial excitatory gradient is reversed by an equal but opposite gradient only if there has been no movement of spins between the two gradients. Moving spins within a vessel become excited by the initial gradient but retain signal if they have moved out of plane before the application of the opposite gradient. Motion in background tissue before the application of the equal and opposite gradient will therefore result in retained signal in background tissues. Phase-contrast techniques have therefore traditionally been employed in the evaluation of stationary body parts, particularly intracerebral vessels. Gating techniques compensating for motion have led to the wider application of phase contrast techniques in nonstationary body parts, such as the renal vessels. Phase contrast techniques are not vulnerable to in-plane flow saturation effects imposed by tortuous vessels.

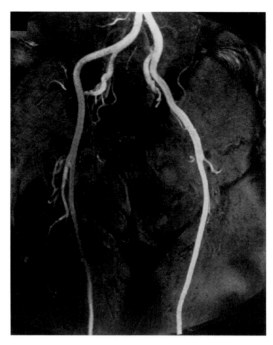

FIG. 27. Coronal MIP reconstruction of pelvic and groin arteries in a patient following pelvic fracture, generated from multiple coronal slices acquired following an intravenous gadolinium bolus (40 cc), with a 30-sec delay, TR 7 msec, TE 2.3 msec, flip angle 70°.

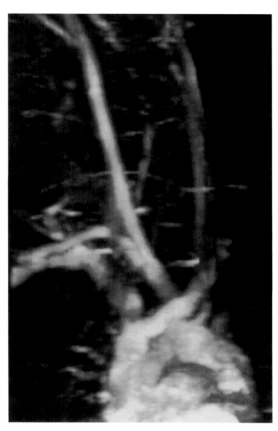

FIG. 29. Coronal MIP reconstruction of superior mediastinal arteries and veins in a patient following posterior dislocation of the medial clavicle.

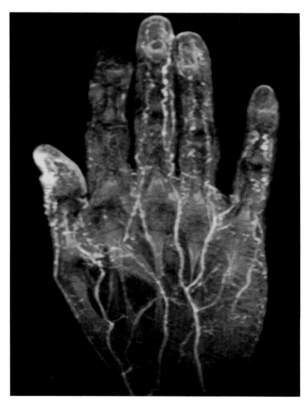

FIG. 28. Coronal MIP reconstruction of digital vessels in a patient with Buergers disease showing corkscrew digital vessels, generated from coronal slices acquired following intravenous injection of 40 cc of gadolinium (as in Fig. 27).

Black Blood

With RARE-based sequences, signal in a slice is rapidly acquired. Spins within a vessel, moving out of the slice before being rephased by a refocusing 180° pulse are devoid of signal. In such a way, unlike time-of-flight angiography, signal is generated in background tissues but lost within vessels. Angiograms using this technique are therefore generated by minimum-intensity projections. Because images are generated by signal loss within vessels, focal stenosis leading to dephasing (which would lead to signal loss at TOF angiography and hence overestimation of stenosis) is not problematic (28).

Routine Magnetic Resonance Angiographic Techniques

Time of Flight: TR 30 msec; TE 6.6 msec; Flip 50—70°

Dynamic Gadolinium: 40 ml Gd DTPA; TR 7; TE 2.3, Flip 50—70°

DIFFUSION IMAGING

Diffusion describes the process by which molecules undergo random motion under the influence of heat. Induced random motion of water molecules is partially impaired by adjacent complex macromolecules, particularly when the water is in a partially bound state.

Diffusion imaging is a technique employed to detect relative motion of unbound protons or water molecules, allowing indirect determination of macromolecular structure.

Organized tissues in which macromolecules are tightly bound allow minimal diffusion of water; in contrast, loosely bound or poorly organized tissues allow greater diffusion of fluid. This technique (similar to phase-contrast angiography) is based on the application of equal and opposite gradients on either side of a 180° refocusing pulse, the time between and strength of applied gradients dictating the sensitivity of the technique to subtle movement or diffusion of water (B value).

Although the clinical role for diffusion imaging in the musculoskeletal system is under evaluation, increased diffusion in degenerate cartilage, increased diffusion at sites of bone injury or bruising, and decreased diffusion as fractures heal provide the current foci for clinical research (29) (Fig. 30).

Potential Musculoskeletal Applications of Diffusion Imaging

Evaluation of Degenerate Cartilage
Detection of Bone Bruises Otherwise Occult by Conventional Techniques
Evaluation of Fracture Healing
Noninvasive Characterization of Synovial Fluid (Degenerate Effusions Viscous, Inflammatory Posttraumatic Effusions Aqueous)

DYNAMIC GADOLINIUM PERFUSION TECHNIQUES: KEYHOLE ACQUISITION

In an attempt to determine vascular integrity of fracture fragments, rapid image acquisition is required following gadolinium injection to serially follow fracture fragment enhancement (bolus tracking).

The keyhole technique involves acquisition of a mask image generated by complete filling of k-space. Subsequent images of the same slice are rapidly acquired by using a keyhole in which only the center (20%) of k-space is filled (responsible for contrast), and the outer portion of k-space is filled or borrowed from the mask image. Such a technique reduces acquisition time by a factor of five per slice. Because the center of k-space is repeatedly sampled, contrast varies in each image; because the periphery of k-space is not sampled, changes in edge enhancement or high-frequency information pass undetected (30) (Fig. 31). In practice, all displaced fracture fragments are devascularized, and it is therefore inappropriate to determine vascular integrity following acute injury. Absent vascularity at 6 weeks, at which time bridging callus is formed and should lead to revascularization, is considered to be pathologic.

Application of Keyhole Imaging Technique

Dynamic Gadolinium-Enhanced TOF Angiography: Bolus Tracking
Evaluation of Fracture Fragment Vascular Integrity: Scaphoid, Femoral Head, Humerus, Talus

---

IMAGING POSTOPERATIVE PATIENTS WITH METALLIC HARDWARE *IN SITU*

Although MR imaging has had a dramatic impact on preoperative evaluation of orthopedic injuries, because of metal-induced artifacts, the use of MR imaging in postoperative patients following hardware fixation has been limited.

The biocompatibility of metallic alloys—stainless steel,

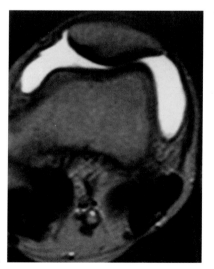
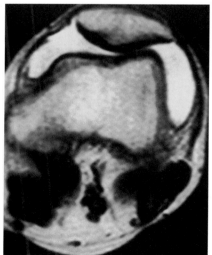
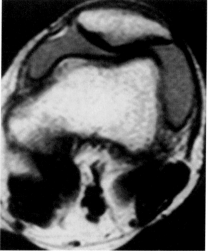

A
B,C

FIG. 30. Axial images of a suprapatellar effusion acquired with a spin-echo navigator-corrected diffusion sequence. Images acquired **(A)** without application of diffusion gradient showing signal hyperintensity, **(B)** with a B value of 256 showing relative preservation of signal within synovial fluid, and **(C)** at a diffusion B value of 512 showing loss of signal within synovial fluid.

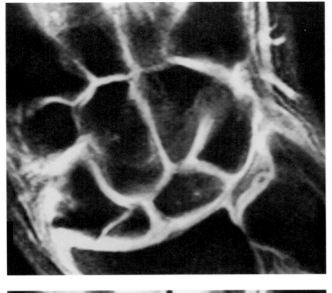

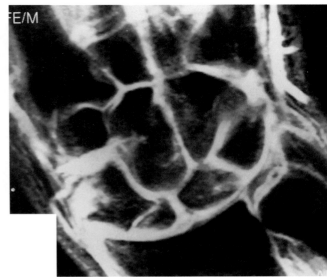

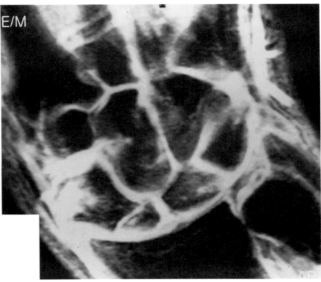

FIG. 31. Dynamic gadolinium enhanced perfusion images serially acquired using keyhole technique **(A)** precontrast, **(B)** 30 sec following contrast injection, **(C)** 45 sec following contrast injection, demonstrating enhancement and therefore vascular integrity of both the proximal and distal fragments. Reproduced with permission from Eustace (39).

cobalt chrome, and titanium alloy—is based on the presence of a constituent element within the alloy that has the ability to form an adherent oxide coating that is stable, chemically inert, and hence biocompatible. The type of metal used in orthopedic fixation devices has traditionally been dictated by the availability of the metal, cost, and mechanical qualities, which include the yield strength (the amount of elastic strain that may be applied to the metal before producing a permanent deformation), the fatigue strength (the ability of the metal to resist axial loading), and the modulus of the metal (the inherent mechanical property of the metal). Although stainless steel is most frequently used for fixation, its low yield stress, rapid metal fatigue, and low modulus, leading to plate and prosthesis failure, have promoted the use and development of other alloys. In this regard, cobalt chrome is favored if tensile and fatigue strength are required, titanium is favored if load sharing with adjacent bone (unce-

mented prostheses) is required (titanium has a similar modulus to cortical bone).

In relation to imaging, titanium alloys are less ferromagnetic than both cobalt chrome and steel, induce less susceptibility artifact, and result in less marked image degradation.

Metallic components placed in a magnet acquire the property of induced magnetism. Protons or water molecules adjacent to the metal become influenced by the field induced by the hardware component, and, rather than precessing under the influence of the main field (relative to a gradient established by the parent field), they precess under the influence of the local field (31). The higher the parent magnetic field strength, the stronger the induced magnetism in the metal component, and hence the greater the local field distortion (Fig. 32) (32).

Signal, when created at MR imaging, is localized in space by frequency and phase. Spins adjacent to the hardware com-

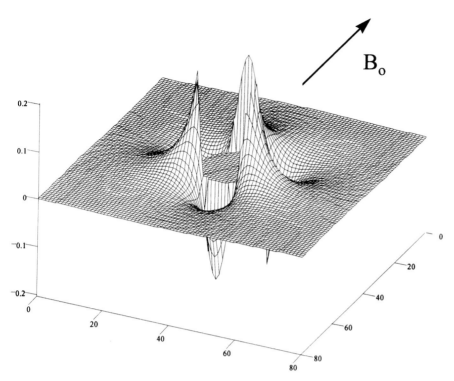

B_o

FIG. 32. Diagrammatic representation of field distortion induced by ferromagnetic components most marked in the frequency-encoding domain. Courtesy of H. Jara, Ph.D.

ponent, precessing under its influences rather than the parent field, either precess at a radically different frequency or rapidly dephase following excitation, resulting in erroneous mapping of signal or distortion in shape, an effect described as metal susceptibility artifact (33). A rim of high signal at the margin of the artifact occurs secondary to mismapping of a disproportionate number of spins to that location as a result of frequency changes (34).

The shape of the induced distortion is a function of the geometry of the hardware component. A fixed loss of signal is created by magnetism within the metal component (35), and a time-dependent signal loss is created by loss of phase coherence, which increases in time (milliseconds) in spins adjacent to the metal component, the dephasing being enhanced by proximity to the metal component, decreasing exponentially in spins progressively further from the primary metal component. The earlier the signal is acquired (short TE, 10 to 15 msec), the less artifact is observed. A delay in acquisition of signal (long TE, 80 to 100 msec) results in more marked artifact or signal loss adjacent to the metal component as spins (within millimeters) progressively further from the metal component dephase, an effect termed metal susceptibility blooming (36). Eddy currents induced in metal components by excitatory radiofrequency pulses produce local heating, effect proton diffusion, and have a further unpredictable effect on observed artifact (37). Signal void or loss within the metal component cannot be recovered. Imaging techniques are therefore employed to limit time-varying field distortion (38).

Two-dimensional MR imaging pulse sequences, as discussed in Chapter 1, use three different methods for localiz-

ing the MR signal produced by soft tissues surrounding the orthopedic component. These methods—slice selection, phase encoding, and frequency encoding—use pulsed magnetic field gradients, which are applied at predetermined times during the MR imaging pulse sequence. Most vulnerable to distortion by magnetism induced in metal components are the slice-selection and frequency-encoding gradients. The phase-encoding method is less prone to produce susceptibility-induced geometric distortions because all the phase-encoding steps are affected equally by the field disturbance induced by an orthopedic component (Fig. 33).

Resonance is achieved only when spins within a slice precess at the same frequency as the frequency of the applied excitatory radiofrequency pulse, the Larmor frequency. If

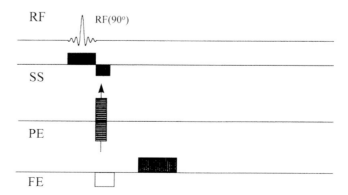

FIG. 33. Diagrammatic representation of MR pulse sequence demonstrating sequential application of excitatory pulse (RF), slice-select gradient (SS), phase-encoding gradient (PE), and then the frequency or readout gradient (FE).

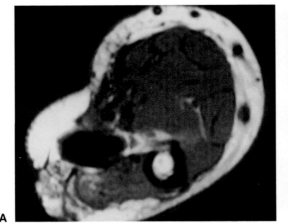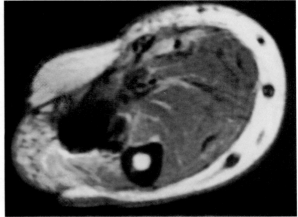

A **B**

FIG. 34. Axial image of the forearm following plate fixation acquired **(A)** with frequency gradients oriented right to left and **(B)** with frequency gradient oriented from superior to inferior.

an imaging slice or plane is selected crossing a metal component, the slice-select gradient becomes locally distorted by the induced magnetic field adjacent to the metal. Spins in the region of the distortion precess at a radically different frequency from the excitatory pulse and when it is applied do not acquire resonance and hence do not generate signal. By selecting an imaging plane (often oblique) that minimizes or avoids the hardware component as much as possible, distortion of the slice select gradients is markedly reduced. If the condition of resonance is not satisfied, all techniques subsequently applied in an attempt to limit both dephasing and signal loss are in vain. Appropriate selection of slice orientation may limit observed artifact around hardware. An awareness of the importance of limiting distortion of slice-select gradients explains the difficulty encountered when trying to image hardware components with complex geometry, such as ankle fixation plates with screws in multiple axes.

Signal adjacent to a metal component is rapidly lost, particularly in the axis of the frequency-encoding gradients, artifact or signal loss acquiring an oval configuration. Selection of the axes of both phase and frequency encoding before imaging allows artifact to be oriented away from the tissue of interest (Figs. 34 and 35).

Although artifact may be reduced by decreasing field of view and increasing readout gradient strength, the imaging field of view is usually dictated by the component being imaged; similarly, increase in readout gradient strength decreases image signal to noise.

Gradient-recalled echo-pulse sequences such as gradient echo and fast field echo are known to be the most vulnerable to magnetic field inhomogeneities because they do not use a 180° RF refocusing pulse, which partially reverses spin dephasing (see Chapter 1). T1-weighted conventional spin echo (CSE) benefits by employing a 180° RF refocusing pulse and the shortest possible echo time. Because it is faster than proton density conventional spin-echo images (long TR), which also uses the shortest possible echo time, it represents the best possible conventional technique to reduce susceptibility artifact. Turbo spin-echo (TSE) pulse sequences use a train of 180° RF refocusing pulses, thus reducing even further the dephasing induced by metal hardware (Fig. 36). Both increasing the number (echo train length) and decreasing the time between successive pulses (the echo spacing) decrease the time available for signal to decline before refocusing (38) (Fig. 37).

Improved MR Imaging of Postoperative Patients

Low-Field Magnets
Titanium Components
Hardware with Simple Geometry
Slice Select Gradient Orientation
Frequency Encode Gradient Orientation
Short-TE Acquisition
Decreased Field of View
Increased Readout Bandwidth
RARE-Based Sequences (Turbo Spin Echo, Haste)

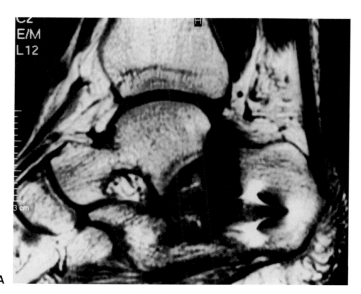
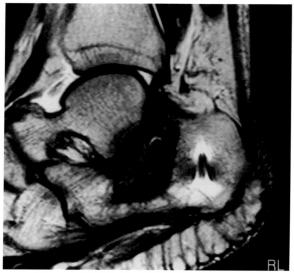

FIG. 35. Sagittal T1-weighted image of the calcaneus following plate fixation acquired **(A)** with frequency gradients oriented in a right-to-left axis and **(B)** with frequency gradients oriented from superior to inferior.

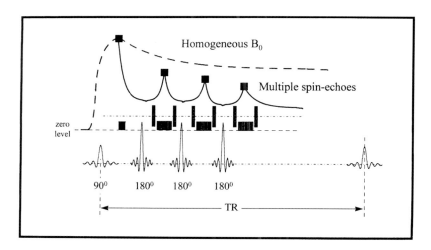

FIG. 36. Diagrammatic representation of the turbo spin-echo sequence. *Interrupted arrow* indicates gradual loss of signal without metallic artifact. *Black line* demonstrates metal-induced dephasing resulting in signal loss with regeneration of signal by serial refocusing 180° pulses.

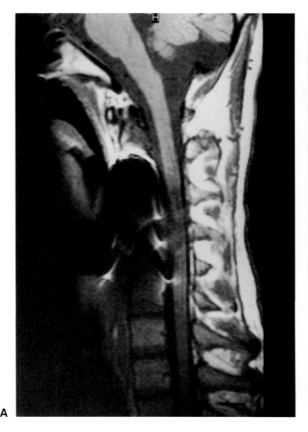

A

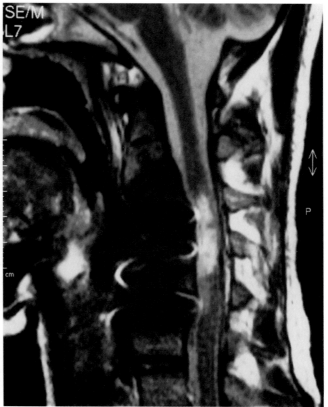

B

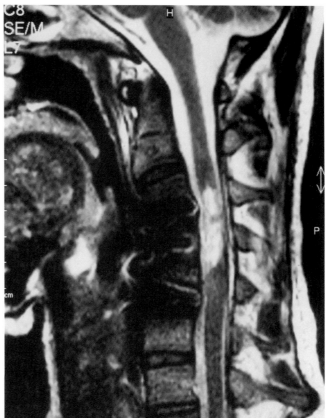

C

FIG. 37. **(A)** Sagittal T1-weighted image of a patient following plate fixation of an acute fracture of the cervical spine shows extensive metal-induced artifact. **(B)** Sagittal image of the same patient acquired with a T2-weighted turbo spin-echo sequence showing marked reduction in artifact. **(C)** Sagittal image of the same patient acquired with same T2-weighted turbo spin-echo sequence with ultrashort echo spacing shows more marked reduction in artifact, allowing clear visualization of pedicle screws and of cord hemorrhage. Reproduced with permission from Eustace et al. (40).

REFERENCES

1. Beltran J, Rosenberg ZS, Kawelblum M, Montes L, Bergman AG, Strongwater A. Pediatric elbow fractures: MRI evaluation. *Skel Radiol* 1994;195:855–859.
2. Buckwalter JA, Rosenberg LC, Hunziker EB. Composition, structure, response to injury and methods of facilitating repairs. In Ewing JW, ed. *Articular Cartilage and Knee Joint Function: Basic Science and Arthroscopy.* New York: Raven Press, 1990:19–54.
3. Waldschmidt JG, Rilling RJ, Kajdacsy-Balla AA, Boynton MD, Erickson SJ. *In vitro* and *in vivo* MR imaging of hyaline cartilage: zonal anatomy, imaging pitfalls, and pathologic conditions. *Radiographics* 1997;17:1387.
4. Peterfy CG, Genant HK. Emerging applications of magnetic resonance imaging in the evaluation of articular cartilage. *Radiol Clin North Am* 1996;34:195.
5. Seo GS, Aoki J, Moriya H, Karakida O, Sone S, Hidaka H, Katsuyama T. Hyaline cartilage: *in vivo* and *in vitro* assessment with magnetization transfer imaging. *Radiology* 1996;201:525.
6. Carey J, Spence L, Blickman H, Eustace S. MR imaging of pediatric growth plate injury: Correlation with plain film radiographs and clinical outcome. *Skel Radiol* 1998;27:250.
7. Yao L, Gentili A, Thomas A. Incidental magnetization transfer contrast in fast spin echo imaging of cartilage. *J Mag Res Imag* 1996;6:180.
8. Winalski CS, Palmer WE, Rosenthal DI, et al. Magnetic resonance imaging of rheumatoid arthritis. *Radiol Clin North Am* 1996;34:243.
9. Tamai K, Yamato M, Yamaguchi T, et al. Dynamic magnetic resonance imaging for the evaluation of synovitis in patients with rheumatoid arthritis (abstract). *Radiology* 1995;194:295.
10. Reiser MF, Naegele M. Inflammatory joint disease: static and dynamic gadolinium enhanced MR imaging. *J Mag Res Imag* 1993;3:307.
11. Singon RD, Zalduondo FM. Value of unenhanced MR imaging in distinguishing between synovitis and effusion of the knee. *Am J Roentgenol* 1992;159:569–571.
12. Li KCP, Hopkins KL, Moore SG, et al. Magnetization transfer contrast MRI of musculoskeletal neoplasms. *Skel Radiol* 1995;24:21.
13. Taccone A, Oddone M, Occhi M, et al. MRI road map of normal age related bone marrow: 1. Cranial bone and spine. *Pediatr Radiol* 1995; 25:588.
14. Steiner RM, Mitchell DG, Rao VM, Schweitzer ME. Magnetic resonance imaging of diffuse bone marrow disease. *Radiol Clin North Am* 1993;31:383–409.
15. Richardson ML, Patten RM. Age related changes in marrow distribution in the shoulder. *Radiology* 1994;192:209.
16. Deely DM, Schweitzer ME. MR imaging of bone marrow disorders. *Radiol Clin North Am* 1997;35:193.
17. Outwater E, Siegelman ES, Huang AB, Birnbaum BA. Adrenal masses, correlation between CT attenuation value and chemical shift ratio at MR imaging with in phase and opposed phase sequences. *Radiology* 1996;200:749.
18. Eustace S, Tello R, DeCarvalho V, Carey J, Wroblicka JT, Melhem ER, Yucel EK. A comparison of whole body turbo short tau inversion recovery MR imaging and planar technetium 99m methylene diphosphonate scintigraphy in the evaluation of patients with suspected skeletal metastases. *Am J Roentgenol* 1997;169:1655–1661.
19. Tirman PFJ, Applegate GR, Flannigan BD, et al. Shoulder MR arthrography. *MRI Clin North Am* 1993;1:125–142.
20. Tirman PFJ, Steinbach LS, Belzer JP, Bost FW. A practical approach to imaging of the shoulder with emphasis on MR imaging. *Orthop Clin North Am* 1997;28:483–515.
21. Winalski CS, Aliabadi P, Wright RJ, Shortkroff S, Sledge CB, Weissman BW. Enhancement of joint fluid with intravenously administered gadopentate dimeglumine:technique, rationale, and implications. *Radiology* 1993;187:179.
22. Palmer WE, Caslowitz PL, Chew FS. MR arthrography of the shoulder: Normal intra-articular structures and common abnormalities. *Am J Roentgenol* 1995;164:141–146.
23. Tirman PFJ, Stauffer AE, Crues JV III, Turner RM. Saline magnetic resonance arthrography in the evaluation of glenohumeral instability. *Arthroscopy* 1993;9:550–559.
24. Palmer WE, Caslowitz PL. Anterior shoulder instability: Diagnostic criteria determined from prospective analysis of 121 MR arthrograms. *Radiology* 1995;197:819–825.
25. Montgomery KD, Potter HG, Helfet DL. The use of magnetic resonance imaging to evaluate the deep venous system in the pelvis in patients with acetabular fractures. Paper presented at Surgery of the Pelvis and Acetabulum: the Second International Consensus, Pittsburgh, 1993.
26. Snidow JJ, Aisen AM, Harris VJ, Trerotola SO, Johnson MS, Sawchuk AP, Dalsing MC. Iliac artery MR angiography: comparison of three dimensional gadolinium enhanced and two dimensional time of flight techniques. *Radiology* 1995;196:371.
27. Krinsky G, Rofsky NM, Flyer M, et al. Gadolinium enhanced three dimensional MR angiography of acquired arch vessel disease. *Am J Roentgenol* 1996;167:981.
28. Simonetti OP, Finn JP, White RD, Laub G, Henry DA. Black blood T2 weighted inversion recovery MR imaging of the heart. *Radiology* 1996;199:49.
29. Trouard TP, Sabharwal Y, Altbach MI, et al. Analysis and comparison of motion corrected techniques in diffusion weighted imaging. *J Mag Res Imag* 1996;6:925.
30. Miyati T, Banno T, Mase M, et al. Dual dynamic contrast enhanced MR imaging. *J Mag Res Imag* 1997;7:230.
31. Laakman RW, Kaufman B, Han JS, et al. MR imaging in patients with metallic implants. *Radiology* 1985;157:711–714.
32. Petersilge CA, Lewin JS, Duerk JL, Yoo JU, Ghaneyem AJ. Optimizing imaging parameters for MR evaluation of the spine with titanium pedicle screws. *Am J Roentgenol* 1996:166:1213–1218.
33. Heindel W, Friedmann G, Thomas B, Firsching R, Ernestus RI. Artifacts in MR imaging after surgical intervention. *J Comput Assist Tomogr* 1986;10:596–599.
34. Bellon EM, Haacke EM, Coleman PE, Sacco DC, Steiger DA, Gangarosa RE. MR artifacts: a review. *Am J Roentgenol* 1986;147:1271–1281.
35. Mueller PR, Stark DD, Simeone JF, et al. MR guided aspiration biopsy: needle design and clinical trials. *Radiology* 1986;161:605–609.
36. Ludeke KM, Roschmann P, Tischler R. Susceptibility artifacts in NMR imaging. *Mag Res Imag* 1985;3:329–343.
37. Farahani K, Sinha U, Sinha S, et al. Effect of field strength on susceptibility artifacts in magnetic resonance imaging. *Comput Med Imag Graph* 1990;14:409–413.
38. Tartaglino LM, Flanders AE, Vinitski S, Friedman DP. Metallic artifact on MR images of the post operative spine: reduction with fast spin echo techniques. *Radiology* 1994;190:565–569.
39. Eustace S. MR imaging of acute orthopedic trauma to the extremities. *Radiol Clin North Am* 1997;35(3):615–629.
40. Eustace S, Jara H, Goldberg R, et al. A comparison of conventional spin-echo and turbo spin-echo imaging of soft tissues adjacent to orthopedic hardware. *Am J Roentgenol* 1998;170(2):455–458.

CHAPTER 4

General Principles

Stephen J. Eustace

This short chapter outlines the basic physiology of bone, reviews basic concepts of bone injury, correlates patterns of bone bruising or edema with mechanism of injury, and finally reviews MR imaging during fracture healing.

BASIC STRUCTURE

Bone is primarily composed of osteoid, which is an organic matrix composed of collagen fibers on which apatite mineral (calcium and phosphate) is deposited and embedded in a gel of protein polysaccharide. In health, collagen fibers in osteoid are oriented parallel to the axis of applied stress. This structure makes bone strength a function of the concentration or amount of osteoid and mineral apatite and a function of the alignment of the collagen fibers.

In adulthood, long bones are hollow structures in which dense cortical bone surrounds central marrow. At the ends of long bones, marrow becomes intermingled with internal osseous seams or trabeculae to form cancellous bone. Although cortical bone typically thins in the metaphysis, structural integrity in this part of long bones is afforded by oriented trabeculae within cancellous bone (1).

The shaft of long bones is lined by periosteum, which is composed of an outer fibrous sheath and an inner layer of undifferentiated pluripotent mesenchymal cells. In a similar way, mesenchymal cells line the inner margin of the cortex, the endosteum, and internal trabeculae. Under the influence

of stress, trauma, or infection, undifferentiated mesenchymal cells may develop into either osteoblasts or osteoclasts, which respectively generate and remodel new bone. Stress reaction may promote differentiation of mesenchymal cells lining trabecular seams. Induced osteoblasts lead to thickening and to an increase in the visibility of the trabecular markings (2).

In contrast to cancellous bone, compact bone of the cortex is a tightly bound organized series of haversian systems or osteons producing lamellae. Following injury to compact cortical bone, healing occurs over 6 weeks to 3 months, essentially dictated by vascular supply. Healing of cancellous bone, with a rich vascular supply, occurs more rapidly and, unlike cortical bone, is infrequently complicated by either delayed or nonunion.

Normal bone undergoes a constant remodeling process, a balance between osteoblasts generating new bone and osteoclasts replacing or removing existing bone or osteons. In response to stress, osteoblastic activity predominates. In areas relieved of normal stress, osteoclastic activity predominates, and osteoporosis results (3) (Fig. 1).

CLASSIFICATION OF FRACTURES BY MECHANISM

Fractures are generally classified by mechanism of injury into fractures secondary to direct trauma and fractures secondary to indirect trauma.

Direct trauma may produce three types of fracture: a *tapping* fracture when a small force is applied to a small area, a *crush* fracture when a large force is applied to a large area,

S. J. Eustace: Department of Radiology, Section of Musculoskeletal Radiology, Boston University School of Medicine and Boston Medical Center, Boston, Massachusetts 02118.

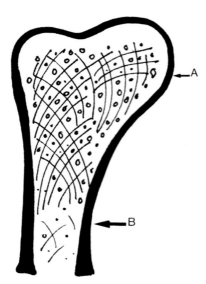

FIG. 1. Diagram showing thick cortical bone in the diaphysis, with relative thinning of cortex in the metaphysis, where structural integrity is maintained by internal trabeculae and bone becomes cancellous in type.

and *penetrating* fractures when a large force is applied to a small area.

Indirect trauma is the term employed when a remote force is transmitted to the fracture site. *Traction* fractures are fractures in which applied forces pull bone apart, resulting in fractures of the patella, olecranon, and malleoli. *Angulation* fractures occur when applied forces are unequally distributed across the shaft of a bone, such that one side is compressed and the other is distracted. *Rotational* fractures occur when a torque or rotational force is applied to bone (4,5).

PATHOLOGIC FRACTURES

The term pathologic fracture is employed when fracture occurs through abnormal bone, reflecting generalized disease with bone demineralization (*insufficiency* fracture) or localized disease, either tumor, infection, or bone necrosis (Figs. 2–4).

STRESS FRACTURES

The term stress fracture is employed when excessive persistent or repetitive localized force is applied to bone resulting in fracture. Fatigue fracture is the term employed when force repeatedly applied to normal bone results in fracture. The term insufficiency fracture (itself a form of pathologic fracture) is employed when repetitive forces applied to abnormal demineralized bone result in fracture (6) (Fig. 5).

THE LANGUAGE OF FRACTURES

The term *compound fracture* is employed when a fracture fragment pierces the skin (compound from within) or when applied trauma breaches the skin and then fractures bone (compound from without).

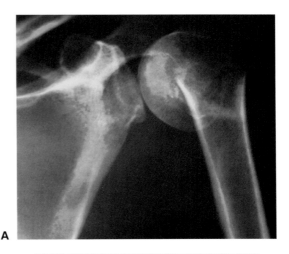

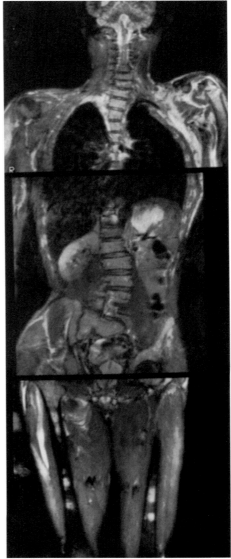

FIG. 2. (A) Radiograph of the left shoulder shows a fracture of the surgical neck of the proximal humerus. **(B)** Whole-body turboSTIR image shows tumor replacing marrow at the site of the fracture, with further focal deposits in the femora and diffuse marrow replacement in the spine. Multiple myeloma.

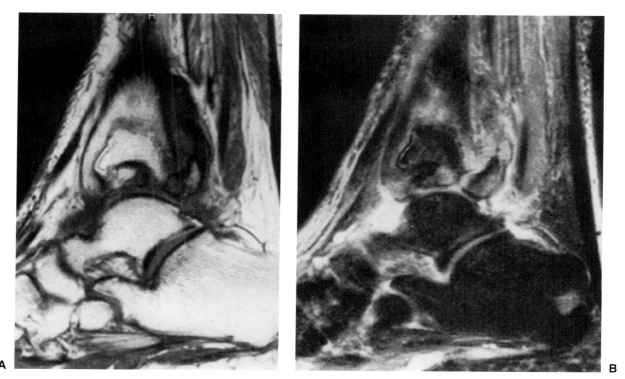

A

B

FIG. 3. Sagittal turbo spin-echo (TSE) T1 **(A)** and turbo inversion recovery (IR TSE) **(B)** images shows a displaced fracture of the posterior malleolus through an underlying bone infarct.

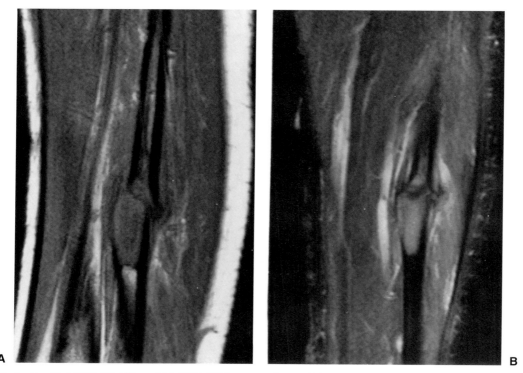

A

B

FIG. 4. Sagittal TSE T1 **(A)** and IR TSE **(B)** images shows delayed union of a fibula fracture at a site of fibrous dysplasia.

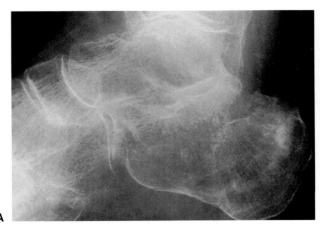
A

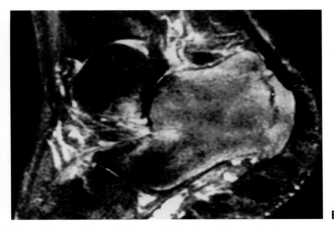
B

FIG. 5. (A) Lateral view of the calcaneus shows oblique linear sclerosis through the dorsal aspect of a demineralized calcaneus. (B) Sagittal IR TSE image shows an undisplaced fracture through an area of diffuse marrow edema.

A *complicated fracture* is a fracture associated with damage to adjacent neurovascular structures or viscera.

A *comminuted fracture* is a fracture in which applied forces result in a complex fracture with more than two fragments.

A *crush fracture* is a fracture, usually of cancellous bone, in which applied forces "concertina" supporting trabeculae, resulting in deformity of bone without discontinuity. Crush fractures usually involve cancellous bone either within the vertebral bodies to produce wedging or in the tibial plateaus at the knee.

A *chondral fracture* is a fracture of cartilage alone; an osteochondral fracture involves both cartilage and underlying bone.

An *avulsion fracture* is a fracture in which traction forces applied to tendon or ligaments result in detachment of bone from the insertion site.

A *greenstick fracture* is a fracture occurring in children whose bones are less brittle than those of adults. Applied forces result in compression or buckling of cortex on one side (torus or buckle fracture) of the bone and separation on the site of distraction (greenstick).

MAGNETIC RESONANCE IMAGING OF OSSEOUS TRAUMA: BONE CONTUSION VERSUS FRACTURE

A *bone bruise* or *contusion* is a term popularized as a result of widespread use of MRI and its ability to perceive and visualize previously unrecognized sites of marrow edema. When employed, bone bruising is the term used to describe local marrow edema and hemorrhage within cancellous bone occurring secondary to either direct or indirect trauma (7–9). Reflecting extensive microtrabecular injury, traumatic bone bruises generally correspond to sites of clinical tenderness and pain.

Impaction fractures result in dramatic disruption of adjacent trabeculae (a "concertina effect" on trabeculae), extensive hemorrhage and edema, and hence the presence of a readily detectable bruise. Chronic impaction as a result of abnormal weight bearing or loss of protective articular cartilage in osteoarthritis produces similar extensive bruising, although it is usually intimately related to articular surfaces. In contrast, disruption of trabeculae following an applied avulsion force is minimal or localized (extreme tensile forces ultimately result in trabecular disruption at a single point perpendicular to the axis of stress, and therefore bruising is usually minimal), with linearity perpendicular to the axis of avulsion forces (Figs. 6 and 7).

Similar marrow edema within both cortical and cancellous bone indistinguishable from a bone bruise may be identified

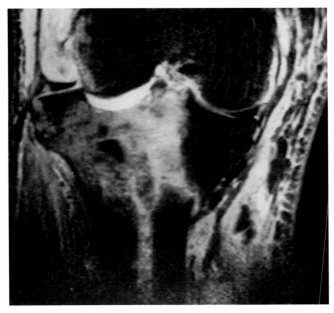

FIG. 6. Coronal IR TSE image of the knee shows a compression fracture of the lateral tibial plateau, with lateral splaying of plateau and meniscus, with extensive subarticular marrow edema at the site of impaction and extensive trabecular trauma. Reproduced with permission from Eustace et al. (22).

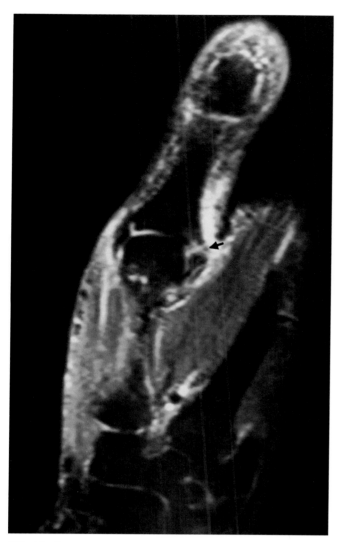

FIG. 7. Coronal IR TSE image of the left thumb shows an undisplaced avulsion *(arrow)* at the insertion of the ulnar collateral ligament (gamekeepers thumb) with minimal marrow edema.

as a result of increased para-articular blood flow in patients with inflammatory synovitis (Fig. 8) or as a result of venous congestion secondary to elevated intramedullary pressure as occurs in patients with avascular necrosis and migratory osteoporosis (Fig. 9). Finally, local marrow edema may occur in response to tumor induced trabecular disruption or secondary to release of prostaglandins by tumors such as, by osteoid osteoma (Fig. 10).

Marrow Edema
Trauma
Tumor Induced
Hyperemic (Synovitis Secondary to Immune Complex Deposition or Infection)
Venous Congestion (Secondary to Elevated Intramedullary Pressure, AVN)

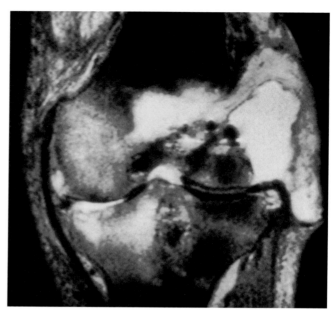

FIG. 8. Coronal IR TSE image of the knee in a patient with septic arthritis complicating reconstruction of the anterior cruciate ligament. There is extensive para-articular hyperemic marrow edema secondary to synovitis and soft tissue inflammation.

At MR imaging, bone bruises are most conspicuous on either fat-suppressed T2-weighted or inversion recovery sequences, manifest as poorly marginated foci of signal hyperintensity within marrow. Bruises are typically hypointense on T1-weighted scans, isointense on density-weighted scans, and hyperintense on T2-weighted scans. With diffusion gradients, and reflecting an increase in free water, bruises are extremely conspicuous and are occasionally identified even in the absence of signal abnormality on other sequences. Following the administration of gadolinium, bruises similar to hyperemic marrow edema typically enhance uniformly. Enhancement in edema secondary to venous occlusion in avascular necrosis is considerably less marked.

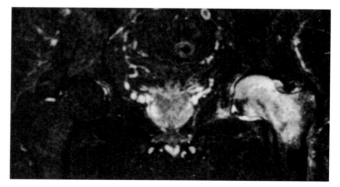

FIG. 9. Coronal IR TSE image of the hips shows extensive marrow edema within the left femoral head secondary to transient osteoporosis, complicating hip trauma (venous congestion). Courtesy of S. Valentine, M.D., Calgary, AB.

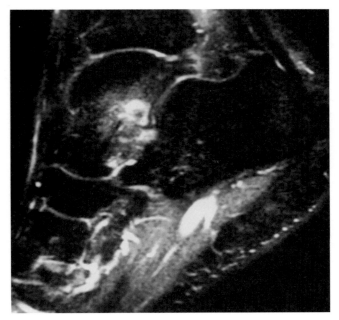

FIG. 10. Sagittal IR TSE image of the foot shows extensive edema within the calcaneus at a site of proven osteoid osteoma (tumorigenic marrow edema).

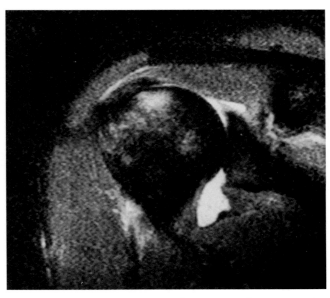

FIG. 12. Coronal oblique IR TSE image of the shoulder shows an extensive impaction bone bruise in the humeral head of a patient immediately following reduction of an anterior shoulder dislocation.

Following trauma, local marrow hemorrhage and edema or bruising often persist unchanged for several months. At 3 months, most bruises begin to resolve and are generally undetectable at 1 year. In one study of 98 patients with anterior cruciate ligament disruption, bruises were identified acutely in 71% but were not identified in any patient at 6 weeks (9,10).

By MR imaging alone, differentiating between a bone bruise and an undisplaced fracture is often difficult (although somewhat academic), as undisplaced cortical disruption may not be perceived. A bone bruise or contusion is the term employed when the configuration of the hemorrhage and edema is globular, most often secondary to impaction forces and diffuse trabecular compression (Figs. 11–13). An undis-

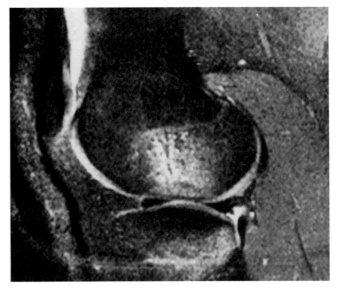

FIG. 11. Sagittal fat-suppressed spin-echo, echo planar image of the knee in a patient with a ruptured anterior cruciate ligament shows *contre-coup* impaction bone bruises in the midlateral femoral condyle and in the posterior margin of the lateral tibial plateau, secondary to rotational torque injury.

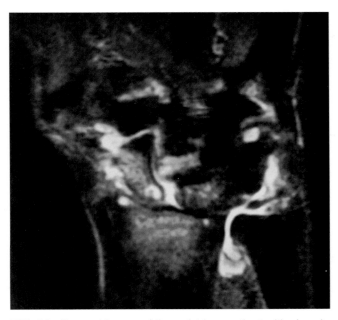

FIG. 13. Coronal image of the wrist in a patient with chronic scapholunate ligament disruption, showing widening of the scapholunate interspace and impaction-type bruising at the radioscaphoid and radiolunate articulations (slack wrist).

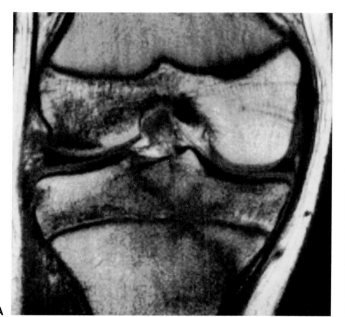

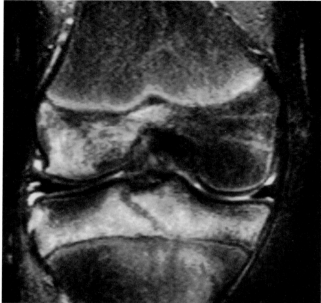

A   B

FIG. 14. Coronal TSE T1 **(A)** and IR TSE **(B)** images of the knee in a patient with a Salter 4 fracture of the medial tibial plateau (hypointense line) secondary to shear forces with associated extensive edema secondary to concomitant impaction forces.

placed fracture is the term employed when bone bruising has a linear configuration and edema is traversed by linear hypointensity on both T1 and on fat-suppressed images, more often the sequel of superimposed shear forces (Fig. 14).

Impaction forces primarily result in globular poorly marginated bone bruising when trabeculae within cancellous bone are diffusely disrupted (Fig. 15). Severe impaction forces result in extensive bruising. When bruise is accompanied by disruption of cortex and trabeculae, structural integrity is dramatically reduced, and bone collapses to produce a wedge compression fracture, particularly in vertebral bodies and in the tibial plateaus. Fracture or trabecular disruption secondary to a *distraction force* (avulsion fracture) most frequently results in local disruption of trabeculae without dissipation of forces to adjacent bone and therefore minimal marrow edema. Marrow edema is uncommon in the avulsed bone fragment (see Fig. 7). Chronically applied traction forces produce chronic microtrabecular trauma without healing. Such nonunion or impaired healing at these sites results in the development of small cysts, termed traction cysts, frequently identified at the insertion of the ACL tendon in the knee and in the supraspinatus tendon in the shoulder (Fig. 16). *Shearing* or *penetrating forces* tend to produce either marrow edema with linearity (often accompanied by a hypointense line on all sequences), termed undisplaced fracture rather than bone bruise, or disrupt cortex and trabeculae in a linear pattern (at a single point in each trabeculum) and produce minimal edema (Figs. 17 and 18 and Table 1).

In summary, bone contusion is a term unique to MR imag-

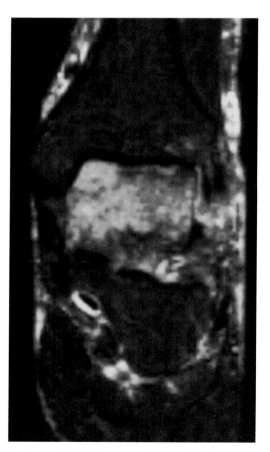

FIG. 15. Coronal IR TSE image of the ankle shows extensive impaction-induced edema throughout the body of the talus secondary to diffuse microtrabecular trauma following a fall.

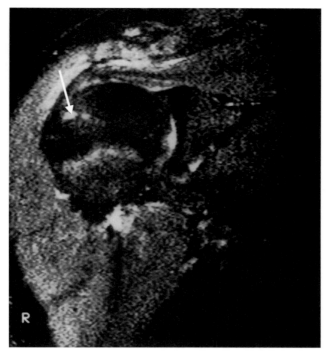

FIG. 16. Coronal oblique IR TSE image of the shoulder shows traction cysts *(arrow)* at the insertion of the supraspinatus tendon, complicating long-standing avulsion forces.

TABLE 1. *Patterns of injury on MRI by mechanism*

Impaction injury	
Bone bruise	Diffuse marrow edema and hemorrhage
Undisplaced fracture	As above with cortical disruption
Wedge or compression	As above with altered anatomic fracture Configuration
Distraction injury	
Undisplaced avulsion	Minimal marrow edema and hemorrhage at insertion of tendon or ligament
Displaced avulsion	As above with displacement of osseous fragment
Chronic avulsion	Minimal edema at tendon or ligament insertion often associated with local cystic change
Shear or penetrating injury	
Undisplaced fracture	Bone bruising with linearity, often with a definite hypointense line on T1-weighted scans
Displaced fracture	Minimal bone bruising with linearity and displacement of bone fragment

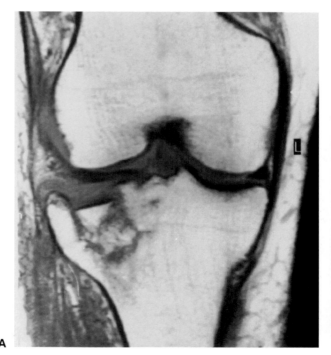

A

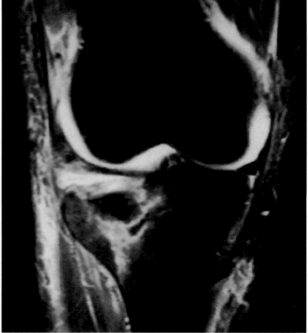

B

FIG. 17. Compression fracture of the lateral tibial plateau complicating an acute valgus injury. Note absent marrow edema within the depressed fragment, with extensive marrow edema at the site of impaction.

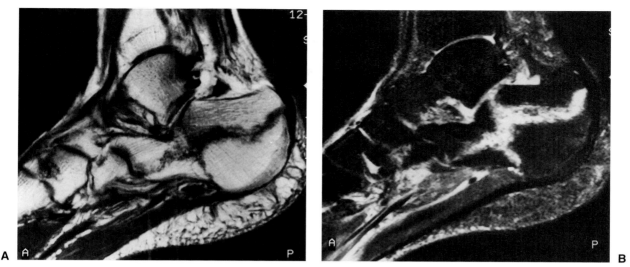

FIG. 18. Sagittal TSE T1 **(A)** and IR TSE **(B)** images of the ankle in a patient with a fracture of the calcaneus. Impaction forces have resulted in discrete disruption of trabeculae in primary vertical and secondary horizontal planes. Applied forces are therefore locally dissipated rather than being diffusely distributed to adjacent trabeculae.

ing and represents the first event in a continuum of traumatic injury to bone (Figs. 19 and 20).

EPIPHYSEAL INJURIES

The physis consists of four longitudinally arranged zones of cartilage—the germinal zone, the proliferating zone, the hypertrophic zone, and the zone of provisional calcification. The perichondrial ring, which is contiguous with adjacent periosteum, encircles the periphery of the physis.

In general, vascular supply to the growth plate is through nutrient arterial branches in the metaphysis and through branches from the periosteum and perichondrial ring. In the proximal femur and radial epiphysis, epiphyseal supply is

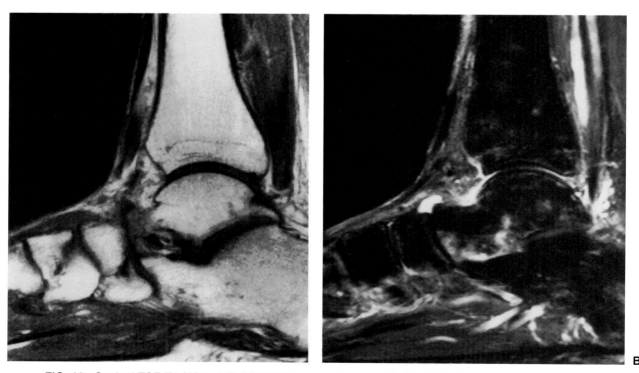

FIG. 19. Sagittal TSE T1 **(A)** and IR TSE **(B)** images show speckled periarticular marrow edema, best identified on the fat-suppressed image secondary to reflex sympathetic dystrophy.

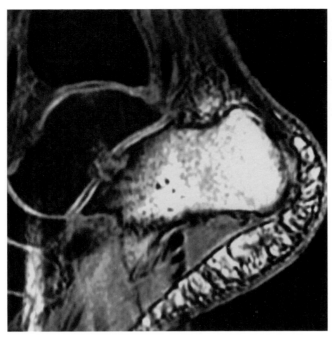

FIG. 20. Bone bruise pitfall. Inhomogeneous frequency-selective fat saturation resulting in spurious signal hyperintensity within the calcaneus and adjacent soft tissues.

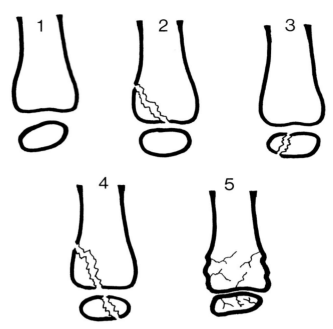

FIG. 21. Diagrammatic representation of the Salter Harris classification of growth plate injuries, types 1 to 5.

from the metaphysis coursing in the perichondrial ring. Following trauma, rupture of these vessels may impair growth plate development and hence growth. Up to 50% of epiphyseal injuries involve the hand and distal radius; involvement of the elbow occurs in approximately 10% of cases (11,12).

The Salter and Harris classification describes five types of growth plate injury (13) (Fig. 21):

Type 1. Epiphyseal separation confined to the physis. This type of injury occurs in up to 10% of cases and is most frequently a sequel to birth trauma or is superimposed on abnormal bone (scurvy, rickets).

Type 2. A fracture through the epiphysis extending to a corner of the metaphysis (the corner sign). This injury is the most common form, occurring in up to 75% of cases. The distal radius is most frequently affected.

Type 3. A fracture vertically through the epiphysis and horizontally through the physis. Such an injury tends to occur in adolescence and reflects partial closure of the growth plate. It represents about 5% of cases, most frequently identified in the distal tibia (Tillaux), the distal femur, and the distal interphalangeal joints in the hand (Fig. 22).

Type 4. A fracture extending vertically through the epiphysis, the physis, and the metaphysis occurring in up to 9% of cases. It is most frequently identified at the elbow, involving the lateral humeral condyle, and in the distal tibia.

Type 5. This fracture occurs secondary to a pure compressive injury and accounts for fewer than 1% of cases.

Type 4 and 5 injuries are associated with a worse prognosis.

LIGAMENT SPRAINS AND RUPTURES

Sprain is the term employed to describe trauma to a ligament resulting in local edema and hemorrhage without the development of ligamentous laxity (Fig. 23).

Rupture is the term employed when injury results in clinical laxity. Most commonly, rupture occurs within the substance of the ligament *(intrasubstance rupture)*, which appears stretched and lax but not discontinuous. On MR imaging, intrasubstance rupture is manifest as ligamentous or tendon swelling and edema, hypointense on T1- and hyperintense on T2-weighted sequences.

Complete rupture is uncommon but is manifest by retraction and discontinuity at the site of injury (Fig. 24).

NORMAL FRACTURE HEALING

Immediately following injury, local hemorrhage results in hematoma formation at the fracture margins. Reflecting the presence of both oxyhemoglobin and methemoglobin, MR imaging demonstrates signal hyperintensity on T1- and T2-weighted scans (paramagnetic effect secondary to the presence of unpaired electrons) at the site of hemorrhage (Fig. 25). Within 24 hr, granulation tissue migrates into the fracture site and replaces the hematoma with a poorly organized cellular matrix, raising periosteum away from the bone cortex to form an osteoblastic collar. The MR signal at the site of fracture remains hyperintense secondary to methemoglobin, with edema identified in marrow adjacent to the fracture margins, more marked in compression than avulsion frac-

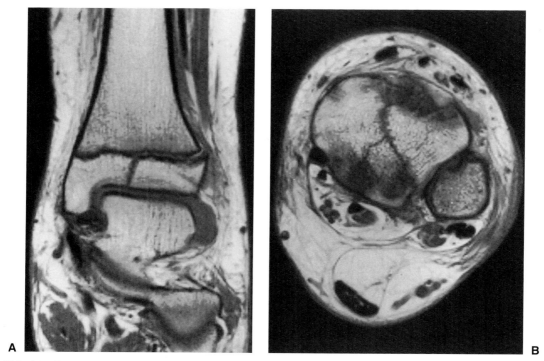

FIG. 22. Coronal **(A)** and axial **(B)** TSE T1-weighted images show a Salter 3 fracture of the distal tibia extending to the tibiotalar articulation.

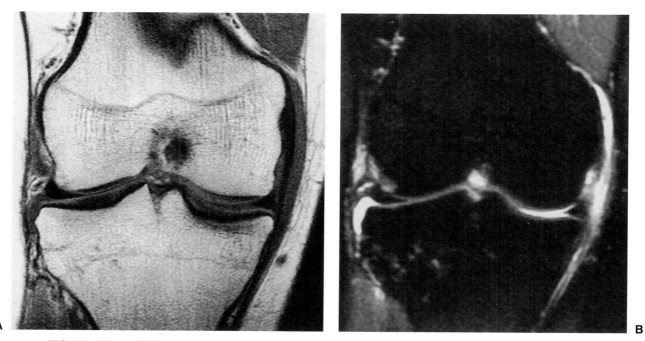

FIG. 23. Coronal TSE T1 **(A)** and IR TSE **(B)** images show edema within and without the fibers of the medial collateral ligament secondary to sprain.

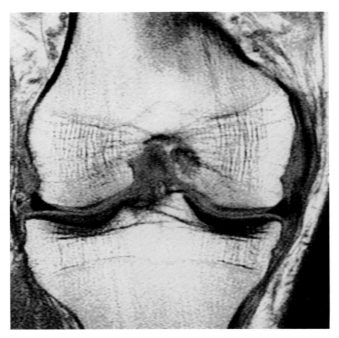

FIG. 24. Coronal TSE T1 image of the knee shows complete disruption of the medial collateral ligament in a patient following an acute valgus injury.

tures (14). Cellular differentiation with cartilage formation is responsible for early callus at the fracture margins, which is relatively isointense on T1-weighted and hyperintense on T2-weighted scans. Osteoblast differentiation with forma-

tion of osteoid results in the formation of sticky immature woven bone. In time, remodeling occurs, and the early bridging callus is replaced by primary spongiosa and lamellar bone, at which time signal characteristics begin to mirror those of native bone. Susceptibility effects manifested on gradient- or fast field-echo sequences may lead to obscuration of fractures at this time (15) (Fig. 26). If fluid remains interposed along the fracture margins, fractures remain extremely conspicuous, even on gradient- or fast field-echo sequences. Under the influence of osteoclasts and osteoblasts, the newly formed bone undergoes further remodeling over time until the primary configuration of bone is restored.

Primary union is the term employed when callus bridges apposed fracture margins, leading to healing at the fracture site. *Secondary union* is employed when healing occurs at the margins of the fracture through bridging callus rather than at the apposed fracture surfaces (16).

In health, fracture healing occurs between 6 weeks and 3 months (17). When motion persists at fracture margins, as a result of poor apposition of fracture surfaces or as a result of poor or impaired vascular supply to the fracture site, fracture healing may be delayed or not occur. Union is considered to be delayed when mineralized callus is poorly identified at 6 months and motion persists at the fracture margins. *Nonunion* is employed when healing has not occurred at 1 year. The term *atrophic nonunion* is employed when fracture margins are demineralized, resorbed, and devitalized, most often secondary to impaired vascular supply to the site (Fig. 27). "*Hypertrophic*" *nonunion* is used when exuberant callus is formed, producing an elephant foot configuration, most

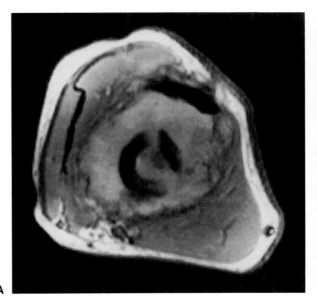
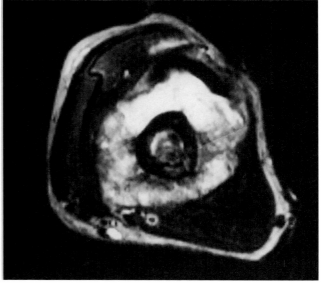

A   B

FIG. 25. Axial SE T1 **(A)** and T2 **(B)** images show relative signal hyperintensity, particularly in the T2-weighted image, at the site of fracture of proximal humerus. Observed signal is secondary to local hemorrhage, with associated paramagnetic extracellular methemoglobin, at the site of early callus formation.

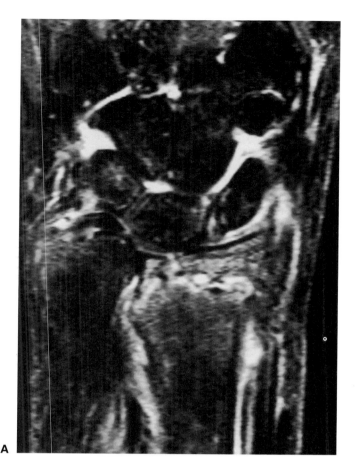

A

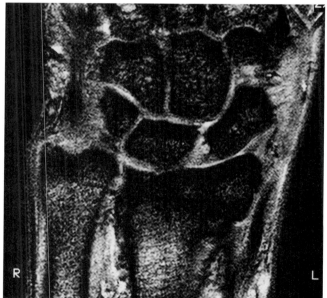

B

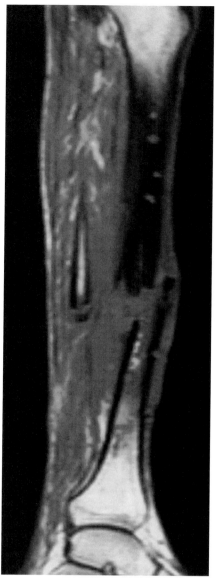

FIG. 27. Sagittal T1-weighted image of the tibia in a patient with nonunion despite previous plate-and-screw fixation shows devitalized fracture margins and soft tissue inflammation secondary to infection.

FIG. 26. **(A)** Coronal IR TSE image shows an ununited intra-articular fracture of the distal radius. **(B)** Susceptibility artifact at the site of fracture in the same patient results in loss of visibility on fast field-echo (gradient-echo) sequences, particularly when T2 weighting (long-TE images) is employed.

frequently secondary to persistent motion at the fracture site. Healing in "atrophic" nonunion is achieved when surgical immobilization is combined with bone grafting; in contrast, healing in hypertrophic nonunion is usually achieved by surgical immobilization alone.

COMPLICATIONS OF FRACTURES

Nerve Injuries

Neurapraxia is the term employed to describe transient disturbance of nerve function secondary to focal contusion and reversible edema. The injury is usually manifest as loss

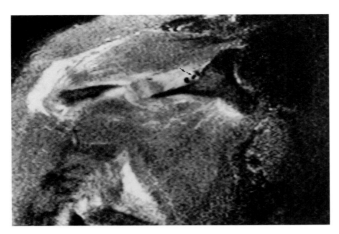

FIG. 28. Coronal oblique IR TSE image shows a fracture through spine of the scapula without encroachment of the suprascapular nerve *(arrow)* within the suprascapular notch.

of motor function with some preservation of sensory function (Fig. 28).

Axonotmesis is the term employed to describe focal nerve contusion, sufficiently severe to result in individual axons to degenerate. Because the endoneural tube remains intact, complete recovery of nerve function generally occurs.

Neurotmesis describes complete disruption of a nerve with discontinuity, or scarring sufficiently extensive to result in complete loss of nerve function, both conditions requiring surgical repair.

Neurapraxia and axonotmesis commonly accompany fractures, and therefore, surgical intervention is rarely required. Neurotmesis is extremely uncommon.

Vascular Injuries

Fracture may result in vessel *transection,* vessel *contusion* accompanied by intimal tear and thrombosis (the most common cause of arterial occlusion following fracture) or reversible arterial *spasm.*

Compartment Syndrome

The deep fascia divides the constituents of a limb into several compartments. Fracture of a limb may result in hemorrhage to muscle and edema, dramatically increasing intracompartmental pressure and impairing vascular supply. Arterial insufficiency is manifest as pallor, paresthesia, paresis, and decreased temperature.

Soft tissue edema primarily involving subcutaneous tissues is secondary to either lymphedema or cellulitis. Edema involving both deep and superficial soft tissues is secondary to either myositis, infection, or deep vein thrombosis.

Soft Tissue Edema Patterns	
Superficial: Lymphedema, Cellulitis Deep and Superficial: Myositis, Fasciitis, Compartment Syndrome, or DVT	

MYOSITIS OSSIFICANS

Heterotopic bone formation within para-articular soft tissues is a well-recognized complication of hip trauma. Although it is occasionally identified in the absence of trauma, there is a history of isolated or repeated hip trauma in two-thirds of cases. Following muscle trauma, mesenchymal cells proliferate at the site of tissue damage and become mineralized as they differentiate into osteoblastic components and subsequently into mature bone (18).

Mineralization may be seen in the damaged soft tissues as early as 11 days, characterized by focal accumulation of radiotracer (^{99m}Tc-MOP) at scintigraphy or edema and signal hyperintensity at MR imaging.

The complication is most frequently identified in patients with preexisting hyperparathyroidism, Paget's disease, seronegative arthritis, or paralysis. Progressive mineralization may be limited by immediate radiation therapy in patients following its identification. Nevertheless, in most patients, surgical resection is the definitive therapy. Once such a process has been identified, imaging is used to determine both its true extent and the maturity of the process. Surgery before completed ossification may result in incomplete resection and recurrence. No change in the extent of ossification on three serial radiographs, markedly reduced concentration of radiotracer at scintigraphy (similar uptake to adjacent mature bone), and absence of edema surrounding heterotopic bone at MR imaging are used as markers of maturity (Fig. 29) (19,20).

BONE GRAFTING

In patients with atrophic nonunion, bone graft is usually required to promote healing following immobilization.

Autologous grafts may be yielded as strips or chips of cancellous bone from the iliac crest, as blocks from the tibia, or as whole bone from the fibula. Cells in cancellous graft both stimulate local osteoblastic activity and, as some of the graft cells actually survive, directly promote healing. At MR imaging, bone chips of cancellous graft are initially hyperintense. At 6 months, incorporated graft shows similar signal to native bone, whereas failed graft becomes uniformly hypointense (Fig. 30).

Homogeneous grafts are derived from cadavers; the bone cells are dead. These grafts both stimulate host osteoblastic activity and provide a structure or scaffold to which woven bone can become attached. At MR imaging, homogeneous grafts are hypointense on all sequences (21).

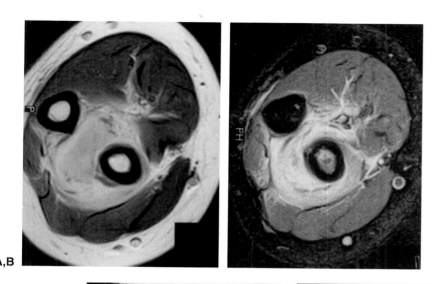

FIG. 29. Axial T1 **(A)** and inversion-recovery **(B)** images of the proximal forearm show extensive inflammation, with signal hyperintensity adjacent to the proximal radius on both sequences at a site of acute posttraumatic myositis ossificans.

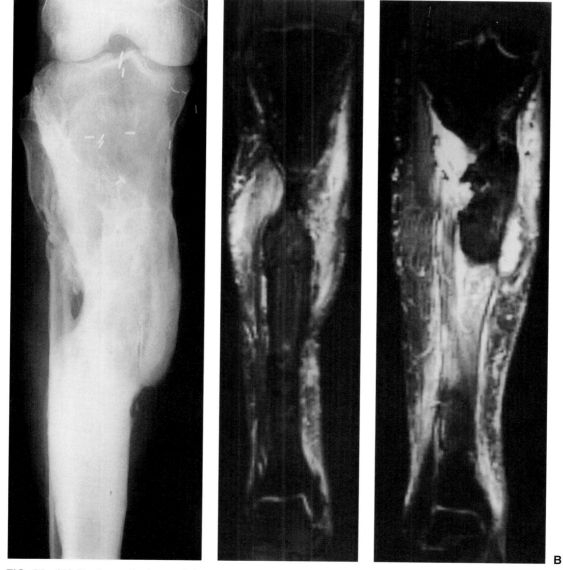

FIG. 30. (A) Radiograph shows deformity of the midtibia at the site of mature bone graft. **(B)** Coronal IR TSE images show normal marrow signal at the site of incorporated graft, with extensive soft tissue edema secondary to cellulitis.

REFERENCES

1. Finnegan MA, Uhtoff HK. Healing of trabecular bone. In: Lang JM, ed. *Fracture Healing*. Edinburgh: Churchill Livingstone, 1987;33–38.
2. McKibbin B. The biology of fracture healing in long bones. *J Bone Joint Surg* 1978;60B:150–162.
3. Hulth A. Current concepts of fracture healing. *Clin Orthop* 1989;249:265–284.
4. Perkins G. *Fractures and Dislocations*. London: Athlone Press, 1958.
5. Alms M. Fracture mechanics. *J Bone Joint Surg* 1961;43B:162–166.
6. Frankel VH, Burstein AH. *Orthopaedic Biomechanics*. Philadelphia: Lea & Febiger, 1970.
7. Berger PE, Ofstein RA, Jackson DW, et al. MRI demonstration of radiographically occult fractures. What have we been missing? *Radiographics* 1989;9:407–436.
8. Mink JH, Deutsch AL. Occult cartilage and bone injuries of the knee. Detection, classification and assessment with MR imaging. *Radiology* 1989;170:823–829.
9. Kapelov SR, Teresi LM, Bradley WG, et al. Bone contusions of the knee. Increased lesion detection with fast spin echo MR imaging with spectroscopic fat saturation. *Radiology* 1993;189:901–904.
10. Graf BK, Cook DA, De Smet AA, et al. Bone bruises on magnetic resonance imaging evaluation of anterior cruciate ligament injuries. *Am J Sports Med* 1993;21:220–223.
11. Ogden JA. Injury to the growth mechanisms of the immature skeleton. *Skel Radiol* 1981;6:187–192.
12. Salter RB, Harris WR. Injuries involving the epiphyseal plate. *J Bone Joint Surg [Am]* 1963;45:587–622.
13. Mizuta T, Benson WM, Foster BK, et al. Statistical analysis of the incidence of physeal injuries. *J Pediatr Orthop* 1987;7:518–523.
14. Palmer WE, Levine SM, Dupuy DE. Knee and shoulder fractures: association of fracture detection and marrow edema on MR images with mechanism of injury. *Radiology* 1997;204:395.
15. Eustace S. MR imaging of acute orthopedic trauma to the extremities. *Radiol Clin North Am* 1997;35:615–631.
16. Marsh JL, Buckwalter JA, Evarts CM. Nonunion, delayed union, malunion and avascular necrosis. In: Epps CH, ed. *Complications in Orthopaedic Surgery*. Philadelphia: JB Lippincott, 1994;183–211.
17. Potts WJ. The role of the hematoma in fracture healing. *Surg Gynecol Obstet* 1933;57:318–324.
18. Goldman AB. Myositis ossificans circumscripta: A benign lesion with malignant differential diagnosis. *Am J Roentgenol* 1976;126:32.
19. Norman A, Dorfman HD. Juxtacortical circumscribed myositis ossificans: evolution and radiological features. *Radiology* 1970;96:301.
20. Ehara S, Nakasato T, Tamakawa Y, et al. MRI of myositis ossificans circumscripta. *Clin Imag* 1991;15:130.
21. Simmons DJ. Fracture healing perspectives. *Clin Orthop* 1985;200:101–113.
22. Eustace S, Brophy D, Denison B. Magnetic resonance imaging of acute orthopedic trauma to the lower extremity. *Emerg Radiol* 1997;4:30.

CHAPTER 5

The Foot and Ankle

Stephen J. Eustace

This chapter outlines accepted and evolving applications of MRI in the evaluation of patients with suspected osseous and soft tissue injury involving the foot and ankle.

PATIENT POSITIONING AND IMAGING PROTOCOLS

Positioning

Magnetic resonance imaging of the foot and ankle is usually performed with the patient supine and the foot in the neutral position. If MR imaging is anticipated, referring orthopedists are encouraged either to delay casting or use a half cast that may be removed when the ankle is supported within the imaging coil. In the supine position, the patient is introduced to the bore of the magnet foot first so that claustrophobia has little impact.

As with the wrist, subtle motion can dramatically degrade the acquired images, and therefore, the foot is routinely stabilized with sandbags (Fig. 1).

Receiver Coil

In order to optimize signal acquisition, imaging either requires a molded or tightly apposed surface coil or the use of a quadrature coil. In routine practice, many radiologists employ the quadrature knee coil to image the ankle (see Fig. 1). When focal areas are to be evaluated and high-resolution imaging is required, a dedicated surface coil allowing routine imaging below an 8-cm field of view is applied. To improve signal acquisition when imaging with low-field dedicated extremity units, phased-array ankle surface coils are employed, decreasing the number of excitations required to yield signal-rich images.

Volumetric coils are used to image patients following cast fixation, as loss of apposition secondary to the presence of cast dramatically decreases received signal from flexible surface coils.

S. J. Eustace: Department of Radiology, Section of Musculoskel-etal Radiology, Boston University School of Medicine and Boston Medical Center, Boston, Massachusetts 02118.

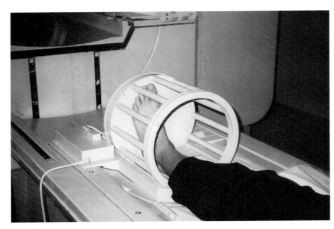

FIG. 1. Supine imaging with foot-first introduction to the bore of the parent field, decreasing impact of claustrophobia.

Imaging Plane

An incorrectly prescribed imaging plane is a frequently encountered practical error. In most cases, tendons are evaluated in the axial plane, and because alteration in axial diameter of tendons is used as a marker of tear (particularly of the tibialis posterior tendon), it is imperative that the acquired images be axial to the tendon and not the foot (Fig. 2). Because flexor and peroneal tendon tears are most common at the malleoli as they arc to enter the foot, directly acquired axial images at this level tend to elongate the perceived diameter of the tendons and misleadingly suggest tendon disruption. Axial images are therefore obliqued, i.e., set up off a sagittal localizer so that they bisect an angle created between the long axis of the tibia and the long axis of the foot (see Fig. 2). Coronal images are prescribed off an axial localizer parallel to a line between medial and lateral malleoli. Sagittal images are directly perpendicular to the plane of the acquired coronal images, which is of importance for imaging the achilles tendon.

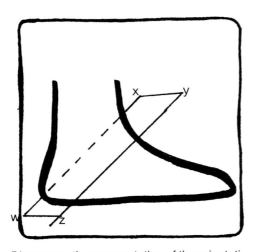

FIG. 2. Diagrammatic representation of the orientation of the axial obliques, bisecting an angle between the tibia and midfoot, to facilitate image acquisition perpendicular to the extrinsic tendons as they round the malleoli.

To image the lateral collateral ligament, direct axial images are acquired to evaluate anterior and posterior talofibular ligaments, followed by axial oblique images prescribed perpendicular to the plantar flexed foot to image the calcaneofibular ligament.

When syndesmotic injury is suspected, conventional imaging may be performed in the direct axial plane with the foot stressed in either inversion or eversion as tolerated.

Field of View

Similar to other sites, a preliminary image, usually a coronal fast inversion recovery image, is acquired with extended coverage, or a field of view of 15 to 20 cm before dedicated imaging. Such an approach allows global perception of the extent of trauma before the high-resolution imaging of internal joint structures is done.

To image patients with suspected ankle fractures or soft tissue injury to either tendons or ligaments, a 14-cm field of view is employed, although this is dictated by the size of the patient. To image patients with suspected calcaneal fractures, the field of view is increased slightly to 16 cm in the sagittal plane.

In patients with trauma to the forefoot, axial images are acquired obliqued in the coronal and in the sagittal plane, with a 20-cm field of view, in order to facilitate visualization of the long axes of the metatarsals.

Slice Thickness

Detailed evaluation of collateral ligaments of the ankle necessitates imaging with a slice thickness not greater than 3 mm. By use of magnets with gradient strengths up to 26 mT/m, 1-mm slices may be routinely acquired. With 13 mT/m systems, thin slices may be yielded by reconstructing three-dimensional data acquired with gradient-echo sequences.

To image osseous abnormality, 3-mm contiguous slices are employed, although an interslice gap of up to 1 mm may be necessary when extended coverage is required (such as coronal images of the midfoot).

Motion Suppression

Immobilization of the foot using sandbags facilitates the acquisition of motion-free images. The use of fast imaging sequences and adequate preprocedural analgesia improves patient tolerance, decreasing gross movement, particularly following ankle fractures.

Imaging Protocol

Following acute trauma, a turbo inversion recovery sequence is usually employed to determine the extent of injury (1 min 15 sec acquisition time). A turbo spin-echo T1-weighted sequence is then applied in coronal, sagittal, and axial planes (1 min 5 sec for each acquisition), allowing detailed evaluation of patient anatomy.

Turbo spin-echo T1 imaging is achieved using a repetition

TABLE 1. *Protocols to image the foot following trauma*

Sequence	Image plane	FOV	TR	TE	ETL	Mapping scheme
Occult or documented fracture evaluation						
IR TSE	Cor direct	14	2,000	20	6	Linear
TSE T1	Cor direct	14	500	15	4	Low—high
+ or − additional planes						
Lateral collateral ligament disruption						
TSE T and IR TSE in axial planes (anterior and posterior talofibular ligaments) and TSE T1 and IR TSE in the axial oblique plane (calcaneofibular ligament)						
+ or − MR arthrography						
Syndesmotic injury						
TSE T1	Direct axial	14	500	15	4	Low—high
+ or − MR arthrography						
Achilles tendon						
TSE T2 fat sat	Sagittal and axial	16	2,000	20, 80	6	Linear
Flexor and peroneal tendons						
TSE T2 fat sat	Axial oblique	16	2,000	20, 80	6	Linear

time of 500 msec, an echo time of 15 msec, a short echo train of up to six, and a low-high echo to view mapping profile. Use of a short echo train facilitates the use of a short repetition time, enhancing T1 weighting and further decreasing acquisition time. With such parameters, images are acquired in 1 min 5 sec. Turbo inversion recovery sequences are acquired using an inversion time of 160 msec, a repetition time of 2,000 msec, an echo time of 20 msec, an echo train of six, and a linear echo to view mapping profile. Such images are acquired in 1 min with a single excitation. Multiple excitations are unnecessary using inversion recovery sequences, as diagnosis is made in most cases on the basis of contrast afforded by fat suppression and signal rescaling.

When collateral ligament injury is suspected, the site of edema is initially localized using an IRTSE image in the coronal plane; turbo T1-weighted images are then acquired in the direct axial plane to evaluate the anterior and posterior talofibular ligaments and in an axial oblique plane to evaluate the calcaneofibular ligament (or in the direct axial plane with the ankle plantar flexed) (1,2). In this setting, when plantarflexion is not possible, a three-dimensional (3D) gradient-echo image is acquired in the coronal plane, which allows thin 1-mm section reconstruction in multiple obliqued planes.

To image suspected extrinsic tendon disruption (flexor, extensor, or peroneal tendons), a dual-echo turbo spin-echo T2-weighted image with fat suppression is acquired in an axial oblique plane perpendicular to the tendons as they round the malleoli. T2 weighting is achieved by employing a repetition time of 2,000 to 3,000 msec (actual TR a function of the coverage required), echo times of 20 and 80 msec, an echo train of six, and linear echo-to-view mapping.

When a patient is referred with a suspected osteochondral abnormality, a coronal turbo inversion recovery sequence is acquired parallel to a line between both malleoli, followed by a T2-weighted fast field- or gradient-echo sequence with off-resonance presaturation. T2 weighting is achieved with a low flip angle of 30°, a long repetition time of 500 msec, and an echo time of 15 msec. Some authors routinely favor the use of fat-saturated dual-echo turbo T2-weighted images to evaluate internal joint structures.

In most patients, because of the impact on acquisition time and need for rapid imaging, a matrix with 256 phase encode steps is employed, and images are acquired with no more than two excitations.

Similar to the knee and shoulder, both GraSE and multishot EPI images with fat saturation may be employed to image internal joint structures, although in our experience neither sequence offers a real advantage to turbo spin-echo T1-weighted images. HASTE images, although rapidly acquired (as little as 15 sec), are heavily T2-weighted.

Magnetic resonance arthrography, with single contrast injection to the tibiotalar joint space, improves visibility of articular cartilage and may improve both the evaluation of the lateral collateral ligament and syndesmosis. Lateral collateral ligament disruption is indicated by communication and free flow of contrast to the peroneal tendon sheaths. Syndesmotic injury is indicated by extension of contrast above the inferior tibiofibular articulation on coronal images. When employed, we inject 4 to 5 cc of a gadolinium, 1% lidocaine, and renografin solution to the tibiotalar joint space alone (0.1 ml of gadolinium DTPA to 5 ml of 1% lidocaine and 15 cc of renografin 60) (Table 1).

BIOMECHANICS OF THE FOOT AND ANKLE

The biomechanics of the foot are complex, involving the integrated motion of 57 articulating surfaces during normal locomotion. In health, the gait cycle is divided into weight-bearing and non-weight-bearing phases in which impaction forces are distributed to either one or both feet.

The weight-bearing cycle is divided into heel-strike, planted-foot, and toe-off phases. On heel strike, the hindfoot is everted, and the midfoot articulations are aligned and mo-

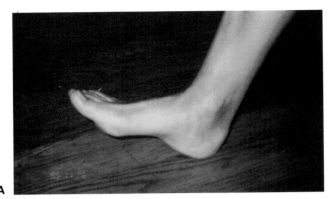

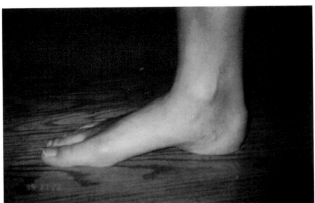

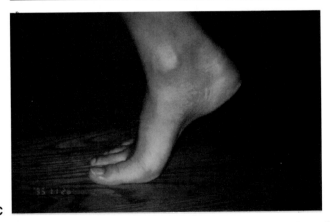

FIG. 3. The normal gait cycle: **(A)** heel strike; **(B)** the planted foot; **(C)** the toe-off phase.

bile, allowing even distribution of impaction forces. As the foot is planted, the long flexors of the calf begin to contract, elevating the medial longitudinal arch and drawing the calcaneus to neutral or varus. Such movement disrupts alignment of midfoot articulations, and the foot becomes rigid or locked in preparation for the final toe-off phase in which all forces are transmitted to the base of the first toe, propelling the foot forward.

Injury to bones, collateral ligaments, and both intrinsic and extrinsic muscle groups will manifest as alterations in this normal pattern, affect gait, and produce compensatory stress on adjacent soft tissue or osseous structures, potentially manifest as tendinitis, tendon tear, bone bruises, or stress fractures. In effect, in interpreting images of the foot, identified abnormalities should be interpreted as a whole rather than as a series of individual abnormalities, in many cases leading to a single unifying diagnosis (Fig. 3) (3,4).

SOFT TISSUE INJURY TO THE FOOT AND ANKLE

The Ankle Ligaments

There are four major ligamentous stabilizers in the foot and ankle, including the lateral collateral ligament, the medial collateral ligament (the deltoid ligament), the syndesmotic complex, and the interosseous ligament (talocalcaneal ligament) in the sinus tarsi.

The Lateral Collateral Ligament

The lateral collateral ligament, which provides lateral stability to the tibiotalar articulation, is composed of five components: the anterior and posterior talofibular ligaments, the calcaneofibular ligament, and the anterior and posterior tibiofibular ligaments.

Injury to the lateral collateral ligament, reported to accompany up to 85% of ankle sprains, reflecting the most common mechanism, inversion with plantar flexion, tends to occur in an orderly sequence from anterior to posterior. In such a way, rupture of the anterior talofibular ligament is followed by rupture of the calcaneofibular and then, extremely rarely, the posterior talofibular ligaments. If the calcaneofibular ligament is ruptured, it is always accompanied by rupture of the anterior talofibular ligament (Fig. 4) (5,6).

The Anterior Talofibular Ligament

The normal anterior talofibular ligament is readily visualized in the direct axial plane running anteromedially from the tip of the lateral malleolus (at the level of the malleolar fossa identified on the inner aspect of the malleolus) to the anterolateral aspect of the talus. In health, the ligament is a fine linear structure, homogeneously hypointense on all sequences. Following injury, intrasubstance hemorrhage may result in ligamentous swelling and signal abnormality, often accompanied by incomplete tear of superior fibers. Complete rupture with retraction is always accompanied by joint effusion and leakage of fluid to neighboring soft tissues. The partially retracted ligament is often noted to billow freely within adjacent joint effusion (Fig. 5) (2,5,6).

In most patients (80%), immobilization without surgical intervention yields complete healing of the injured ligament. However, in a small number of patients, scarring impairing

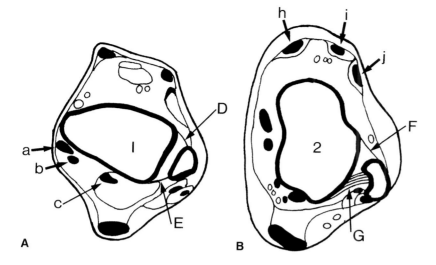

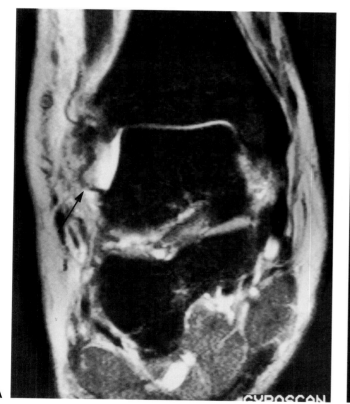

FIG. 4. Diagrammatic representation of the anatomy of the ankle in the direct axial plane (A) at the syndesmosis and (B) below the syndesmosis; a, tibialis posterior; b, flexor digitorum; c, flexor hallucis; D, anterior tibiofibular ligament; E, posterior tibiofibular ligament; F, anterior talofibular ligament; G, posterior talofibular ligament; h, tibialis anterior; i, extensor hallucis; j, extensor digitorum tendons. Adapted from Erickson and Johnson (83).

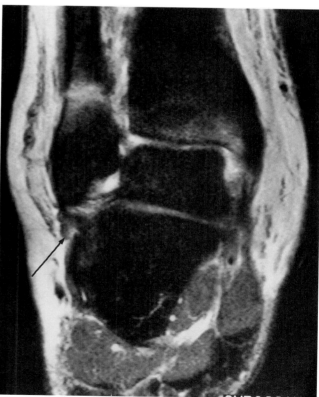

FIG. 5. (A) Coronal IR TSE image showing extensive periarticular soft tissue edema following ankle injury, with disruption of the anterior talofibular ligament *(arrow)* billowing in joint effusion. Similar edema is identified in the anterior tibiotalar ligament. (B) Coronal IR TSE image in the same patient shows a Weber C fracture with complete disruption of the syndesmosis and passage of fluid to the inferior tibiofibular articulation. The calcaneofibular ligament is intact *(arrow)*. Image shows impaction bruise of the tibial plafond rather than the talar dome, markedly decreasing the likelihood of posttraumatic osteochondral abnormality of the talar dome.

mobility, a retracted fibrosed ligament (a meniscoid lesion) resulting in impingement, or persistent clinical instability requires surgical repair.

The Calcaneofibular Ligament

The normal calcaneofibular ligament is readily visualized on images acquired in an axial oblique plane prescribed perpendicular to the posterior subtalar joint or in the axial plane acquired in a plantarflexed foot. The ligament is identified as a fine linear structure deep to the peroneal tendons uniformly hypointense on all sequences (2,5,6). Following injury, intrasubstance hemorrhage and edema produce swelling and signal abnormality in the ligament enhancing its conspicuity. Communication with peroneal tendon sheaths results in frequently identified associated peroneal tendon sheath fluid and occasionally subluxation.

Magnetic resonance arthrographic images in patients following rupture show free communication between the tibiotalar joint space and the peroneal tendon sheaths (Fig. 6).

The Posterior Talofibular Ligament

This is a fan-shaped isointense structure, usually identified on the same image as the anterior talofibular ligament in the direct axial plane. The ligament runs from the malleolar fossa on the inner aspect of the lateral malleolus to the posterior tibial tubercle of the talus. Because of its fan-shaped configuration, the ligament is extremely strong and is rarely injured.

The Medial Collateral (Deltoid) Ligament

The medial collateral ligament has five components including the anterior and posterior tibiotalar, the tibiocalcaneal, the tibiospring, and the tibionavicular ligaments. Classically the ligament is divided into deep and superficial components. The superficial layer arises from the anterior margin of the medial malleolus and branches to the navicular, the sustentaculum, the calcaneus, and to the medial tubercle of the talus. The deep layer arises from the posterior margin of the malleolus and attaches to the medial aspect of the talus.

On MRI, the fan-shaped components of the superficial medial collateral ligament are only visualized in multiple oblique planes. In contrast, the deep component is routinely identified on direct coronal images as a short striated structure. In general, injury to the medial collateral ligament accompanies complex ankle trauma, invariably associated with disruption of the lateral collateral ligament or the syndesmosis (2,7–10) and sometimes fracture of the fibula.

The Syndesmosis

The syndesmosis is the term used to describe the three stabilizing components of the inferior tibiofibular articulation, the anterior and posterior tibiofibular ligaments (ATIF, PTIF) and the interosseous membrane. Injury to the syndesmosis is extremely uncommon in the absence of a fracture.

The ligaments of the syndesmosis are readily visualized on direct axial images just proximal to the tibiotalar articulation (identification of the malleolar fossa on the inner aspect of the lateral malleolus is used to differentiate between the anterior and posterior talofibular and anterior and posterior tibiofibular ligaments when any doubt exists) (see Fig. 4).

The ATIF ligament is a linear hypointense structure running from the anterior tibial tubercle laterally along the anterior margin of the inferior tibiofibular articulation to the fibula. Often the ligament courses slightly inferiorly and therefore can only be fully appreciated by reviewing serial

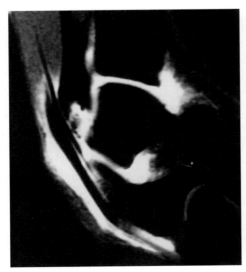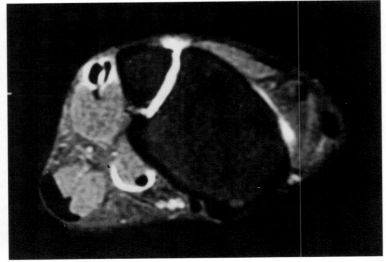

FIG. 6. Magnetic resonance arthrogram following direct intra-articular gadolinium shows disruption of the lateral collateral ligament with communication to the peroneal tendon sheath. Axial image shows associated disruption of the anterior tibiofibular ligament, and of the peroneous brevis tendon.

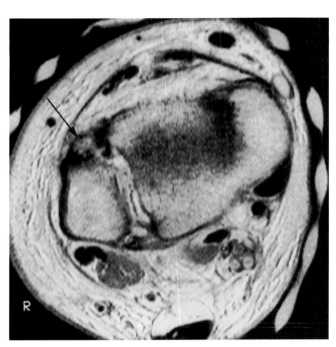

FIG. 7. Axial image shows disruption of the anterior tibiofibular ligament (arrow).

images. The PTIF has both similar signal characteristics and orientation to the ATIF and runs along the posterior margin of the tibiofibular articulation (Fig. 7).

Injury to the syndesmosis usually involves rupture of the anterior tibiofibular ligament and spares the posterior. The posterior ligament is stronger, and therefore, when it is stressed, the result is an avulsion fracture at its insertion more often than soft tissue rupture. An ATIF injury may result in intrasubstance hemorrhage and edema or complete disruption accompanied by widening of the anterior joint space (see Fig. 7). Occasionally, if untreated, chronic tear may produce ATIF thickening and fibrosis to produce a meniscoid lesion and secondary syndesmotic impingement (10,11).

The Ligaments of the Sinus Tarsi

The sinus tarsi is a cone-shaped space interposed between the inferolateral border of the talus and the superolateral surface of the calcaneus. In health, the sinus tarsi is predominantly filled with fat, allowing the space to narrow slightly on eversion. On inversion, widening of the space and hence stability between the talus and calcaneus is maintained by both the cervical and interosseous ligaments (12,13). Minor trauma, either inversion or eversion, may manifest as hemorrhage, edema, and secondary compression of neurovascular structures within the space, and hence acute pain (the sinus tarsi syndrome). Acute inversion may occasionally result in disruption of ligamentous structures and gross subtalar insta-

bility. Occasionally disruption of the ligaments precedes or is a part of subtalar dislocation (Fig. 8).

Because the sinus tarsi is richly vascularized, ruptured ligaments readily heal without surgical intervention, although scarring and persistent laxity may result in long-term instability.

At MR imaging, the sinus tarsi is readily visualized on direct coronal images, fat-suppressed inversion recovery images facilitating the detection of edema and hemorrhage, and turbo spin-echo T1-weighted images allowing the evaluation of interosseous and cervical ligaments (14).

In practice, when a patient presents following inversion injury, coronal imaging should be extended through the sinus tarsi to the base of the fifth metatarsal. Such an approach, in addition to facilitating evaluation of the tibiotalar articulation, facilitates detection of injury within the sinus tarsi and at the base of the fifth metatarsal.

Impingement Syndromes

Three impingement syndromes are described causing chronic pain following ankle trauma: the anterolateral, syndesmotic, and posterolateral impingement syndromes. The anterolateral impingement syndrome describes soft tissue impingement with associated pain between anterolateral osseous structures of the ankle joint (the lateral gutter). Most commonly, fibrous overgrowth or synovitis following chronic tear of the anterior talofibular ligament is responsible, rarely tear resulting in a hyalinized connective tissue meniscoid lesion (15). The syndesmotic impingement syndrome describes the acute pain incurred when soft tissue is impinged between the osseous structures of the syndesmosis, usually manifest by thickening and synovitis at the site of a chronic tear of the anterior tibiofibular ligament (16). Posterior impingement describes impingement of a posterior soft tissue structure between posterolateral osseous structures of the ankle. In most cases, the syndrome reflects impingement of a hypertrophied posterior inferior tibiofibular ligament or the posterior intermalleolar ligament (17).

Tendon Injuries

Although flexor and extensor tendon injuries usually reflect chronic trauma, injury to both the achilles and peroneal tendons often accompanies acute trauma, acute traumatic injury to the flexor hallucis and tibialis posterior tendons is less common (18).

The Achilles Tendon

The achilles tendon, formed by merging of the gastrocnemius and soleus tendons, is the most commonly injured tendon in the foot.

The tendon is readily visualized on both sagittal and axial images at MRI. It is readily identified as a hypointense struc-

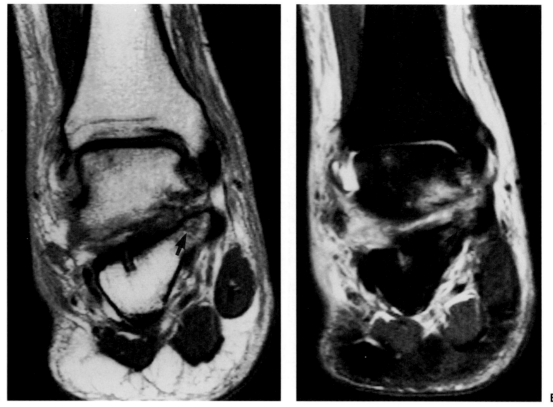

FIG. 8. (A) Coronal TSE T1 and **(B)** IR TSE images show rupture of the interosseous ligament within the sinus tarsi in a patient following acute inversion injury. There is *contre-coup* impaction bruising of the sustentaculum and undersurface of the talus, with undisplaced fracture of the sustentaculum *(arrows)*.

ture, conspicuity being enhanced by adjacent hyperintense fat.

Injury to the achilles is usually divided into insertional and noninsertional types. Insertional injury usually occurs following chronic trauma, impingement by a bony spur (Haglund's syndrome), or chronic local synovitis (Fig. 9). Noninsertional injury usually occurs following acute, often innocuous trauma.

Noninsertional injury typically occurs 3 to 6 cm proximal to the tendon insertion in the region of the myotendinous junction. At this location, tendon fibers interwine and create a zone of relative ischemia. Injury, although more common in patients with gout, in patients on steroids, and in chronic renal failure, typically occurs in poorly conditioned athletes in the third and fifth decades following unaccustomed exercise (19–21).

Noninsertional injury may result in either partial tear (Fig. 10), which may be clinically difficult to diagnose (and should be differentiated from tear of the medial head of the gastrocnemius), or complete tear, readily detected clinically (impaired plantar flexion and a palpable gap in soft tissues behind the ankle). In the former, MR imaging is undertaken for diagnosis; in the latter, it is undertaken for surgical planning, to determine the extent of tendon retraction.

At MR imaging, the achilles tendon is uniformly hypointense, with a semilunar configuration in the axial plane. Injury is manifest as tendon enlargement, with development of a convex rather than concave anterior margin in the axial plane secondary to intrasubstance hemorrhage and edema. Subtle foci of signal abnormality within the tendon, particularly on short-TE sequences, may be observed secondary to magic angle phenomenon. Partial tear is manifest by partial rather than complete discontinuity of tendon fibers and is best detected in the sagittal plane. Following conservative management, signal abnormalities gradually resolve, although they may persist for at least a year (22,23).

Peroneal Tendon Injury

The peroneal muscle bellies within the lateral compartment of the calf give rise to the peroneus brevis and longus tendons at the ankle. The peroneal tendons, peroneus brevis anterior to the peroneus longus, course around the lateral malleolus within its slightly concave aspect called the fibular groove.

The peroneus brevis tendon passes along the lateral margin of the foot to insert at the base of the fifth metatarsal; the peroneus longus tendon courses beneath the cuboid to

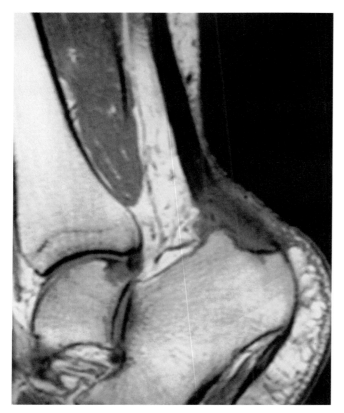

FIG. 9. Sagittal T1-weighted image acquired with a dedicated low-field extremity magnet shows insertional achilles partial tear with associated dorsal calcaneal spur (Haglund's syndrome). (Courtesy of Lunar Artoscan.)

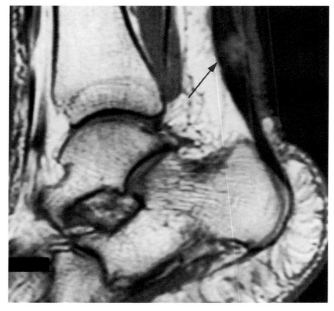

FIG. 10. Sagittal T1-weighted image shows an incomplete tear of the achilles tendon at the musculotendinous junction (6 cm proximal to calcaneal insertion) characterized by local signal abnormality and swelling.

insert at the base of the first metatarsal and medial cuneiform.

Functioning to plantarflex and evert the foot, the tendons, if unrestrained, would freely bowstring at the lateral malleolus. Normally, the position within the fibular groove is maintained by a tight retinaculum, which prevents both tendon subluxation and dislocation or bowstringing (24).

Because the primary functions of these tendons are eversion and plantarflexion, it is not surprising that injury is usually a sequel to forced dorsiflexion or forced inversion. When it is secondary to distraction forces of inversion, tendon injury is commonly accompanied by disruption of the superior peroneal retinaculum (with avulsion of a small fibular fragment at its site of attachment), fractures of the fibula, osteochondral lesion of the lateral talar dome, lateral collateral ligament injury, sinus tarsi disruption, and fractures of the base of the fifth metatarsal.

Peroneus brevis tendon injury is more common than injury to the peroneus longus (25). It is postulated that laxity of the superior peroneal retinaculum allows the brevis tendon to sublux and interpose between the longus and the fibrous edge of the fibula, resulting in shear-induced longitudinal tendon splits (Fig. 11).

At MR imaging, the tendons are best evaluated in either the axial or axial oblique planes. Tendinitis is manifest as peritendinous fluid and alteration in the transverse caliber of the tendon. In most cases, reflecting mechanism, tears are longitudinal and manifest as a split or pseudothird tendon in the axial plane (Fig. 12), although complete transverse tears are occasionally observed.

Following retinacular disruption, tendons may sublux or completely dislocate, which often can be demonstrated only by imaging the foot in eversion or dorsiflexion (26).

Tibialis Posterior Tendon Injury

The tibialis posterior tendon is the second most commonly injured tendon in the foot. The tendinous continuation of the muscle belly within the deep posterior compartment of the calf rounds the medial malleolus and passes forward to a dominant insertion at the base of the navicular, and to six further lesser insertions in the forefoot, at the bases of the cuneiforms and the bases of metatarsals two through four. The tibialis posterior tendon provides major support to the medial longitudinal arch during the planted-foot phase of the gait cycle and is responsible for both plantarflexion and inversion (27).

Although acute injuries to the tibialis posterior tendon have been described following forced dorsiflexion with eversion in young athletes, in most cases injury occurs as a result of chronic overuse or trauma in middle-aged women.

Chronic tear results in collapse of the medial arch or acquired flatfoot with progressive hindfoot valgus, posterior subtalar joint subluxation, and arthritis. Medial arch collapse may result in impaction bone bruising between the anterior

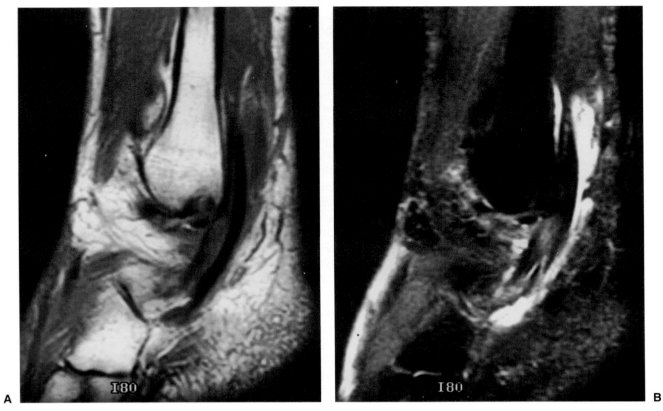

A   B

FIG. 11. Sagittal TSE T1 **(A)** and IR TSE **(B)** images show interposition of the peroneus brevis tendon as it rounds the malleolus associated with a longitudinal tendon split.

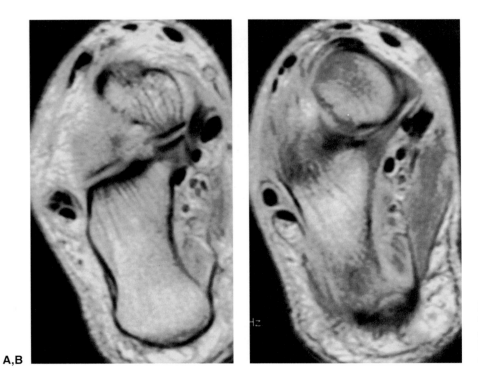

A,B

FIG. 12. Axial oblique proton-density-weighted image shows the appearance of an accessory tendon secondary to a longitudinal split in the peroneus brevis **(A)** with distal reconstitution **(B).**

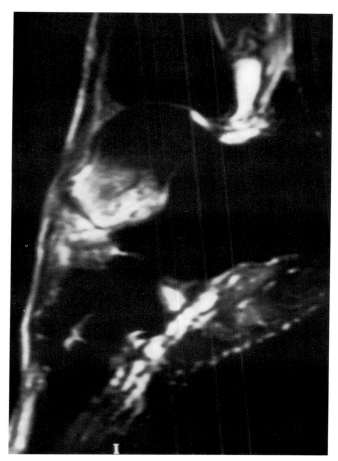

FIG. 13. Acquired medial arch collapse with impaction of anterior talar process and extensive secondary marrow edema.

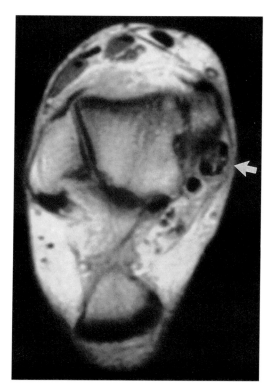

FIG. 14. Axial oblique image shows central split within the tibialis posterior tendon posterior to the medial malleolus *(arrow),* transverse diameter up to four times the size of the other flexor tendons.

talar process and the navicular or between the calcaneus and the cuboid (Fig. 13).

At MR imaging, the tibialis posterior tendon is twice the transverse diameter of the other flexor tendons on images acquired perpendicular to the long axis of the tendon. Following injury, intrasubstance hemorrhage and edema result in tendon swelling to up to four times the transverse diameter of the other flexors, or type 1 tear, often accompanied by tendon sheath inflammation, peritendinous fluid, or tenosynovitis (Fig. 14). In chronicity, disrupted fibers become stretched and attenuated, and the transverse diameter decreases to less than that of other flexors, type 2 tear, finally progressing to complete disruption with discontinuity, type 3 tear (Fig. 15) (28,29).

Flexor Hallucis Longus Injury

The flexor hallucis is a dominant flexor and inverter of the foot, with an extensive course to insert at the base of the distal phalanx of the great toe.

Injury to the flexor hallucis may occur proximally, usually secondary to chronic overuse at the level of the medial malle-

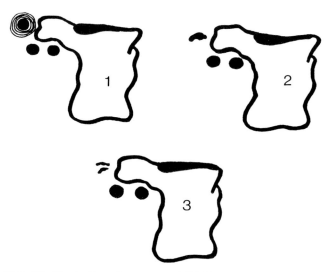

FIG. 15. Illustration of patterns of tibialis posterior tendon injury. Type 1 injury manifest by intrasubstance edema and swelling of the tendon; type 2 manifest by tendon atresia; type 3 injury manifest by attenuation and tendon rupture. Adapted from Rosenberg et al. (28).

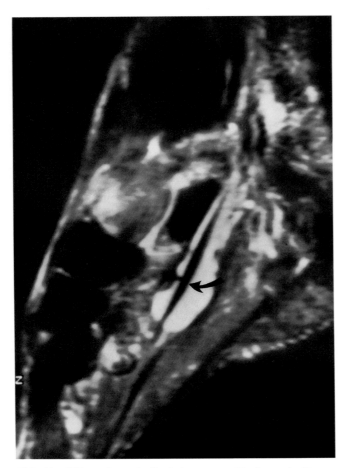

FIG. 16. Diffuse flexor hallucis tenosynovitis *(arrow)* with associated impaction bruising of the anterior talar process secondary to secondary imposed stress on the medial longitudinal arch.

olus (Fig. 16) or the musculotendinous junction, as occurs in ballet dancers (30,31), or distally, which is usually acute and secondary to stubbing the toe attempting to kick a football, hence the term "turf toe" (Fig. 17) (32–34).

Similar to other tendon or ligamentous injuries, intrasubstance rupture initially leads to tendon swelling before attenuation and rupture.

The flexor hallucis tendon runs in a fibro-osseous tunnel along the posterior aspect of the talus, which may be a site of friction leading to tear in ballet dancers, accentuated by an accessory os trigonum (35).

Although peritendinous fluid is a useful marker of tendon insult and tenosynovitis, communication to the tibiotalar articulation in up to 20% of the normal population may account for this observation in the absence of symptoms (36).

Tibialis Anterior Tendon Injury

The tibialis anterior muscle arising in the anterior compartment of the calf originates its tendon at the level of the tibiotalar articulation; the tendon passes to the foot deep to the extensor retinaculum before inserting on the medial cuneiform and the medial base of the first metatarsal. The tibialis anterior thus is a dominant flexor and inverter of the foot, and injury is therefore induced acutely by forced extension and eversion. In most cases, rupture is the sequel of chronic trauma, with repeated encroachment on the tendon by the extensor retinaculum over time (37).

The tibialis anterior tendon is best visualized in the axial oblique plane with sections just distal to the medial malleolus.

Os Trigonum Syndrome

The os trigonum represents a congenital nonunion of the lateral tubercle of the posterior process of the talus, to which it remains intimately related in adulthood. During flexion-extension, synovial tissue may interdigitate between it and the posterior tibia, resulting in capsular entrapment, local pain, and inflammation. Inflammatory changes are usually

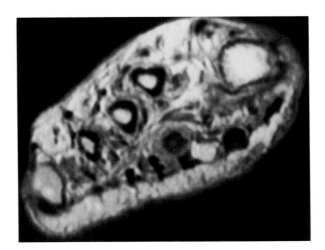

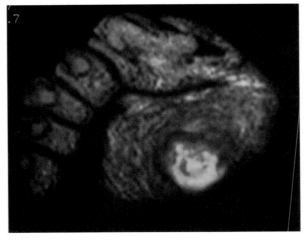

FIG. 17. Acute tear of the flexor digitorum longus tendon to the second toe complicating a cock-up toe deformity.

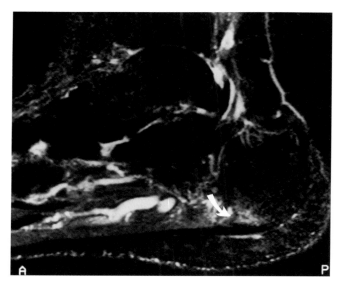

FIG. 18. Sagittal IR TSE image shows local inflammatory change at the insertion of the plantar aponeurosis on the dorsal calcaneus in a patient with early plantar fasciitis *(arrow).*

clearly visualized in the sagittal plane intimately related to the posterior tibiotalar joint recess. The relationship between the inflammatory process and the medially located flexor hallucis tendon sheath is best achieved in the axial plane (31,35).

Plantar Fasciitis

Plantar fasciitis is the term used to describe inflammation of the plantar fascia at its insertion on the medial calcaneal tuberosity. The inflammation is thought to be the result of repetitive microtrauma or avulsive traction forces applied at this site, primarily in joggers and athletes (the presence of a heel spur is not a predisposing factor). Weight-bearing forces repeatedly stress the medial arch during jogging, and its configuration is maintained by contraction of both intrinsic and extrinsic flexors and the plantar aponeurosis.

In acute plantar fasciitis, sagittal fat-suppressed turbo spin-echo or turbo inversion recovery sequences show signal hyperintensity within and adjacent to the insertion of the plantar aponeurosis, often extending to adjacent subcutaneous tissues (Fig. 18). In chronic plantar fasciitis, inflammatory changes extend to the midbelly of the aponeurosis, which often becomes markedly thickened, reflecting extensive fibrous replacement, and signal hyperintensity is less marked (38–40).

OSSEOUS INJURY TO THE TIBIA, FOOT, AND ANKLE

Tibial Fractures: Infected Nonunion

Numerous classification systems for fractures of the tibia have been proposed in attempts to predict fracture outcome and appropriate mode of treatment, although in most cases classification systems lack both reproducibility and sensitivity.

Reviewing the impact of closed reduction, Nicoll (41) reported that over 90% of fractures without displacement, without comminution, and without a soft tissue wound underwent rapid healing; in contrast, in displaced comminuted fractures with an associated soft tissue wound, nonunion occurred in up to 40% of cases.

Nonunion occurs more commonly in fractures of the distal tibia, as these fractures more commonly involve poorly vascularized compact diaphyseal cortical bone rather than cancellous bone of the metaphyses. It is more likely to occur in high-velocity injuries rather than low-velocity, in displaced rather than undisplaced fractures, in comminuted rather than simple fractures, in fractures that develop an infection (compound fractures or following open reduction), and in fractures poorly immobilized or with persistent distraction by an intact fibula.

Although MRI has little role in the evaluation of undisplaced fractures of the diaphysis, it is of particular value in patients in whom complicating infection is suspected. Diffusion imaging, based on changes in water content of callus at fracture margins, may be a method allowing early triage of patients into those who are and are not likely to develop nonunion, although this is under investigation at the time of this writing.

When diaphyseal fractures are compound, infection may become superimposed on devitalized bone fragments, stripping periosteum and impairing the healing process, even if fragments are adequately immobilized.

Triple-phase bone scan can differentiate superficial cellulitis from osteomyelitis, although spatial resolution, sensitivity, and specificity are poor, even when it is performed in conjunction with an ^{111}In-labeled white cell study.

With MRI, fat-suppressed sequences may show bone destruction and both soft tissue and marrow edema in patients with both cellulitis and osteomyelitis. Although it may be difficult to differentiate posttraumatic edema at fracture margins from edema induced by infection, the identification of progressive marrow edema on serial scans, soft tissue, or osseous fluid collections and focal enhancement on gadolinium-enhanced images suggest the presence of superimposed infection (42–46).

Fatigue Versus Insufficiency Fractures of the Tibia: Medial Tibial Stress Syndrome

Fatigue fractures represent fractures through well-mineralized bone secondary to abnormal biomechanical forces applied repetitively over time. In contrast, insufficiency fractures represent fractures through abnormal bone secondary to an inability to resist the forces induced by normal function of locomotion and weight bearing.

In military recruits, fatigue fractures occur in the proximal tibia secondary to repetitive stresses applied in marching and involve the posteromedial cortex more frequently than the anteromedial cortex. In young athletes, fractures most frequently involve the anteromedial cortex at the junction of the middle and lower third of the tibia; in ballet dancers they involve the middle third of the tibia; and in long-distance runners they tend to involve the distal fibula.

Insufficiency fractures tend to occur in elderly osteoporotic women, commonly with complicating medical diseases necessitating chronic steroid use. Insufficiency fractures typically occur at three sites: the junction of the proximal metaphysis and diaphysis, the junction of the distal metaphysis and the diaphysis, and the distal fibula (47–49).

Medial tibial stress syndrome is the term employed to describe the syndrome of multiple fatigue fractures or shin splints along the anteromedial cortex of the tibia identified in young adult athletes.

The mechanism for the development of the stress fractures is unclear, although most now believe that they are a sequel to chronic traction effects imposed by muscle insertions (dif-ferent muscle groups are employed by militiary recruits, athletes, and ballet dancers). Frequently, fatigue fractures occur at the insertion of the flexor digitorum longus and deep crural fascia along the distal half of the anteromedial border of the tibia. Repeated contraction of flexor muscle groups initially produces multifocal localized periosteal blistering and edema within the adjacent soft tissues. Although at this stage no radiographic abnormality is usually identified, induced osteoblastic activity at sites of traction results in increased uptake at scintigraphy and subtle soft tissue and periosteal signal hyperintensity at MRI (50), so-called stage 1 disease (Figs. 19 and 20). As disease progresses, periosteal blistering is accompanied initially by focal marrow edema and then by diffuse edema, stages 2 and 3, during which time the diagnosis usually becomes apparent on conventional radiographs. In chronicity, as a result of either hyperemia-induced demineralization or ischemia, periosteal blistering is accompanied by cortical break extending through marrow as a true fracture, stage 4.

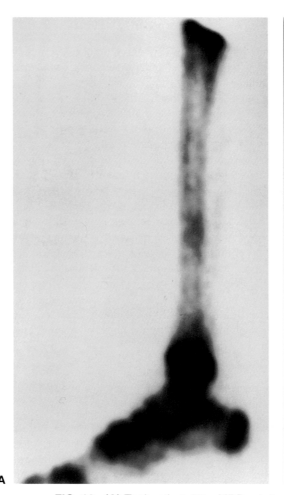
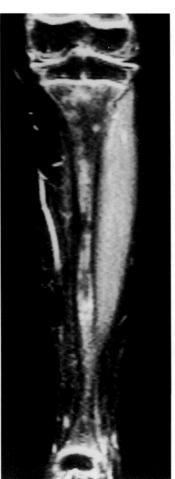
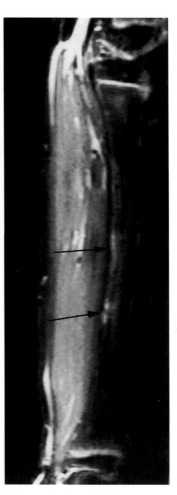

A

B

FIG. 19. (A) Technetium-99m-MDP scintiscan shows focal accumulation of radiotracer in the midtibia, suggestive of a shin splint. (B) Coronal *(left)* and sagittal IR TSE MR images in the same patient show diffuse marrow edema throughout the diaphysis of the tibia with foci most marked posteriorly *(arrows)* at sites of shin splints.

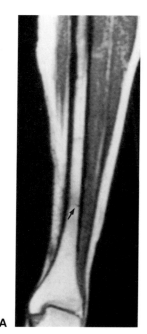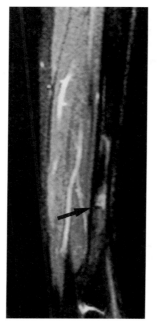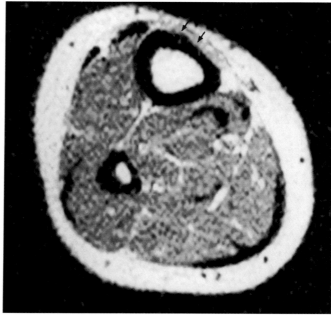

A   B,C

FIG. 20. Coronal T1 **(A)**, sagittal **(B)**, and axial images **(C)** show transverse hypointense lines with adjacent edema in the distal tibia corresponding to shin splints in a young athlete.

As a result of the site of insult and mechanism (traction or avulsion) (see Chapter 4), observed marrow edema in this injury is often extremely limited and may be overlooked if not specifically sought.

Medial Tibial Stress Syndrome
Stage 1. Periosteal and Soft Tissue Edema.
Stage 2. Periosteal Blistering and Subtle Adjacent Marrow Edema.
Stage 3. Periosteal Blistering and More Marked Marrow Edema.
Stage 4. Cortical Disruption Extending Through Marrow Perpendicular to Long Axis of Tibia.

Ankle Fractures

Three classifications are commonly employed to describe fracture at the ankle: the Lange Hansen classification (51) is by mechanism, the Henderson classification (52) is based purely on radiographic anatomy, and the Danis Weber classification (53) is based on the level of the fracture of the fibula (an attempt to triage patients into those who are and are not likely to have disruption of the syndesmosis).

The Lange Hansen Classification

Understanding the Lange Hansen classification (52) allows a directed search for specific abnormalities when reviewing MR images following ankle trauma. In simple terms, supination (inversion) injuries, which occur more frequently than eversion injuries, are associated with lateral traction and either tear of the lateral collateral ligament or transverse fracture of the distal fibula associated with oblique impaction fracture of the medial malleolus. Pronation (eversion) injuries result in medial traction manifest as either transverse fracture through the medial malleolus or disruption of the medial collateral ligament accompanied by oblique impaction fracture through the fibula.

The Lange Hansen classification recognizes that pronation or supination may be complicated by superimposed external rotation forces. When supination is accompanied by adduction (essentially simple inversion), the lateral collateral ligament usually tears while the syndesmosis remains intact. When supination is accompanied by external rotation (the leg rotates internally on the planted supinated foot), both the lateral collateral ligament and the anterior syndesmosis tend to rupture, and torque forces tend to produce an oblique fracture of the fibula extending superiorly from anteroinferior to posterosuperior.

When pronation is accompanied by abduction (essentially simple eversion), traction produces medial collateral disruption or medial malleolar transverse fracture accompanied by disruption of the syndesmosis. Additional lateral displacement of the talus produces an oblique fracture at or above the syndesmosis. When pronation is accompanied by external rotation, following medial malleolar or ligamentous injury, the anterior syndesmosis tears, and the fibula fractures in a spiral or oblique manner from anteroinferior to posterosuperior. If torque forces are transmitted to the neck of the fibula, the term *Maisonneuve fracture* is applied. When the fracture remains in the distal third, it is termed a Dupuytren fracture. Vertical forces driving the talus into the distal tibia results in impaction fracture, the location of which is dictated by the position of the foot and amount of loading to produce the injury (Fig. 21).

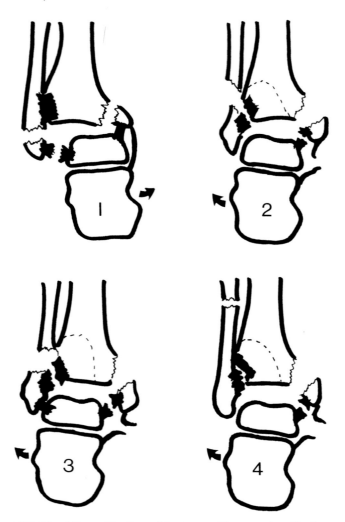

FIG. 21. AO modification of the Lange Hansen classification of ankle fractures. The higher the fibular fracture, the greater the likelihood of syndesmotic disruption. Type 1 injury following inversion with a transverse fracture of the distal fibula without syndesmotic disruption; type 2 injury following eversion commonly associated with both syndesmotic and medial collateral ligament injury; type 3 injury following eversion associated with a higher fibular fracture, invariably associated with disruption of the syndesmosis; type 4 injury is the most severe.

The Danis Weber Classification

This classification divides ankle fractures into three groups: type A, in whom fibula fracture is below the syndesmosis secondary to supination; type B, in whom fibula fracture begins at or near the syndesmosis secondary to supination external rotation (the syndesmosis is disrupted in 50% of cases); and type C, in whom fibula fracture begins above the syndesmosis secondary to pronation with external rotation. In type C injuries, fibula fracture may be diaphyseal or in the proximal fibula (Maisonneuve fracture) (Fig. 22) (52).

Magnetic Resonance Imaging in Ankle Fractures

Although conventional radiographs demonstrate osseous injury, overlapping bone structures may obscure subtle ab-

normality. When fine detail is sought, computed tomographic imaging is now usually undertaken rather than conventional planar tomography. Magnetic resonance imaging represents an alternative to CT for osseous evaluation as it allows direct multiplanar imaging in contiguous thin slices. Refocusing pulses inherent in the turbo or fast spin-echo sequence minimize susceptibility effects of trabeculae, while increased receiver bandwidth (32 kHz) using the same sequence (used to decrease echo spacing and accelerate acquisition of signal) decreases the effects of chemical shift and improves the evaluation of cortex and cartilage.

The primary advantage of MR imaging is the ability to image soft tissue injury directly rather than to infer its presence on the basis of secondary signs on radiographs. Because integrity of both collateral ligaments and syndesmosis is used to triage patients into surgical and nonsurgical groups, direct visualization of these structures is of considerable importance. In Weber B fractures, an inability to directly visualize the syndesmosis wing plan radiographs frequently results in unnecessary surgical fixation (syndesmotic disruption occurs in only 50% of cases) (see Figs. 5, 23, and 24) (52).

Magnetic resonance arthrography improves evaluation of syndesmotic and collateral ligament integrity, with extension of contrast 1 cm above the inferior tibiofibular articulation suggesting syndesmotic injury and extravasation to the peroneal tendon sheath indicating calcaneofibular ligament disruption (Fig. 25) (11).

Magnetic resonance imaging is useful in the evaluation of patients with suspected posttraumatic osteochondral injury. Lateral osteochondral lesions are invariably secondary to trauma, complicating inversion injuries. Forced inversion results in impaction of the lateral talar dome against the fibula. Early MRI identification of an osteochondral injury or subarticular bruising allows triage of patients into groups in whom

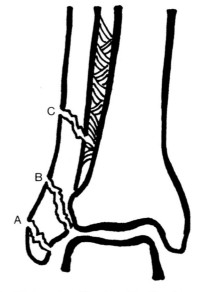

FIG. 22. The Weber classification classifies fractures according to location into one of three types: A, B, and C. The limitation of this classification is the fact that 50% of patients with Weber B fractures will have an intact syndesmosis.

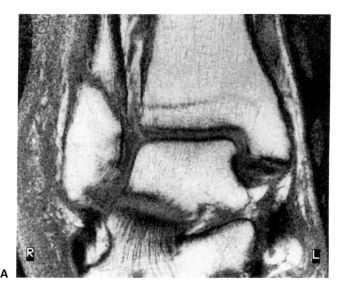

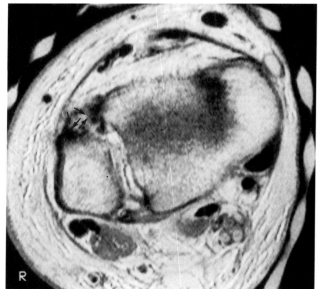
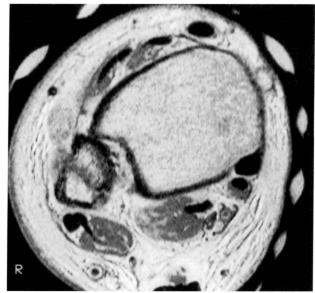

FIG. 23. (A) Coronal TSE T1-weighted image showing an oblique Weber B fracture of the distal fibula extending to the syndesmosis. (The syndesmosis is intact in 50% of cases). **(B)** Axial TSE T1 images at the syndesmosis *(left)* show disruption of the anterior tibiofibular ligament *(small arrows);* images *(right)* 1 cm above the syndesmosis show minimal anterior subluxation of the distal fibular from the tibiofibular articulation.

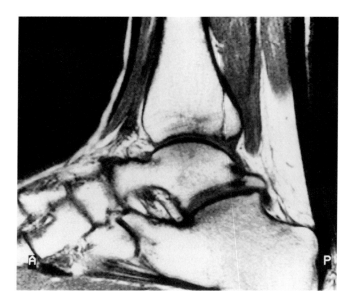

FIG. 24. Sagittal TSE T1-weighted image shows an occult undisplaced fracture of the posterior malleolus.

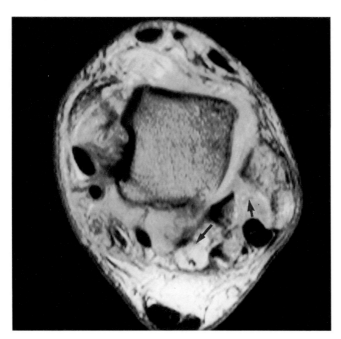

FIG. 25. Axial proton-density-weighted image shows an oblique vertical split through the lateral malleolus *(arrow)* with interposition of peroneal tendons between fracture fragments *(arrow).*

additional avoidance of weight bearing should be undertaken to prevent progression of the injury. Similar to atraumatic osteochondral injury, conservative management is initially undertaken in all patients unless a free fragment is identified (Fig. 26) (54,55).

Berndt and Harty (56) have staged osteochondral injuries according to relative stability of the osteochondral fragment, with stage 1 characterized by a subchondral bone bruise or fracture, stage 2 by a single rent in the overlying cartilage and partial detachment of the fragment, stage 3 by rents on either side of the subchondral contusion with detachment without displacement, and stage 4 by the presence of a displaced detached fragment.

Soft tissue foreign bodies, which may complicate ankle trauma, are readily identified within the adjacent soft tissues. When these are clinically suspected, gradient-echo sequences are used to enhance susceptibility blooming of both metal and wooden soft tissue foreign bodies (Fig. 27) (57).

Ankle Dislocations

Ankle dislocations are extremely uncommon and usually complicate axial loading with rotation to a plantarflexed foot. Attempted reduction is undertaken acutely, and therefore, when patients are referred for MR imaging, it is to assess residual soft tissue injury (58).

Pilon Fractures

Pilon fractures represent impaction fractures of the distal tibia occurring secondary to gross axial loading (59). Undis-

placed fractures may be treated conservatively; displaced fractures usually require surgical reconstruction and immobilization. Although computed tomography is routinely used in these cases to document the number and position of the fragments, MR imaging may serve a similar function, although severe comminution may be better evaluated by computed tomography.

Growth Plate Injuries at the Ankle

Similar to other sites, growth plate injuries are classified using the Salter Harris classification discussed in Chapter 4. The presence of an unfused growth plate is a site of biomechanical weakness, and, although it is subject to the same mechanism as in adults, similar forces may produce quite different fractures.

The Triplane Fracture

The triplane fracture of the distal tibia, complicating external rotation of the foot at the ankle, occurs most frequently

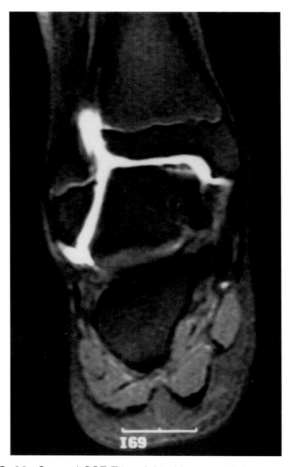

FIG. 26. Coronal CSE T1-weighted image with fat suppression following direct intra-articular injection of gadolinium shows an undisplaced osteochondral lesion of the medial talar dome 3 months following minor ankle trauma. (Courtesy of M. Barish, M.D., Boston Medical Center, Boston, MA).

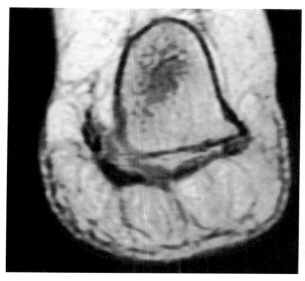 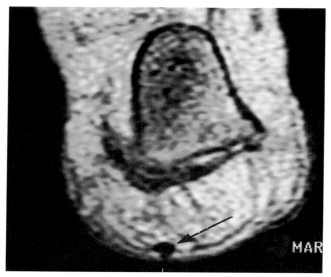

FIG. 27. (A) Coronal T1-weighted spin-echo image of the dorsal calcaneus in a patient with a suspected soft tissue body following trauma. **(B)** Coronal fast field- or gradient-echo image shows susceptibility blooming at the site of subcutaneous metal fragment *(black arrow)*.

during an 18-month period of asymmetric growth plate closure in the distal tibia between 13 and 15 years in boys and between 12 and 14 years in girls (60). The fracture is characterized by three distinct fracture planes: a vertical fracture through the epiphysis, a horizontal fracture through the physis, and an oblique fracture through the metaphysis in such a way as to constitute a Salter 4 fracture. In most cases, imaging reveals lateral displacement of the epiphyseal fragment. Direct multiplanar MR imaging represents an alternative to computed tomographic reconstructions in the evaluation of this injury. With magnetic resonance, relative displacement of bone fragments may be documented in three planes, with turbo spin-echo T1-weighted images, in little more than 3 min. Undisplaced fractures may be treated conservatively, but displaced fractures usually require screw fixation (Fig. 28).

The Tillaux Fracture

Described by Tillaux in 1848 (61,62), this fracture is a subtle avulsion from the anterolateral growth plate of the distal tibia, which, like the triplane fracture, results from the stress imposed by extreme external rotation. In adolescence, the growth plate of the distal tibia closes from medial to lateral. In that period, traction on the anterior tibiofibular ligament in external rotation, rather than rupturing the ligament, is transmitted to bone and results in an avulsion at the junction of fused and unfused growth plate, a Salter 3 type fracture. Untreated, the fracture fails to heal, as traction from the anterior tibiofibular ligament draws fracture surfaces apart. Early diagnosis and either immobilization or surgical repair in displaced fractures must be undertaken (Figs. 29 and 30).

Although the diagnosis is usually apparent on conventional radiographs, particularly oblique mortice views, occa-

sionally they are identified only when patients with persistent symptoms are referred for MRI. Because these are predominantly traction rather than impaction in origin, adjacent marrow edema is usually limited.

The Chaput Fracture

The Chaput fracture (62) is a less common mirror fracture of the posterolateral margin induced by traction effect of the posterior tibiofibular ligament.

The Lefort-Wagstaffe Fracture

The Lefort-Wagstaffe fracture (63) is a further extremely uncommon avulsion occurring in slightly older patients following closure of the distal tibial growth plate in which avulsion occurs at the fibula insertion of the anterior tibiofibular ligament.

Calcaneal Fractures

The calcaneus is the most commonly fractured tarsal bone, its fracture usually being of compression in nature following a fall from a height. Thus, fractures are often bilateral and are commonly accompanied by compression fractures at the dorsolumbar junction. Rowe classifies calcaneal fractures 1 through 5 ranging from extra-articular stage 1 through to intra-articular comminuted stage 5 fractures (64) (Fig. 31).

Most compression fractures, accounting for almost 75% of cases, result in marked comminution, loss of height, and extension of fracture to the articular surfaces of the posterior subtalar joint. In contrast, extra-articular fractures involving the margins of the calcaneus, accounting for 25% of cases, are usually a sequel to rotational injury.

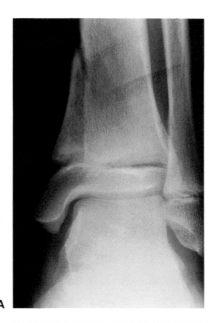

A

FIG. 28. (A) Anteroposterior radiograph shows a Salter 2 fracture of the distal tibia. (B) Sagittal TSE T1 *(left)* and IR TSE *(right)* images show a vertical oblique fracture extending through the distal tibia to the growth plate, where there is anterior extension of the fracture in the axial plane. (C) Coronal IR TSE *(left)* and TSE T1-weighted images show additional sagittal extension of the fracture through the epiphysis completing the Triplane fracture.

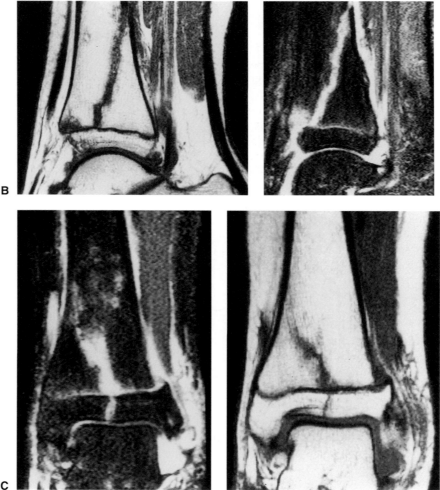

B

C

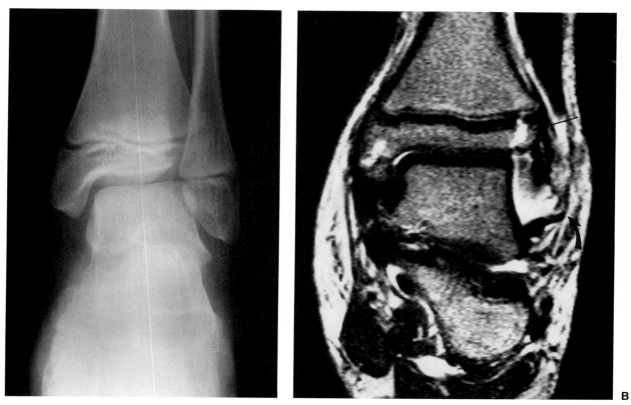

A

B

FIG. 29. (A) Radiograph shows normal bony outlines. (B) Coronal TSE T2-weighted image shows an undisplaced fracture of the lateral epiphysis (Tillaux fracture) *(straight arrow)* with associated undisplaced transverse fracture of the medial malleolus. Incidental note is made of disrupted anterior talofibular ligament billowing within lateral recess joint fluid *(curved arrow)*.

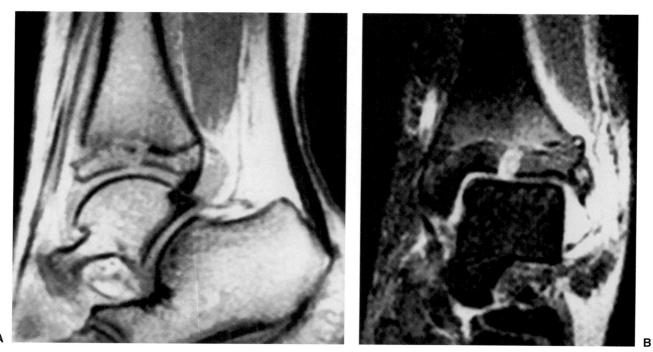

A

B

FIG. 30. (A) Sagittal T1-weighted image shows an epiphyseal fracture. (B) Coronal inversion recovery image shows extension through the midportion of the epiphysis (Tillaux type fracture, Salter 3). (Courtesy of Lunar Artoscan, Madison, WI.)

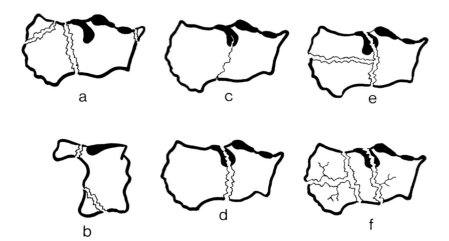

FIG. 31. Modified Rowe classification of calcaneal fractures: a,b, extra-articular fractures; c, intra-articular fracture of posterior subtalar articulation without displacement; d, displaced intra-articular fracture to the posterior subtalar articulation; e, comminuted undisplaced intra-articular fracture with secondary horizontal component; f, comminuted impaction intra-articular fracture of the calcaneus.

Although most extra-articular fractures are readily identified on conventional radiographs, occasionally they remain occult before MR imaging is undertaken to evaluate persistent foot pain (39).

In contrast, intra-articular fractures are routinely referred for tomographic imaging to evaluate fragment number and position. Specifically, tomographic imaging is undertaken to assess amount of step-off or distraction at posterior subtalar articulations, amount of rotation and displacement of bone fragments, and the size and position of the fixed sustentacular fragment (used for pin fixation) (65,66). Both computed tomography and MR imaging facilitate identification of entrapped peroneal and flexor hallucis tendons (67).

Computed tomography with reformatted imaging is now

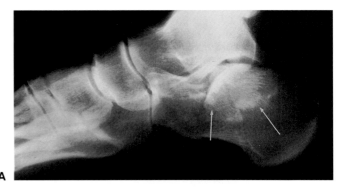

FIG. 32. Lateral radiograph **(A)** shows a subtle undisplaced compression fracture *(white arrows)*. Sagittal TSE T1-weighted **(B)** and IR TSE **(C)** images show an undisplaced intra-articular fracture with secondary horizontal component.

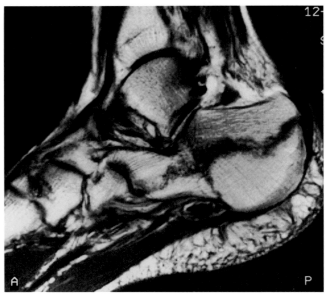

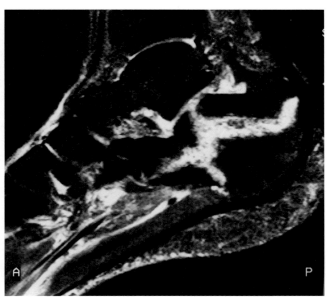

most frequently employed to evaluate these complex fractures, resulting in the abandonment of planar tomography. Nevertheless, MR imaging allows similar evaluation of osseous injury, except in severely comminuted cases, in multiple directly imaged planes and improves evaluation of associated soft tissue injury (unlike many other fractures, soft tissue injury around the calcaneus is not subtle and may be equally perceived at CT) (Fig. 32).

Talus Fracture and Subtalar Dislocations

Fractures of the talus occur secondary to axial loading on a hyperextended foot such as occurs as a driver slams his foot onto the brakes during a motor vehicle accident. The injury was so common in World War I pilots that talar neck fracture was termed aviator's astragalus.

Radiologic interest in talar fractures reflects its important biomechanical function of distributing weight during gait, as 60% of talar surfaces are covered by articular cartilage, and because of its susceptibilty to ischemic necrosis following trauma (68).

Almost a third of fractures of the talus involve the neck. When displaced, fractures at this site disrupt supply from both the dorsalis pedis artery and from the sinus tarsi (the major vascular supply to the talus), invariably resulting in osteonecrosis (69).

Hawkins (70) describes four types of talar neck fracture: type 1, a nondisplaced fracture of the talar neck in whom osteonecrosis rarely occurs (Fig. 33); types 2 and 3, a displaced fracture of the talar neck with subluxation (type 2) or dislocation (type 3) of the subtalar joint in whom osteonecrosis occurs in up to 50% of cases; and type 4, a displaced fracture of the talar neck with complete dislocation of the body of the talus from the subtalar and tibiotalar articulations in whom osteonecrosis occurs in up to 100% of cases (Fig. 34).

Although osteonecrosis is usually self-limiting and eventually heals with avoidance of weight bearing, it is a significant cause of delayed union following fracture.

Although identification of subchondral atrophy on a radiograph at 6 weeks (Hawkins' sign) excludes osteonecrosis, MR imaging is the only definitive diagnostic tool allowing diagnosis as early as 3 weeks.

Talar fractures are also identified involving the talar body, the talar head, and the medial and posterior talar processes.

Subtalar Dislocation

Subtalar dislocation is more often medial than lateral. Following inversion with medial subtalar dislocation, the talonavicular and talocalcaneal ligaments are disrupted, allowing displacement of the calcaneus and all the distal bones of the foot medially relative to the talus and the tibiotalar articulation. Occasionally, following restoration of anatomic alignment, MR imaging is undertaken to determine the integrity of the interosseous ligament. In cases where the ligament is disrupted, surgical fixation is undertaken. When the inter-

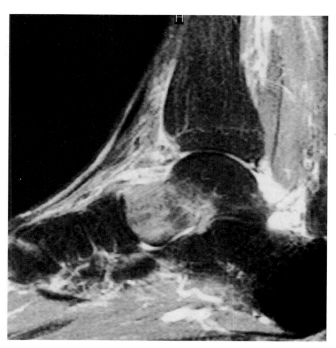

FIG. 33. Sagittal IR TSE image shows extensive edema throughout the anterior talar process at a site of an undisplaced Hawkins type 1 anterior talar process fracture. Note the typically associated edema within the dorsal soft tissues immediately above the fracture reflecting the impaction nature of the injury (commonly associated with *contre-coup* bruising in the anterior margin of the distal tibia).

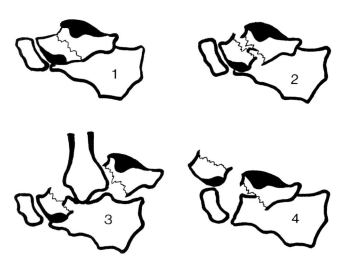

FIG. 34. Modified Hawkins classification of fractures of the anterior talar process. Type 1 injury is an undisplaced fracture. Type 2 injury is a minimally displaced anterior talar process fracture. Type 3 fracture is an anterior talar process fracture with posterior subtalar dislocation (frequently complicated by avascular necrosis). Type 4 injury is characterized by fracture of the anterior talar process and both subtalar and tibiotalar dislocation.

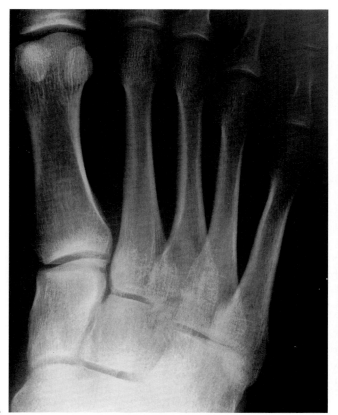

A

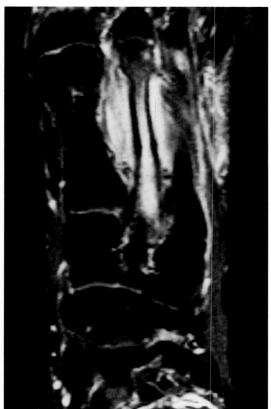

B

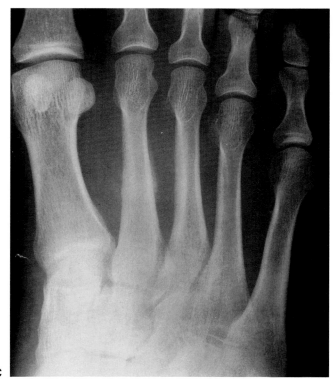

C

FIG. 35. (A) Radiograph in a male jogger with foot pain. **(B)** Axial IR TSE image acquired the same day in the same patient shows extensive edema both within the metatarsal and in the adjacent soft tissues at site of stress fracture. **(C)** Radiograph 3 weeks later shows typical radiographic changes of a stress fracture with marginal callus and sclerosis.

osseous ligament is intact, closed reduction and stabilization are attempted. The outcome following lateral subtalar dislocations is generally worse (68).

Stress Fractures

Repetitive trauma to normal bones either as a result of primary overuse or as a result of secondary overuse in an attempt to compensate for adjacent injury may lead to stress fractures. In such a way, biomechanical stress imposed by primary repetitive trauma, most often jogging, may account for fractures in the metatarsals (the most common site), the proximal shaft of the fifth metatarsal (Jones fracture, with a propensity to result in nonunion), and fractures in the sesamoids, navicular, and calcaneus (although fractures in this site are usually insufficiency in type). As a result of primary disease in soft tissues (tendon rupture) or in the bones of the foot or as a result of neuropathy, alterations in gait cycle may lead to secondary stress fractures.

Metatarsals

The metatarsals are the most common sites of stress fractures, most commonly occurring in athletes (71–73), and triggered by impaction are commonly associated with extensive marrow edema (Fig. 35). Imposed stress during jogging, promoting central plantar bowing of the metatarsal in the toe-off phase, initially induces acute local pain. Local periosteal disruption results in the development of marginal periosteal reaction with new bone formation parallel to the long axis of the bone. Persistent stress ultimately leads to bone fatigue and the development of a linear break traversing the shaft perpendicular to its long axis.

Although all changes are ultimately visualized on conventional radiographs, many patients present with symptoms in the absence of radiographic abnormality. Extensive marrow edema within the shafts of the affected bones is readily identified on fat-suppressed MR images up to 4 weeks before the

development of periosteal reaction, in many cases associated with extensive mass-like circumferential soft tissue edema. Early diagnosis and forced avoidance of weight bearing may promote early healing (72).

The Calcaneus

The calcaneus is predominantly cancellous bone and is therefore vulnerable to the changes imposed by metabolic bone disease (73). In this setting, insufficiency fractures are therefore more common than stress fractures. In patients with both osteoporosis and, more commonly, osteomalacia, repeated heel strike as part of the gait cycle results in calcaneal impaction, initially resulting in microtrabecular trauma and bruising, ultimately leading to compression fracture with curvilinear configuration concave posteriorly (Fig. 36).

As compression injuries, stress and insufficiency fractures of the calcaneus result in extensive marrow edema, readily identified at MRI. At the onset of symptoms, MR imaging allows the identification of bone bruise long before any radiographic change can be detected. If this is untreated, further compression leads to progression from bone bruise to impaction fracture.

Sesamoid Fracture

The tibial sesamoid is particularly vulnerable to the impaction forces imposed by weight bearing, as forces are referred to the great toe before projecting the foot forward. Because the sesamoids lie within the two heads of the flexor hallucis brevis and tend to bowstring (with the hallucis brevis) across the first metatarsophalangeal joint during the toe-off phase of the gait cycle, more weight is transferred to the tibial sesamoid (75).

Affected patients often complain of excruciating pain. In most cases fractures are undisplaced and stellate and, in the absence of dedicated views, are radiographically occult. Inversion recovery images in the sagittal and coronal planes

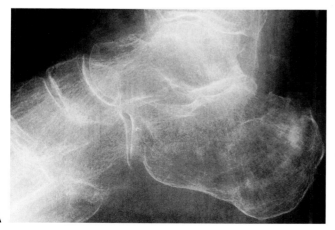
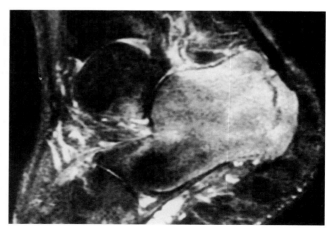

A   B

FIG. 36. (A) Lateral radiograph shows curvilinear sclerosis in the posterior body of a demineralized calcaneus. **(B)** Sagittal IR TSE image shows hypointense curvilinear insufficiency fracture with extensive adjacent edema.

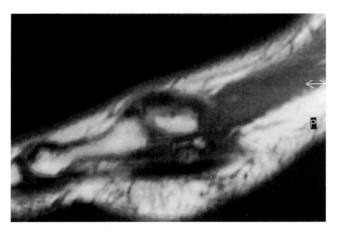

FIG. 37. Sagittal TSE T1-weighted image shows a stellate undisplaced occult fracture of the tibial sesamoid.

and turbo spin-echo T1-weighted images facilitate diagnosis at MRI.

Untreated, stellate fractures ultimately distract, at which time surgical excision is the only therapeutic option (Fig. 37).

Further gait-related stress fractures have been identified in the anterior talar process (76), the navicular (through the midbody parallel to the long axis of the foot) (77), the cuboid, the cuneiforms, and in accessory ossicles (Fig. 38).

Cuneiform fractures are commonly identified in patients with peripheral neuropathy in whom differentiation from infection may be difficult.

Fracture of the os naviculare or the os peroneii may accompany chronic stress on either the tibialis posterior or peroneus brevis tendons.

Stress fractures of the anterior talar process and of the navicular are occasionally identified secondary to impaction accompanying medial longitudinal arch collapse and tibialis posterior tendon rupture. In each case, fractures are readily identified at MR imaging as a result of the associated extensive marrow edema, often in the absence of radiographic change.

Because of their reactive osteoblastic activity, stress fractures are readily identified at scintigraphy, which is often used as an alternative to MR imaging in diagnosis. Phosphate analogs, used for bone scan, are chemisorbed to the surface of cells actively secreting hydroxyapatite, resulting in focal accumulation or hot spots at the site of fractures. Fractures through the dorsal calcaneus, involving cancellous bone, are often more conspicuous at MRI.

Insufficiency Fractures

Normal forces applied to abnormal bone may result in fracture. In such a way, demineralized bone, biomechanically weak or insufficient, may fracture secondary to the impact of normal weight bearing. Fractures through insufficient bone are therefore termed insufficiency fractures.

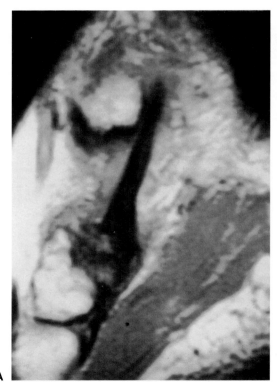

A

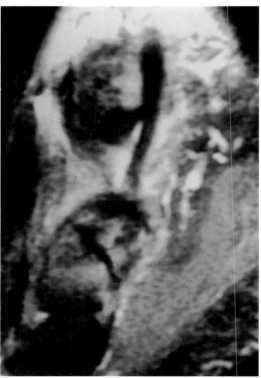

B

FIG. 38. Sagittal TSE T1 **(A)** and IR TSE **(B)** images show a stress fracture in the os peroneii perpendicular to the axis of the avulsion forces imposed by the peroneus brevis tendon.

The dorsal calcaneus is a site particularly susceptible to demineralization and is therefore the most common site of insufficiency fracture in the foot (see Fig. 36) (74).

Neuropathic Fractures Versus Infection: Lisfranc Fracture Dislocation

Neuropathic fractures in the foot are common and classically involve the Lisfranc tarsometatarsophalangeal articulations. Dislocation at this site, either homolateral or divergent, may be associated with destruction and debris with soft tissue swelling. Because of their conspicuous and extensive marrow and soft tissue edema at the site of dislocation, differentiation from infection may be difficult (78,79). Both infection and trauma produce extensive radiographic destruction and sclerosis, and both produce extensive soft tissue and bone marrow edema on MR imaging (Fig. 39). Although differentiation is difficult, the identification of an adjacent ulcer, sinus tract, or fluid collection suggests infection. Although both forms of edema enhance following administration of gadolinium, focal enhancement within bone and in adjacent soft tissues suggests infection (78,79).

Plantar Plate

Similar to the small joints of the hand, hyperextension of metatarsophalangeal and intertarsal joints of the feet is resisted by a ligamentous thickening of the dorsal capsule. The plantar plate or plantar accessory ligament of the first metatarsophalangeal joint is formed by fibers from the tendons of the flexor hallucis longus, adductor hallucis, and abductor hallucis tendons, which combine with the deep transverse ligament to form a fibrocartilaginous plate along the plantar aspect of the metatarsophalangeal joint capsule.

The plate is clearly visualized using a local surface coil. Following hyperextension injury, MR images show intense local edema, synovitis, and flexor hallucis longus tenosynovitis, all features of turf toe (32–34).

COMPLICATIONS OF TRAUMA TO THE FOOT

Reflex Sympathetic Dystrophy

Reflex sympathetic dystrophy, algodystrophy, Sudek's atrophy, causalgia, and shoulder hand syndrome are all terms used to describe a syndrome characterized by posttraumatic vasomotor instability, hyperemia, pain, and bone demineralization. Although it has been described to occur after myriad injuries including chest wall zoster and even myocardial infarct, direct trauma is the trigger in most cases.

Affected patients initially complain of severe pain at the site of involvement, most frequently an extremity, which may last up to 6 months. After 2 to 3 months, patients enter the dystrophic phase characterized by local swelling, edema, restricted motion, and radiographic evidence of demineralization. In chronicity, affected patients complain of persistent pain, persistent joint immobility, skin and muscle atrophy, and show extensive patchy demineralization on radiographs.

On radiographs, endosteal resorption (slow process) and cortical tunneling (focal lucencies within the cortex) may be dominant with less marked mild subperiosteal resorption (rapid process). The changes are often most marked adjacent to joints, where they may be accompanied by synovitis.

On three-phase bone scan, increased uptake is noted diffusely on all phases, reflecting hyperemia and diffuse osteoblastic activity.

Although soft tissue changes, soft tissue edema, predominate at MR imaging, occasionally, fat-suppressed images

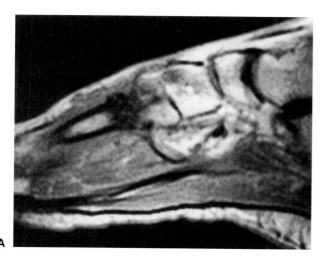
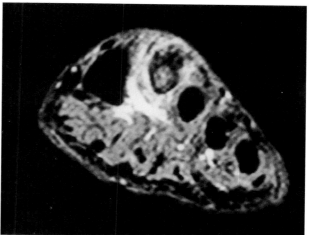

A   **B**

FIG. 39. Sagittal T1 **(A)** and axial inversion recovery **(B)** images show delayed union of a fracture at the base of the second metatarsal with extensive hypointense sclerosis **(A)** and circumferential edema **(B)**.

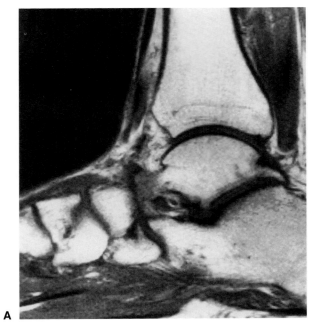 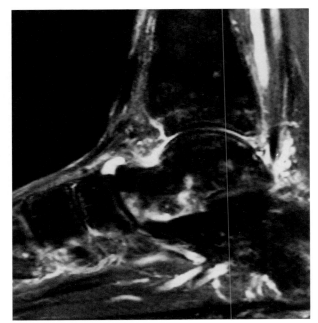

A
B

FIG. 40. Sagittal TSE T1 **(A)** and IR TSE **(B)** images show patchy speckled periarticular marrow edema in a patient with posttraumatic reflex sympathetic dystrophy.

shows heterogeneous miliary foci of marrow edema or signal hyperintensity, usually most prominent in subarticular regions. When identified, miliary marrow changes at MRI often precede radiographic evidence of demineralization and are usually a marker of severe disease (Fig. 40) (80).

Compartment Syndrome

The plantar aspect of the foot, although divided into four muscle layers, is divided surgically into compartments de-

marcated by septa or fascia (81). Although a complex classification recognizes nine separate compartments, most foot surgeons recognize four compartments, the medial, deep central, superficial central, and lateral (Fig. 41). The central compartment communicates directly with the central compartment of the leg.

Although compartment syndrome in the foot is of particular importance when dealing with deep space infection, compartment syndrome with neurovascular compression may occasionally complicate acute foot trauma.

Synostosis

Occasionally, heterotopic bone is formed at the level of the syndesmosis following trauma; when extensive, it may impair motion and may be corrected only by surgical resection (82). Identifiable marrow edema within the heterotopic bone is used to indicate immature bone and, similarly to heterotopic bone at other sites, may delay surgical intervention.

FIG. 41. Coronal TSE T1-weighted image of the midfoot shows division of the sole into four compartments: M, medial; C, central; I, interosseous; L, lateral.

REFERENCES

1. Kier R, Dietz MJ, McCarthy SM, et al. MR imaging of the normal ligaments and tendons of the ankle. *J Comput Assist Tomogr* 1991;15: 477.
2. Rubin DA, Towers JD, Britton CA. MR imaging of the foot: Utility of complex oblique imaging planes. *Am J Roentgenol* 1996;166:1079.
3. Mann RA, Inman VT. Phasic activity of intrinsic muscles of the foot. *J Bone Joint Surg* 1964;46A:469–481.
4. Mann RA. Biomechanics. In: Jahss MH, ed. *Disorders of the Foot,* 2nd ed, vol 1. Philadelphia: WB Saunders, 1991.
5. Beltran J, Munchow AM, Khabin H, et al. Ligaments of the lateral aspect of the ankle and sinus tarsi: An MR imaging study. *Radiology* 1990;177:455.

6. Erickson SJ, Smith JW, Ruiz ME, et al. MR imaging of the lateral collateral ligament of the ankle. *Am J Roentgenol* 1991;156:131.
7. Klein MA. MR imaging of the ankle: Normal and abnormal findings in the medial collateral ligament. *Am J Roentgenol* 1994;162:377.
8. Link SC, Erickson SJ, Timind ME. MR imaging of the ankle and foot: Normal structures and anatomic variants that may stimulate disease. *Am J Roentgenol* 1993;161:607.
9. Rule J, Yao L, Seeger L. Spring ligament of the ankle: Normal MR anatomy. *Am J Roentgenol* 1993;161:1241.
10. Schneck CD, Mesgarzadeh M, Bonakdarpoor A, et al. MR imaging of the most commonly injured ankle ligaments: II. Ligament injuries. *Radiology* 1992;184:507.
11. Chandnani VP, Harper MT, Fickle JR, et al. Chronic ankle instability: Evaluation with MR arthrography, MR imaging and stress radiography. *Radiology* 1994;192:189.
12. Aerts P, Disler DG. Abnormalities of the foot and ankle: MR imaging findings. *Am J Roentgenol* 1995;165:119.
13. Klein MA, Spreitzer AM. MR imaging of the tarsal sinus and canal: Normal anatomy, pathologic findings, and features of the sinus tarsi syndrome. *Radiology* 1993;186:233.
14. Trattnig S, Breitenseher M, Haller J, et al. Sinus tarsi syndrome: MRI diagnosis. *Radiologe* 1995;35:463.
15. Liu SH, Raskin A, Osti L, et al. Arthroscopic treatment of anterolateral ankle impingement. *Arthroscopy* 1994;10:215.
16. Bassett FH, Gates HS, Billys JB, et al. Talar impingement by the anterior tibiofibular ligament. *J Bone Joint Surg* 1990;72A:55.
17. Ferkel RD, Scranton PE. Arthroscopy of the ankle and foot. *J Bone Joint Surg* 1993;75A:1233.
18. Daffner RH, Riemer BL, Lupetin AR, et al. Magnetic resonance imaging in acute tendon ruptures. *Skel Radiol* 1986;15:619.
19. Inglis AE, Scott WN, Sculco TP, et al. Ruptures of the tendo achillis: An objective assessment of surgical and nonsurgical treatment. *J Bone Joint Surg* 1976;58A:990.
20. Keene JS, Lash EG, Fisher DR, et al. Magnetic resonance imaging of achilles tendon ruptures. *Am J Sports Med* 1989;17:333.
21. Lien MD, Zegel HG, Balduini FC, et al. Repair of achilles tendon ruptures with a polylactic acid implant: Assessment with MR imaging. *Am J Roentgenol* 1991;156:769.
22. Panageas E, Greenber S, Franklin PD, et al. Magnetic resonance imaging of pathologic conditions of the achilles tendon. *Orthop Rev* 1990;19:975.
23. Quinn SF, Muray WT, Clark RA, et al. Achilles tendon: MR imaging at 1.5 T. *Radiology* 1987;164:767.
24. Cheung Y, Rosenberg ZS, Magee T, et al. Normal anatomy and pathologic conditions of ankle tendons: Current imaging techniques. *Radiographics* 1992;12:429.
25. Thompson FM, Patterson AH. Rupture of the peroneus longus tendon. Report of three cases. *J Bone Joint Surg* 1989;71A:293.
26. Khoury NJ, El Khoury GY, Saltzman CL, et al. Peroneus longus and brevis tendon tears. MR imaging evaluation. *Radiology* 1996;200:833.
27. Mann RA. Flatfoot in adults. In: Mann RA, Coughlin MJ, eds. *Surgery of the Foot and Ankle, ed 6*. St Louis: Mosby, 1993;757–784.
28. Rosenberg ZS, Cheung Y, Jahss MH, et al. Rupture of posterior tibial tendon: CT and MRI imaging with surgical correlation. *Radiology* 1988;169:229.
29. Conti SJ, Cox IH, Hyde JS, et al. Clinical significance of magnetic resonance imaging in preoperative planning for reconstruction of posterior tibial tendon ruptures. *Foot Ankle* 1990;13:208.
30. Hamilton WG. *Foot and Ankle Injuries in Dancers*. New York: Raven Press, 1987;127.
31. Marotta JJ, Micheli LJ. Os trigonum impingement in dancers. *Am J Sports Med* 1992;20:23.
32. Yao L, Do HM, Cracchiolo A, et al. Plantar plate of the foot: Findings on conventional arthrography and MR imaging. *Am J Roentgenol* 1994;163:641.
33. Tewes DP, Fischer DA, Fritts HM, et al. MRI findings of acute turf toe. A case report and review of anatomy. *Clin Orthop* 1994;304:200.
34. Rodeo SA, O'Brien S, Warren RF, et al. Turf-toe: An analysis of metatarsophalangeal joint sprains in professional football players. *Am J Sports Med* 1990;18:280.
35. Karasick D, Schweitzer ME. The os trigonum syndrome: Imaging features. *Am J Roentgenol* 1996;166:125.
36. Schweitzer ME, van Leersum M, Ehrlich SS. Fluid in normal and abnormal ankle joints: amount and distribution as seen on MR images. *Am J Roentgenol* 1994;162:111.
37. Khoury NJ, El Khoury GY, Saltzman CL, et al. Rupture of the anterior tibial tendon. diagnosis by MR imaging. *Am J Roentgenol* 1996;167:351.
38. Berkowitz JF, Kier R, Ridcel S. Plantar fasciitis: MR imaging. *Radiology* 1991;179:665.
39. Hall RL, Erickson SJ, Shereff MJ, et al. Magnetic resonance imaging in the evaluation of heel pain. *Orthopedics* 1996;19:225.
40. Kier R. Magnetic resonance imaging of plantar fasciitis and other causes of heel pain. *MRI Clin North Am* 1994;2:97.
41. Nicoll EA. Fractures of the tibial shaft: a survey of 705 cases. *J Bone Joint Surg* 1964;46B:373–387.
42. Erdman WA, Tamburro F, Jayson HT, et al. Osteomyelitis: Characteristics and pitfalls of diagnosis with MR imaging. *Radiology* 1991;181:533.
43. Morrison WB, Schweitzer ME, Bock GW, et al. Diagnosis of osteomyelitis: Utility of fat-suppressed, contrast-enhanced MR images. *Radiology* 1993;189:251.
44. Seabold JE, Flickinger FW, Kao SCS, et al. Indium-111-leucocyte/technetium-99m-MDP bone scanning and magnetic resonance imaging: Difficulty of diagnosing osteomyelitis in patients with neuropathic osteoarthropathy. *J Nucl Med* 1990;31:549.
45. Mason MD, Zlatkin MB, Esterhai JL, et al. Chronic complicated osteomyelitis of the lower extremity: Evaluation with MR imaging. *Radiology* 1989;173:355.
46. Unger E, Moldofsky P, Gatenby R, et al. Diagnosis of osteomyelitis by MR imaging. *Am J Roentgenol* 1988;150:605.
47. Tyrrell PNM, Davies AM. Magnetic resonance imaging appearances of fatigue fractures of the long bones of the lower limb. *Br J Radiol* 1994;67:332.
48. Umans HR, Kaye JJ. Longitudinal stress fractures of the tibia: Diagnosis by magnetic resonance imaging. *Skeletal Radiol* 1996;25:319.
49. Sterling JC, Edelstein DW, Calvo RD, et al. Stress fractures in the athlete: diagnosis and management. *Sports Med* 1992;14:336.
50. Fredericson M, Bergman AG, Hoffman KL, et al. Tibial stress reaction in runners: Correlation of clinical symptoms and scintigraphy with a new magnetic resonance imaging grading system. *Am J Sports Med* 1995;23:472.
51. Lauge-Hansen N. Ligamentous ankle fractures. Diagnosis and treatment. *Acta Chir Scand* 1949;97:544–550.
52. Muller ME, Allgower M, Schneider R, Willenegger H. *Manual of Internal Fixation: Techniques Recommended by the AO Group, 3rd ed.* New York: Springer Verlag, 1991.
53. Henderson MS. Trimalleolar fracture of the ankle. *Surg Clin North Am* 1932;12:867–872.
54. Anderson JF, Crichton KJ, Grattan-Smith T, et al. Osteochondral fractures of the dome of the talus. *J Bone Joint Surg* 1989;70A:1143.
55. De Smet AA, Fisher DR, Burnstein MI, et al. Value of MR imaging in staging osteochondral lesions of the talus (osteochondritis dissecans): Results in 14 patients. *Am J Roentgenol* 1990;154:555.
56. Berndt AL, Harty M. Transchondral fractures (osteochondritis dessicans) of the talus. *J Bone Joint Surg [Am]* 1959;41A:988.
57. Monu JU, McManus CM, Ward WG, et al. Soft tissue masses caused by long standing foreign bodies in the extremities: MR imaging findings. *Am J Roentgenol* 1995;165:395.
58. Fernandes TJ. The mechanism of talo-tibial dislocations without fracture. *J Bone Joint Surg* 1976;58B:364–365.
59. Ruedi T, Allgower M. Fractures of the lower end of the tibia into the ankle joint. *Injury* 1969;1:92.
60. Feldman F, Singson RD, Rosenberg ZS, Berdon WE, Amodio J, Abramson SJ. Distal tibial triplane fractures: diagnosis with CT. *Radiology* 1987;164:429.
61. Landin LA, Danielsson LG. Children's ankle fractures: Classification and epidemiology. *Acta Orthop Scand* 1983;54:634–640.
62. Protas JM, Kornblatt BA. Fractures of the lateral margin of the distal tibia: The Tillaux fracture. *Radiology* 1981;138:55–57.
63. Greenspan A. *Orthopedic Radiology: A Practical Approach.* Philadelphia: JB Lippincott, 1988;7.1–7.34.
64. Rowe CR, Sakellarides HT, Freeman PA, Sorbie C. Fractures of the os calcis: A long term follow up study of 146 patients. *JAMA* 1963;184:920–923,
65. Heger L, Wulff K, Seddig MSA. Computed tomography of calcaneal fractures. *Am J Roentgenol* 1985;145:131–137.
66. Rosenberg ZS, Feldman F, Singson RD, et al. Intra-articular calcaneal fractures: Computed tomographic analysis. *Skel Radiol* 1987;16:105–113.

67. Rosenberg ZS, Feldman F, Singson RD, et al. Peroneal tendon injuries associated with calcaneal fractures. *Am J Roentgenol* 1987;149: 125–129.
68. El Khoury GY, Yousefzadeh DK, Mulligan GM, et al. Subtalar dislocation. *Skel Radiol* 1982;8:99–104.
69. DeLee JC, Curtis R. Subtalar dislocation of the foot. *J Bone Joint Surg* 1982;64A:433–437.
70. Lancaster S, Horowitz M, Alonso J. Subtalar dislocation: A prognosticating classification. *Orthopedics* 1985;8:1234.
71. Matheson GB, Clement DB, McKenzie DC, et al. Stress fractures in athletes, a study of 320 cases. *Am J Sports Med* 1987;130:651–658.
72. Irwin CG. Fractures of the metatarsals. *Proc R Soc Med* 1938;31: 789–793.
73. Richli WR, Rosenthal DI. Avulsion fracture of the fifth metatarsal: experimental study of pathomechanics. *Am J Roentgenol* 1984;143: 889–891.
74. Kathol MH, El Khoury GY, Moore TE, et al. Calcaneal insufficiency avulsion fractures in patients with diabetes mellitus. *Radiology* 1991; 180:725–729.
75. Jahss MH. The sesamoids of the hallux. *Clin Orthop* 1981;157:88–97.
76. Umans H, Pavlov H. Insufficiency fracture of the talus: Diagnosis with MR imaging. *Radiology* 1995;197:439.
77. Pavlov H, Torg JS, Freiberger RH. Tarsal navicular stress fractures: Radiographic evaluation. *Radiology* 1983;148:641–645.
78. Moore TE, Yuh WTC, Kathol MH, et al. Abnormalities of the foot in patients with diabetes mellitus: Findings on MR imaging. *Am J Roentgenol* 1993;157:813.
79. Spaeth HJ Jr, Dardani M. Magnetic resonance imaging of the diabetic foot. *MRI Clin North Am* 1994;2:123–130.
80. Schweitzer ME, Mandel S, Schwartzman RJ, et al. Reflex sympathetic dystrophy revisited: MR imaging findings before and after infusion of contrast material. *Radiology* 1995;195:211.
81. Manoli A, Weber TG. Fasciotomy of the foot—an anatomical study with special reference to release of the calcaneal compartment. *Foot Ankle Int* 1990;10:267.
82. Kaye RA. Stabilization of ankle syndesmosis injuries with a syndesmosis screw. *Foot Ankle* 1989;9:290–293.
83. Erickson SJ, Johnson JE. MR imaging of the ankle and foot. *Radiol Clin North Am* 1997;35:163.

CHAPTER 6

The Knee

Stephen J. Eustace

Widespread use of magnetic resonance imaging (MRI) has dramatically altered perception of knee trauma. Although MRI was initially employed to evaluate patients with suspected internal soft tissue derangement, improved access, decreased imaging costs, and rapid image acquisition have led to widespread MR imaging of patients immediately following trauma to both bone and soft tissues. Although conventional radiographs and planar and computed tomography allow detailed evaluation of osseous structures, simultaneous evaluation of bone and soft tissues in multiple planes makes MR imaging an attractive alternative, obviating the need for multiple costly imaging studies. Deployment of emergency room scanners with rapid image acquisition, paralleled by installation of dedicated low-field extremity magnets (Lunar

Artoscan) in outpatient clinics, is likely to lead to wider use of MR imaging in the evaluation of acute trauma in the years ahead.

PATIENT POSITIONING AND IMAGING PROTOCOLS

Positioning

The patient is usually positioned feet first with the knee in extension. In such a position, the leg tends to rotate externally up to 10° to 15°. Because the anterior cruciate ligament (ACL) runs from posterior to anterior, from lateral to medial, hugging the inner aspect of the lateral femoral condyle in a slightly oblique axis, directly acquired sagittal images in this position actually parallel the anterior cruciate ligament (ACL). However, because patient positioning is inconsistent, a modified technique discussed under imaging planes is now more frequently employed.

S. J. Eustace: Department of Radiology, Section of Musculoskeletal Radiology, Boston University School of Medicine and Boston Medical Center, Boston, Massachusetts 02118.

Receiver Coil

In order to optimize reception of generated signal, imaging requires either a molded or tightly apposed surface coil or the use of a dedicated quadrature coil. Quadrature coils increase image signal to noise 1.4-fold by acquiring signal simultaneously in two perpendicular planes. To improve signal acquisition, dedicated phased-array knee coils are now commercially available, which dramatically alter quality of images yielded with low-field permanent magnet systems (increasing both coverage and image signal). Although plaster cast interposed between target tissues and receiver coil may impair signal to noise in images acquired with simple surface coils, such signal loss is minimized using quadrature-type coils as are used to image the knee (Fig. 1). (Recently molded plaster, within 1 to 2 hr, tends to impair the reception of signal.)

Imaging Plane

Both coronal and sagittal images are generally prescribed off an axial localizer. By use of an axial localizer, sagittal oblique images are acquired to parallel or image the ACL in plane. Sagittal images prescribed off either the inner aspect of the lateral femoral condyle or the anterolateral margin of the lateral femoral condyle consistently allow the ACL to be imaged in plane (Fig. 2) (1). Coronal images are acquired perpendicular to the axis of the femoral condyles. Axial images are prescribed off a sagittal localizer.

Field of View

A preliminary image is often acquired with extended coverage—a field of view of 20 cm—before dedicated images are made with a 14-cm field of view. In such a way, an overview of the extent of trauma is obtained before high-resolution imaging of internal joint structures. Coverage

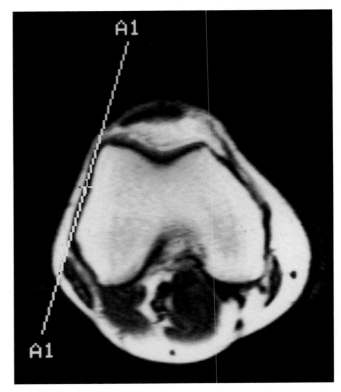

FIG. 2. Axial T1-weighted localizer demonstrating imaging orientation to image the anterior cruciate ligament.

using dedicated extremity systems is currently limited to 11 cm, although extended coverage may be obtained with phased-array coils.

Slice Thickness

Detailed evaluation of menisci requires acquisition of images with a slice thickness not greater than 3 mm. Thick slices not only result in tears being missed but also impair visualization of the ACL. Thick slices may partial volume the inner aspect of the lateral femoral condyle, alter the configuration of the ACL, and misleadingly suggest the presence of an ACL tear. In most cases, sagittal oblique imaging and use of 3-mm slices overcome this potential pitfall. In cases in which the ACL is poorly visualized, thin-slice three-dimensional (3D) acquisitions are undertaken.

Motion Suppression

Pulsation from the popliteal artery may track over the intercondylar notch and obscure abnormality. Orientation of the phase-encode gradients from top to toe on sagittal images or side to side on axial acquisitions overcomes this pitfall. Placing a saturation band above the knee may completely eliminate arterial pulsation. Rapid image acquisition may

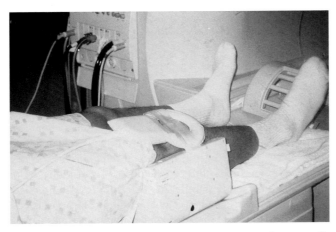

FIG. 1. Typical supine position with encasing quadrature coil. Image shows an additional superficial surface coil for high-resolution imaging of patellofemoral cartilage.

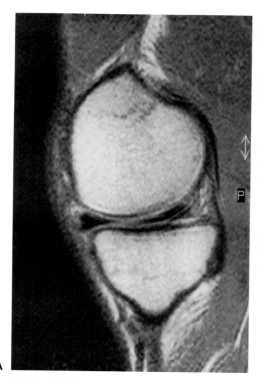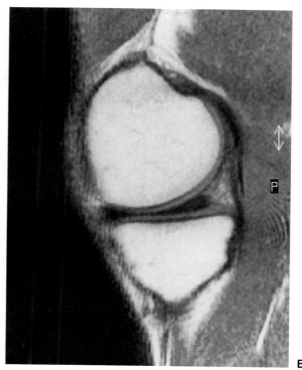

FIG. 3. (A) Sagittal conventional spin-echo T1-weighted image shows pseudotear of the posterior horn of the medial meniscus secondary to motion. **(B)** Sagittal turbo spin-echo T1-weighted image (acquired in 1 min) without motion shows a normal meniscus.

eliminate motion observed on images made by conventional protocols (Fig. 3).

IMAGING PROTOCOL

Following acute trauma, a turbo inversion recovery image is usually acquired in the coronal plane to determine the extent of injury. A turbo spin-echo T1-weighted sequence is then applied in coronal, sagittal, and axial planes. Such a protocol allows rapid evaluation of both osseous and soft tissue structures (approximately 5-min scan time). Collateral ligament injury is easily identified on fat-suppressed short-inversion-time inversion recovery images, and meniscal and cruciate abnormalities are readily visualized on T1-weighted scans (Fig. 4).

When soft tissue injury is suspected, a turbo spin-echo T1 and turbo short-inversion-time inversion recovery image is acquired in the direct coronal plane, a dual-echo turbo spin-echo T2-weighted scan is acquired in the sagittal oblique plane, and finally, an axial T2-weighted fast field-echo image with off-resonance magnetization transfer is acquired to image the patellofemoral articular cartilage.

Turbo spin-echo T1 imaging is achieved using a repetition time of 500 msec, an echo time of 15 msec, a short echo train of four, and a low-high echo to view mapping profile. With such parameters, images are acquired in 1 min 5 sec. Recent studies comparing conventional to turbo spin-echo T1-weighted imaging in acute knee trauma indicate that

turbo images yield improved spatial resolution and signal relative to noise and equivalent contrast relative to conventional spin echo. Turbo images are acquired in less than a third of the acquisition time required to acquire conventional images. Turbo spin-echo T2-weighted imaging is achieved using a repetition time of 3,000 msec, echo times of 20 and 80 msec, an echo train of six, and linear echo-to-view mapping. Potential loss of signal in tendons and menisci using turbo spin-echo sequences as a result of magnetization transfer is not apparent in clinical practice. Although previous authors have concluded that T2*-weighted gradient or fast field-echo images are most sensitive for detection of meniscal tears, Escobedo et al. have validated use of turbo spin-echo imaging in this role using a short echo train (not greater than six) (2). Images acquired with extended echo trains become blurred and lose apparent edge enhancement.

Turbo inversion recovery sequences are acquired using an inversion time of 160 msec, a repetition time of 2,000 msec, an echo time of 20 msec, an echo train of six, and a linear echo to view mapping profile. Such images are acquired in 2 min, with two excitations. Multiple excitations are unnecessary using inversion recovery sequences, as diagnosis is made in most cases on the basis of contrast afforded by fat suppression (Fig. 5).

A T2-weighted fast field (gradient)-echo image is acquired to evaluate the patellofemoral cartilage, employing a flip angle of 30°, a repetition time of 700 msec, and an echo time of 15 msec; images are acquired in 2 min. Contrast

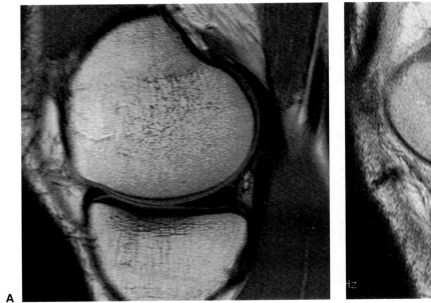
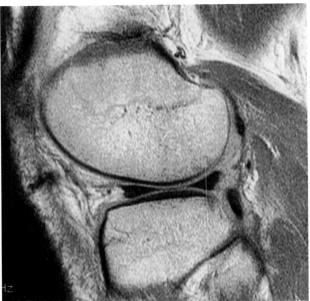

FIG. 4. Sagittal proton-density-weighted images show **(A)** the normal medial meniscus and **(B)** normal lateral meniscus.

between free fluid and cartilage is improved by using an off-resonance magnetization transfer pulse. Although not formally evaluated, such a sequence allows clear visualization of chondromalacia, including cartilage thinning, fibrillation, rents, and osteochondral defects (Figs. 6 and 7) (3,4).

In most patients, images are acquired with 256 phase-encode steps and swayed by need for rapid imaging, with no more than two excitations.

Faster imaging may be obtained with both GraSE, HASTE, and EPI sequences (5). GraSE imaging incorporat-

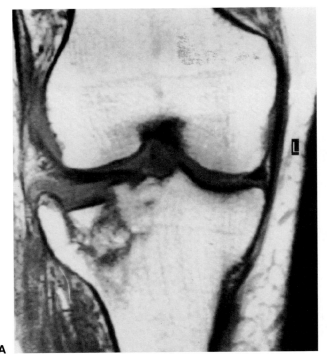
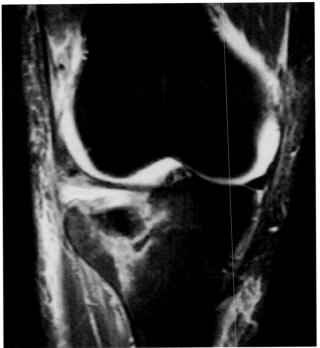

FIG. 5. (A) Coronal TSE T1-weighted image (TE_{eff} 15 msec, TR 500 msec, turbo factor 4) acquired in 1 min in a patient with a lateral tibial plateau fracture. **(B)** Coronal IR TSE (TE_{eff} 20 msec, TR 2,000 msec, turbo factor 6) image in the same patient acquired in 2 min with two excitations.

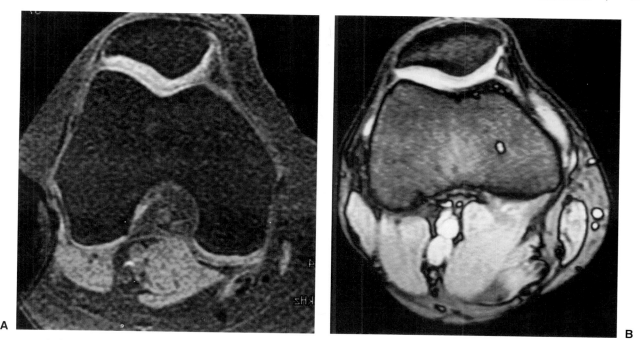

FIG. 6. Axial images of patellofemoral cartilage. **(A)** T1-weighted image with fat suppression. **(B)** T2-weighted image.

ing both gradient-echo and spin-echo information offers the theoretical advantage of providing T2* evaluation of meniscal tears (6), with spin-echo-based evaluation of bone marrow. Combining serial refocusing pulses and gradient rever-

sals (see Chapter 2), the sequence affords further reduction in acquisition time relative to turbo spin echo. GraSE images acquired with low-high mapping suffer from image blur. Images acquired with linear mapping are more T2 weighted.

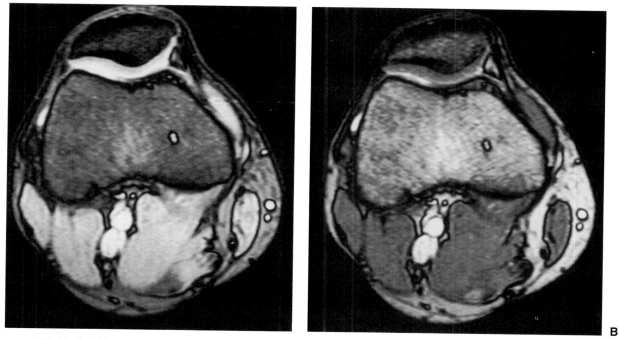

FIG. 7. Axial image demonstrating the effect of an off-resonance pulse. **(A)** T2-weighted fast field-echo image without off-resonance saturation. **(B)** Improved cartilage to synovial fluid discrimination using the same sequence and same imaging parameters following the application of an off-resonance saturation pulse.

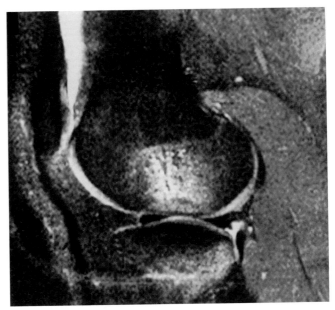

FIG. 8. Sagittal density-weighted GraSE image with additional frequency-selective fat saturation in a patient with bone bruises reflecting an underlying tear of the anterior cruciate ligament.

Similar to echo planar-based sequences, chemical shift artifact is problematic, pixel shift increasing as echo train length (specifically EPI factor) is extended. Improved GraSE images are therefore yielded with frequency-selective presaturation of fat (Fig. 8).

HASTE imaging allows extremely rapid image acquisition with elongated echo trains (k-space is half filled). With extended echo trains, images are heavily T2 weighted, and fine detail, particularly in bone, is obscured. Fast HASTE is achieved by using high readout bandwidths (32 kHz), decreasing echo spacing. When this is done, images acquired with fast HASTE have even less signal relative to noise (7).

Echo planar imaging requires versatile gradients, with speed (rise time less than 200 μsec) and amplitude. Stronger gradients, those with higher amplitudes (23 mT/m) improve image signal. Although enhanced by fast high-amplitude gradients (slew rate greater than 120 mT/m per sec), we have successfully employed spin-echo-based EPI sequences in the knee using 13 mT/m gradients (Philips Powertrack 1000).

Echo planar images may be yielded in a single shot or following a single excitation, in which k-space is filled in entirety after a single acquisition. Such images are extremely noisy and, without fat saturation, may be dramatically distorted by gross chemical shift artifact. Shorter echo trains require multiple excitations or shots to fill k-space, increasing acquisition time. Multiple shots both increase image signal and decrease the amount of pixel chemical shift.

Because of the beneficial effect of the refocusing pulse inherent in the spin-echo sequence, decreasing marrow-based susceptibility artifact, the spin-echo-based EPI multishot technique is often preferred (Fig. 9; Table 1) (8,9).

MAGNETIC RESONANCE IMAGING OF SOFT TISSUE INJURY FOLLOWING ACUTE TRAUMA

The Menisci

Anatomy

The menisci represent C-shaped semilunar rings interposed between the articular surfaces of the femoral condyles and the tibial plateaus. They function to act as a buffer between the two surfaces, protecting articular cartilage, distributing the strain of weight bearing (they support 50% of load sharing), improving stability, and providing lubrication facilitating joint flexion and extension.

The menisci have an organized structure, composed of an outer circumferential zone and an inner transverse zone divided by a middle perforating collagen bundle to superior and inferior leaves (14). Menisci are poorly vascularized: only the outer third of the menisci are vascularized in adulthood via a perimeniscal plexus derived from branches of

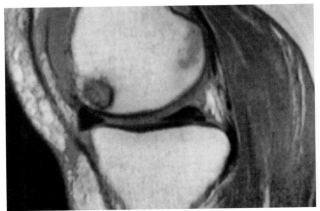

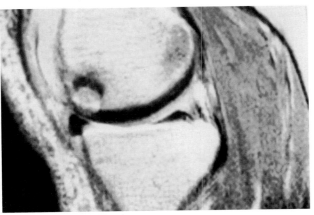

FIG. 9. (A) Sagittal turbo spin-echo T1-weighted image shows an osteochondral defect of the anterior condyle. (B) Multishot spin-echo, echo planar image shows the same osteochondral defect. Note pseudothickening of cortex of distal femur secondary to inherent multidirectional chemical shift artifact.

TABLE 1. *Knee protocol*

Sequence	Image plane	FOV	TR	TE	ETL	Mapping scheme
TSE T1	Cor direct	14	500	15	4	Low–high
IR TSE	Cor direct	14	2,000	20	6	Linear
TSE T2 (fat sat)	Sag oblique	14	2,000	20, 80	6	Linear
FFE T2	Axial	14	700	15		30 degree flip angle

medial and lateral geniculate arteries, and therefore, following injury, meniscal healing is poor (15,16).

The medial meniscus has an open C shape and is attached to the intercondylar notch of the tibia both anteriorly and posteriorly, to the anterior horn of the lateral meniscus through the transverse meniscal ligament in 40%, to the posterior capsule, and to the medial collateral ligament. The lateral meniscus is more circular in shape, has anterior and posterior intercondylar notch attachments, tranverse meniscal attachment to the anterior horn of the medial meniscus, meniscofemoral ligament attachments to the inner aspect of the medial femoral condyle (Wrisberg posteriorly, Humphrey anteriorly), and is loosely attached to the capsule but not the lateral collateral ligament. It is separated from the posterior capsule by the popliteus tendon (14).

Menisci are repeatedly subjected to rotational forces on flexion and extension. In extension, the femur internally rotates as a locking screw-home mechanism. In flexion, the opposite occurs under the influence of the popliteus tendon. As the popliteus contracts, the posterior horn of the lateral meniscus is pulled posteriorly to accommodate the posterior shift in load bearing as part of flexion (17).

Meniscal Tears

At MR imaging, the compact menisci are hypointense on all sequences. Traditionally, sagittal images are primarily used to evaluate their integrity. In the sagittal plane, the posterior horn of the medial meniscus is typically twice the size of the anterior horn. In contrast, the anterior and posterior horns of the lateral meniscus are equal in dimensions. Typically, the bodies of the menisci are seen only on the outer two slices (18,19).

Menisci may tear in the setting of acute trauma or in the setting of minor trauma superimposed on meniscal degeneration.

Following repetitive trauma, as part of the aging process, the central portion of the meniscus undergoes first globular and then progressive linear mucoid degeneration. Such changes have led to the application of a universally accepted grading system (20–22) in which intrasubstance focal signal change (slight T1 and T2 hyperintensity) is classified as grade 1, linear or diffuse globular signal abnormality not extending to a surface is classified as grade 2, and signal abnormality, either linear or globular with definite extension to a surface, is classified as grade 3. Extension of signal abnormality to a surface is the hallmark feature allowing

diagnosis of meniscal tear (20–22) (Fig. 10). Because extension of signal to multiple surfaces or in multiple planes reflects a more serious tear with surgical implications, some advocate use of the term grade 4 to accommodate this scenario, although this is currently not widely employed.

Grade 2 signal abnormality may be seen occasionally in the periphery of normal menisci in children secondary to the presence of perforating vessels (23).

Many descriptive terms are used in the analysis and description of grade 3 signal abnormality. In simple terms, tears (grade 3 signal) may be vertical or horizontal in axis. Vertical tears may be either parallel to the long axis of the meniscus, classified as longitudinal, or may be perpendicular to the long axis, classified as radial (24,25).

Diagnostic Criteria for Meniscal Tears

Signal Abnormality: Grade 1, Focal Signal Abnormality; Grade 2, Linear or Globular Signal Abnormality; Grade 3, Linear Signal Abnormality Extending to a Surface
Signal Orientation: Vertical, Traumatic; Horizontal, Degenerate
Vertical Tears: Radial (Parrot Beak) Versus Longitudinal (Bucket Handle)
Meniscocapsular Separation: Posterior Horn Medial Meniscus Greater Than 5 mm of Exposed Articular Cartilage

---

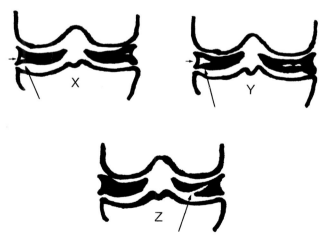

FIG. 10. Meniscal grading system: X, grade 1 signal abnormality within the body of the meniscus; Y, grade 2 globular or linear signal abnormality not extending to a surface; Z, grade 3 linear signal abnormality extending to a surface, consistent with a meniscal tear.

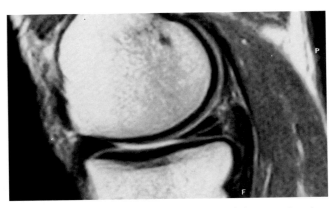

FIG. 11. Sagittal proton-density-weighted image showing oblique linear signal abnormality extending to the inferior surface secondary to an acute tear.

The most common acute traumatic tear affects the posterior horn of the medial meniscus. It is manifest as linear signal abnormality with a predominantly vertical orientation extending to a surface, often with secondary horizontal components. It is important to document to which surface the tear extends: inferior surface tears are poorly visualized at arthroscopy unless specifically sought (Fig. 11) (30).

> **Diagnostic Accuracy of MR Imaging in Meniscal Tears**
>
> Medial Meniscus: 87% to 97% Sensitivities; 82% to 91% Specificities
> Lateral Meniscus: 69% to 92% Sensitivities; 91% to 98% Specificities
> Overall Negative Predictive Value of MR Imaging: 90% (26–29)

The most common tear following acute trauma to a degenerate meniscus is horizontal in axis and often extends through body and both horns, aptly described as horizontal cleavage in type (Fig. 12). Degenerate meniscal tears often follow what is considered to be innocuous trauma, such as squatting or following repetitive flexion extension imposed by climbing stairs (31).

Lateral meniscal injury is less common than medial, as the meniscus is more mobile and has fewer osseous or capsular attachments. Although both vertical and horizontal tears occur, vertical radial tears extending from the free edge to the periphery of the meniscus are considerably more common laterally, where tear occurs at the junction of the horn and body, with a meniscal rent simulating a parrot beak (Figs. 13 and 14). These are manifest as blunting or acute truncation of the meniscal horn on sagittal images. Free-edge tears of the lateral meniscus commonly

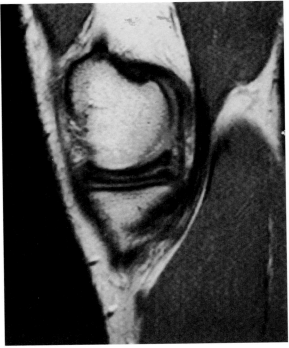
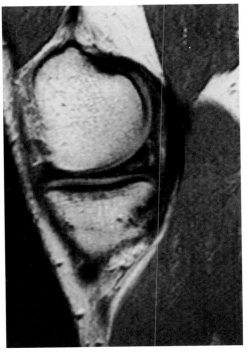

FIG. 12. Horizontal signal abnormality extending through **(A)** the body and **(B)** both horns of the meniscus secondary to acute horizontal cleavage tear.

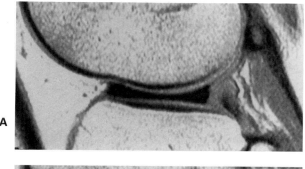

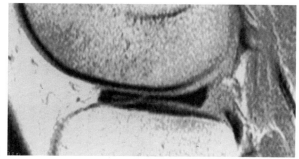

FIG. 13. (A) Discoid lateral meniscus with (B) an associated free edge parrot beak tear. .

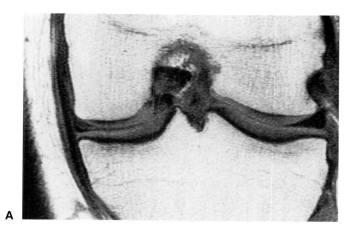

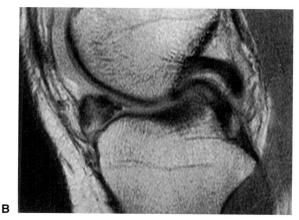

FIG. 15. (A) Bucket-handle tear of the medial meniscus with (B) reflection of fragment or handle to the intercondylar notch, in the sagittal plane producing a double PCL sign.

accompany rotational torque injuries, resulting in disruption of the anterior cruciate ligament (32).

A more severe form of tear, more commonly affecting the medial meniscus, is characterized by longitudinal extension of a vertical tear through both meniscal horns and body with reflection of the medial fragment to the intercondylar notch like a bucket handle, the "bucket handle" tear (Figs. 15 and 16) (33).

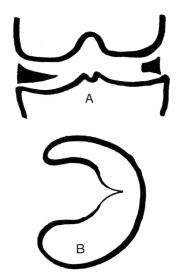

FIG. 14. Diagram showing acute meniscal truncation in (A) the coronal plane and (B) in the axial plane, secondary to a free edge parrot beak tear.

A variant of the bucket handle tear results in pseudohypertrophy of the anterior horn of the lateral meniscus. This injury, when it occurs, accompanies rotational torque with anterior translation of the lateral tibial plateau relative to the femoral condyle. As the lateral tibial plateau rotates back to anatomic alignment, the posterior horn of the lateral meniscus is sheared off the posterolateral plateau and flipped on top of the anterior horn to produce the appearance of a double anterior horn, pseudohypertrophy (Fig. 17) (34).

Meniscocapsular separation or tearing usually involves the relatively immobile medial meniscus at its attachment with the posteromedial tibial plateau through the meniscotibial or coronary ligaments. Although the diagnosis is difficult, it is suggested in the presence of at least 5 mm of uncovered tibial articular cartilage or by fluid interposed between the meniscus and the capsule.

Fluid in the medial collateral ligament bursa (interposed between the deep and superficial fibers of the medial collateral ligament) may simulate detachment of the body on coronal images.

A "discoid" meniscus describes an anatomic variant in which the normal open configuration of the meniscus is ab-

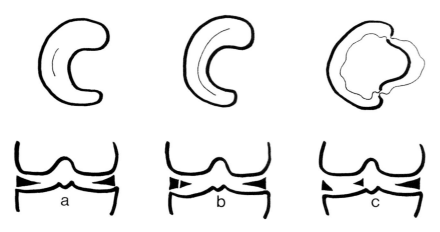

FIG. 16. Diagram showing serial progression of a vertical tear in the longitudinal plane ultimately leading to displacement or reflection of fragment to the intercondylar notch (stage c, corresponding to Fig. 15).

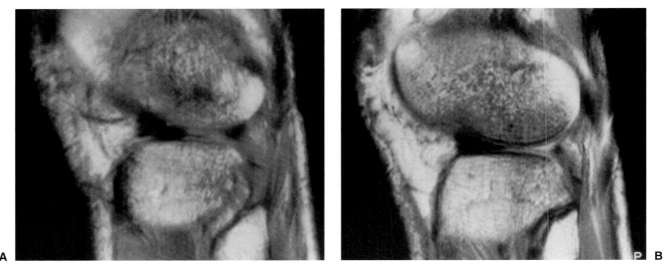

FIG. 17. (A) Pseudohypertrophy of the anterior horn of the lateral meniscus secondary to rotational torque injury, with reflection of the posterior horn on top of the anterior horn to produce **(B)** a double anterior horn appearance.

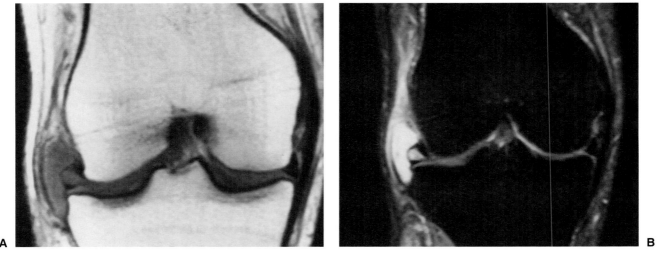

FIG. 18. (A) Coronal TSE T1 and **(B)** IR TSE images showing a meniscal cyst complicating or arising out of a meniscal tear.

sent and the meniscus acquires a solid appearance. The configuration lacks normal biomechanical integrity and is predisposed to tear, and occasionally a painful "snapping knee syndrome."

Criteria for diagnosis on MR images include identification of the body of the meniscus on more than three contiguous sagittal 4-mm slices, lack of rapid tapering from the periphery to the free edge of the meniscus, and an abnormally wide meniscal body on coronal images, encroaching further into the femorotibial compartment without the normal triangular configuration (35).

Occasionally tears of the meniscus are complicated by insudation of synovial fluid and cyst formation, initially intrameniscal but extending to become parameniscal, and finally occasionally extending to adjacent soft tissues (Fig. 18) (36).

Pitfalls in Diagnosis of Meniscal Tears

Popliteus Tendon Mimics Tear in Posterior Horn Lateral Meniscus
Transverse Meniscal Ligament Mimics Tear in Anterior Horn Lateral Meniscus
Vacuum Phenomenon: Susceptibility Blooming of Air Within a Degenerate Meniscus
Chondrocalcinosis: Manifest as Signal Hyperintensity Within Meniscal Body
Lax Meniscus: Meniscal Fold Secondary to Laxity
Concave Meniscal Effect: Pseudohorizontal Cleavage Tear Most Lateral Sagittal Oblique Images
Medial Meniscal Ossicle: Pseudotear of the Posterior Horn
Grade 2 Signal in Children: Penetrating Vessels
Grade 2 Signal in Adult Posterior Horn Medial Meniscus: Magic Angle (37–41)

Collateral Ligaments

The Lateral Collateral Ligament Complex

Lateral knee stability is through the joint capsule and structures of the lateral collateral ligament complex. Traditional descriptions divide the lateral collateral ligament into three layers: an outer layer, comprised of the iliotibial band anteriorly, continuous posteriorly with the biceps femoris tendon; the middle layer, which is composed of the posterolateral fibular collateral ligament, and the deep layer, composed of the popliteus tendon a renate ligament and capsule.

Injury to the lateral collateral ligament is uncommon, usually accompanying acute varus either secondary to motorcycle accident in which the motorcycle falls on the knee, and less commonly complicating an awkward fall.

Evaluation of the lateral collateral ligament is usually made on the basis of coronal images; fat-suppressed images are often used to localize sites of edema or injury; T1-weighted images are most frequently employed to facilitate detailed evaluation of the integrity of the soft tissues (Figs. 19 and 20) (42–44).

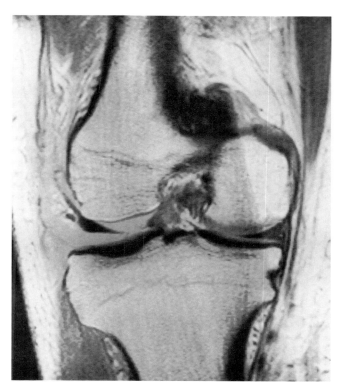

FIG. 19. Coronal TSE T1-weighted image showing disruption of the iliotibial band complicating an acute varus injury.

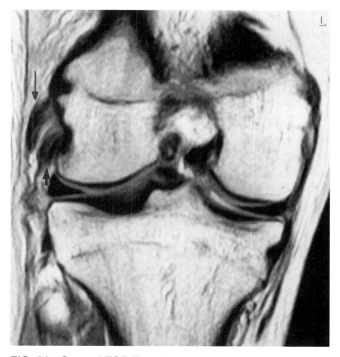

FIG. 20. Coronal TSE T1-weighted image showing complex injury of the conjoined and popliteus tendons with redundancy of the fibula collateral ligament and popliteus *(arrow)* tendons deep to the biceps femoris.

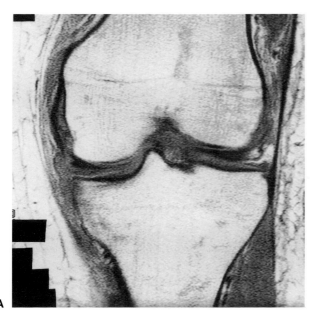 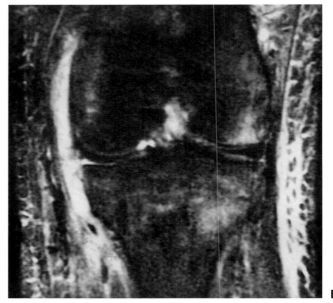

A   B

FIG. 21. **(A)** Coronal TSE T1 and **(B)** IR TSE images showing complete disruption of the medial collateral ligament following acute valgus injury with *contre-coup* kissing impaction bruises of the lateral condyle and tibial plateau.

The Medial Collateral Ligament Complex

Medial knee stability is through subcutaneous fascial investment, the distal sartorius, and the medial collateral ligament.

The medial collateral ligament is composed of deep fibers, which are essentially meniscofemoral and meniscotibial ligamentous attachments, separated from a thick superficial meniscotibial ligament by the medial collateral ligament bursa.

Grading of medial collateral ligament injury follows clinical grades 1 through 3, ranging from joint line tenderness and partial tear through to complete tear. At MR imaging, grade 1 injury is characterized by the presence of fluid on either the inner or outer aspect of the superficial fibers of the MCL; grade 2 is defined by fluid on both sides of the ligament without discontinuity; grade 3 is defined by tendon disruption and complete discontinuity (Fig. 21).

Medial collateral ligament injury usually accompanies an acute valgus injury: as valgus strain widens the medial joint space, it narrows the lateral space and leads to femoral condylar impaction directly on the underlying tibial plateau, resulting in the development of *contre-coup* impaction bone bruises (45,46).

Cruciate Ligaments

The Anterior Cruciate Ligament

The anterior cruciate ligament (ACL) is an intracapsular extrasynovial ligament primarily responsible for restraining anterior displacement of the tibia on flexion extension. The ligament runs in a hand-in-pocket axis from lateral to medial, from posterior to anterior, hugging the inner aspect of the

lateral femoral condyle, inserting anteriorly in the intercondylar notch (47).

Bone Bruise Patterns in the Knee (Fig. 22)

MCL Injury—Kissing Contusion: Midlateral Femoral Condyle and Midlateral Tibial Plateau Bruising
ACL Injury—*Contre-Coup* Contusion: Midlateral Femoral Condyle and Posterolateral Tibial Plateau
Transient Patella Dislocation—*Contre-Coup* Contusion: Medial Patella Facet and High Outer Lateral Femoral Condyle

---

The ligament has two identifiable bands, the anteromedial (AMB) and posterolateral (PLB) bands according to insertion on the tibial spine. The AMB is stronger and, being taut, resists anterior displacement in flexion. The PLB is taut

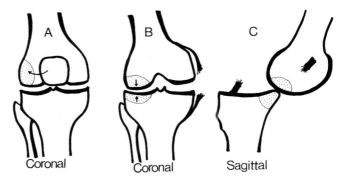

FIG. 22. Diagram demonstrating the site of bone bruises accompanying common knee injuries. **A,** transient patella dislocation; **B,** MCL injury; **C,** ACL injury.

in extension, resisting hyperextension and hence posterior femoral displacement. Being taut throughout the gait cycle, both flexion and extension, the ACL maintains functional isometry (48).

Disruption of the anterior cruciate ligament most frequently follows a rotational torque injury. Acute stretching, particularly of the AMB, which resists anterior tibial displacement in 30° of flexion, leads to ligamentous disruption. Although the AMB is most frequently disrupted in partial tears, most patients with partial tears progress to complete tears within a year. In addition, when a partial tear is suspected on the basis of MR appearances, cadaveric studies indicate that in most cases both bundles are disrupted but retained within an intact synovial sleeve (49).

Clinical systems grade ACL disruption on the basis of ligamentous laxity. A grade 1 injury shows no change in ligament length; a grade 2 injury shows a slight increase in ligament length; a grade 3 injury, complete disruption, shows gross knee instability with anterior draw. At MR imaging, appearances range from diffuse signal hyperintensity throughout the ligament in all imaging planes secondary to interstitial edema or ligamentous strain, to diffuse swelling of and signal abnormality in the ACL on axial, sagittal, and coronal images thought to be caused by partial tear with hemorrhage and edema, to complete ligamentous discontinuity or altered axis consistent with a complete tear (50–55).

Several signs are used to confirm diagnosis of ACL injury at MRI. Swelling, altered axis, and discontinuity are considered to be primary signs of either partial or complete tears (Figs. 23–25). Secondary signs have been widely reviewed in the literature and include anterior draw of the tibia by more than 5 mm relative to the femoral condyle, buckling of the posterior cruciate ligament (PCL), and posterior displacement of the posterior horn of the lateral meniscus. Of all the secondary signs, we rely most heavily on the identification of bone bruises in the midfemoral condyle and posterolateral tibial plateau (see Fig. 8), reflecting anterior translation of the tibia with impaction on the lateral femoral condyle. This sign is present in over 90% of acute ACL injuries. In the absence of bone bruising, primary images are reviewed in all three planes. Specifically, the axis of the sagittal oblique images are reviewed to ensure that poor visualization of the ACL (thought to be a complete tear) is not a function of an incorrect imaging plane. Recognizing bone bruise pattern and potential impaction to the lateral condyle, authors have emphasized the significance of a deep

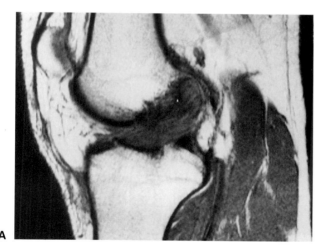

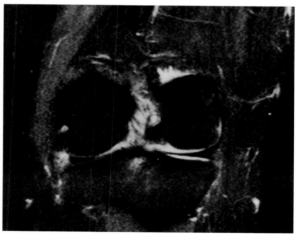

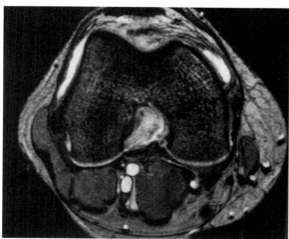

FIG. 23. (A) Sagittal TSE proton-density-weighted image shows increase in the bulk of the ACL worrisome for incomplete tear, intrasubstance rupture. (B) Coronal IR TSE shows edema within the ACL synovial sleeve hugging the inner aspect of the lateral femoral condyle. (C) Axial T2-weighted fast field-echo image shows edema within a swollen ACL hugging the inner aspect of the lateral femoral condyle confirming the presence of a partial tear.

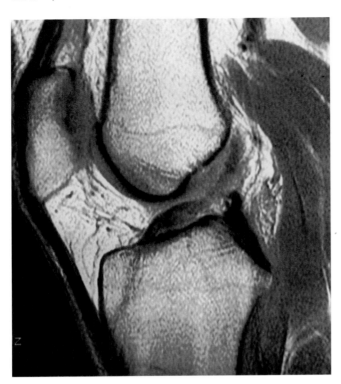

FIG. 24. Midsubstance complete tear of the anterior cruciate ligament.

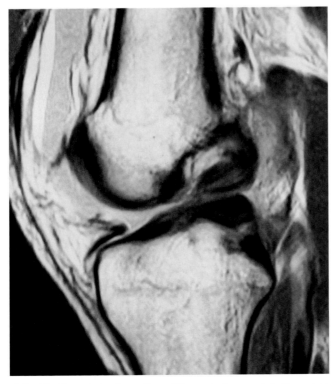

FIG. 25. Complete disruption of the anterior cruciate ligament with complete discontinuity.

lateral femoral condylar notch on both conventional radiographs and MR images (56–59).

Diagnostic Signs of ACL Disruption
Primary Signs: Contour Abnormality, Signal Abnormality, Axis Abnormality, Discontinuity
Secondary Signs: Anterior Translation by 5 mm, Posterior Horn Subluxation, PCL Buckling, Deep Lateral Notch, *Contre-Coup* Bone Bruise

Posterior Cruciate Ligament Disruption

The posterior cruciate ligament (PCL) is, like the ACL, an intrasynovial extracapsular ligament primarily responsible for resisting posterior translation of the tibia. The ligament is on average 13 mm long and is comprised of a dominant anterolateral bundle and a smaller posteromedial band. Arising from the inner aspect of the medial femoral condyle, the ligament runs posteriorly in a C-shaped configuration to attach in a midline depression in the posterior margin of the tibial plateau.

Being tightly bound, the PCL is uniformly hypointense, although some signal hyperintensity is often seen at the apex of the C, where fibers run at the magic angle (55° to the z axis) (60,61).

Injury to the posterior cruciate ligament is uncommon and best visualized in the sagittal plane when it occurs. The ligament functions to resist posterior translation of the tibia, and injury most frequently occurs when posterior tibial translation is forced by impaction injury to the shin or patella, as occurs in a motor vehicle dashboard injury. Acute tears are usually interstitial midsubstance rather than avulsions (Fig. 26). Although these injuries are easily recognized and require major impaction forces to occur, search should always be made for additional intra-articular derangement, includ-

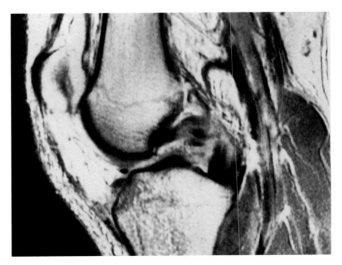

FIG. 26. Sagittal image showing intrasubstance rupture of the posterior cruciate ligament complicating a hyperextension injury.

ing ACL disruption, osteochondral fractures, collateral ligament injury, and outside the knee, for the presence of posterior column hip fractures (62–70).

The Extensor Mechanism

Extension of the knee occurs through contraction of the quadriceps muscle group, forces of which are translated though the quadriceps tendon, the patella, and the patella tendon. Injury to any of the components manifests as impaired extensor function. Although complete disruption is clinically evident as a result of incurred loss of function, most injuries are partial and clinically occult and only diagnosed at MRI (71).

Injuries may be divided into those occurring in young patients, which tend to be complete, frequently as a result of attempted rapid extension incurred by attempted jumping (72,73), and those occurring in older patients, which are often incomplete and often follow innocuous attempted knee extension walking down a curb or downstairs.

Up until skeletal maturity, the apophyses are the weakest point in the extensor mechanism, and so acute injury presents as either complete or incomplete avulsion, most frequently at the patella tendon insertion on the tibial tuberosity. In maturity, extensor mechanism injury is more frequently of the quadriceps muscle group or distal quadriceps tendon (Fig. 27) (74,75).

Although identification of a displaced patella (patella alta) on conventional radiographs suggests patella tendon avulsion in young athletes, the diagnosis is often confirmed only

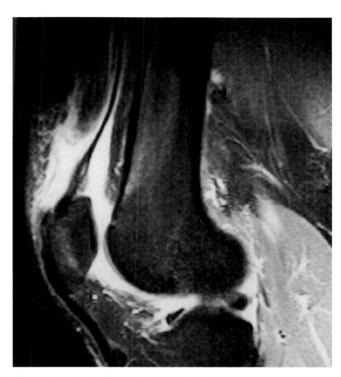

FIG. 28. Sagittal IR TSE image showing nearly complete rupture of the quadriceps tendon above the patella insertion.

at MRI. In adulthood, where incomplete quadriceps tears are common, intact fibers may maintain patella position, and although patients complain of pain, the diagnosis is often clinically occult. In these patients, a wider field of view is employed, allowing visualization of the distal quadriceps muscle bellies and tendon (Figs. 28 and 29).

Popliteus Tendon Injury

The popliteus muscle extends from its inferomedial insertion in the achilles tendon superiorly through the calf and laterally to buttress the posterolateral aspect of the knee at its tendinous insertion in the popliteus recess of the posterolateral aspect of the lateral femoral condyle.

Popliteus injury usually reflects gross rotational torque injury with varus and is therefore rarely identified as an isolated entity but commonly accompanies complex disruption of the lateral collateral ligament, the anterior cruciate ligament, and the menisci.

Popliteus tendon injury is described as type 1, in which rupture occurs at its insertion in the popliteal recess, type 2, in which rupture is in the midsubstance of the tendon, and type 3, in which rupture occurs at the junction of the proximal tendon and muscle belly behind the knee (Fig. 30) (76–78).

Plantaris Tendon Rupture

Plantaris tendon injury is extremely uncommon. Similar to the popliteus tendon, the plantaris tendon extends superi-

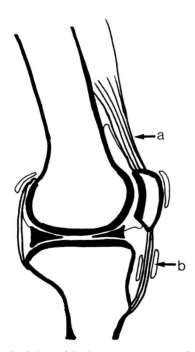

FIG. 27. Sagittal view of the knee extensor mechanism, injury involving the quadriceps **(a)** occurring in adulthood, injury involving the patella tendon **(b)** occurring in childhood.

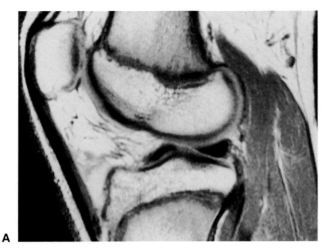 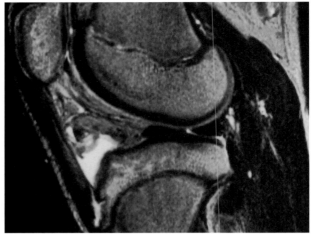

FIG. 29. (A) Sagittal proton-density- and **(B)** T2-weighted images of the knee showing prepatellar fluid and inflammatory change adjacent to the insertion of the patella tendon in a young basketball player.

orly from the achilles to insert on the posterior aspect of the lateral femoral condyle adjacent to the lateral head of the gastrocnemius. Rupture often manifests as hemorrhage and edema adjacent but deep to the medial head of the gastrocnemius in the calf. Because of the rotational torque mechanism of injury, plantaris rupture is often accompanied by disruption of the ACL (79).

MAGNETIC RESONANCE IMAGING OF ACUTE SOFT TISSUE INJURY IN THE CALF

Muscle Injuries

Muscle injury, most frequently involving the calf muscles, may follow a direct blow, contusion, or laceration or follow indirect trauma imposed by function, acutely manifest as tear or strain or as delayed-onset muscle soreness (DOMS) (80).

Although both lacerations and contusions are usually clinically apparent, MR imaging is undertaken following laceration to determine the integrity of neurovascular structures, whereas it is undertaken following contusion when histories are ambiguous, compartment syndrome is suspected, or aspiration is planned (81–84). Intramuscular hemorrhage is manifest by either a walled-off local hematoma or interstitial hemorrhage producing a feathery appearance.

Although a walled-off hematoma develops T1 signal hyperintensity with time secondary to the paramagnetic effects, both deoxy- and methemoglobin, acute interstitial muscle bleed is characterized by persistent signal isointensity on T1-

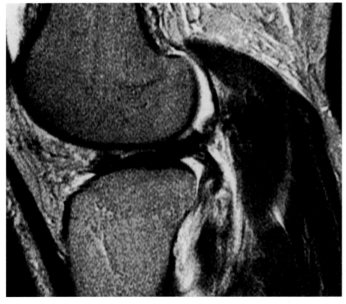 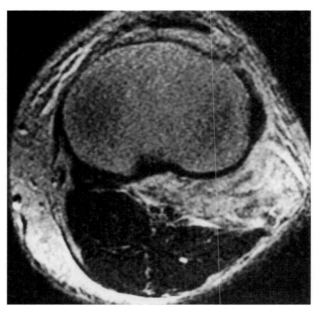

FIG. 30. (A) Sagittal T2-weighted image showing disruption of the popliteus tendon at the musculotendinous junction characterized by extensive hemorrhage and edema. **(B)** Axial image in the same patient shows extension of edema to a swollen muscle belly deep to popliteal vessels.

and signal hyperintensity on T2-weighted scans. Persistent signal characteristics most likely reflect secondary edema as a result of the inflammatory response induced by hemorrhage into interstitial tissues (85).

Muscle strain or tear is graded according to severity, as first degree, manifest as focal signal abnormality without a tear, second degree, manifest as a partial tear, or third degree, characterized by a complete tear with hemorrhage and retraction. The presence of hemorrhage filling in the gap created by muscle tear may lead to obscuration of the injury at clinical examination.

Muscle tears most commonly occur during vigorous exercise. In the calf, tears most frequently involve the gastrocnemius at the junction of either the medial or lateral heads (Fig. 31). The gastrocnemius crosses two joints, has an abundance of fast twitch fibers, and has eccentric muscle contraction (lengthens during contraction), features known to predispose to muscle tear (80–84).

Delayed-onset muscle soreness (DOMS) is also most frequently identified in muscles with eccentric contractions following chronic overuse. Muscles such as the gastrocnemius with eccentric contractions require less oxygen and energy, produce less lactate, and use smaller numbers of muscle fibers than concentric contractions. Following exercise, symptoms of DOMS develop up to 48 hr following exercise and usually resolve within 5 to 7 days without intervention. Symptoms are most frequently referable to the pain-receptor-rich myotendinous junction. In patients with local swelling, physical massage may alleviate symptoms (86).

At MR imaging, DOMS is manifest by local signal abnormality most frequently at muscle or fascial attachments, but occasionally at sites remote from the site of tenderness. In mild cases, MR imaging may show perifascial edema and small fluid collections which usually resolve as symptoms subside over 5 to 7 days. In severe cases, progression of the inflammatory process may lead to the development of myonecrosis manifest as dramatic intrasubstance signal hyperintensity on T2 and inversion recovery sequences (87).

Focal Muscle Herniation

Focal herniation of muscle through a defect in the overlying fascia following blunt trauma is most common in the lower leg, especially in the anterior tibial compartment. Patients usually present with either a local swelling or tenderness.

At MR imaging focal herniation is identified along the anterolateral border of the mid calf often more marked during either contraction or relaxation. Focal bulges retain muscle signal allowing differentiation of the entity from suspected soft tissue tumors. Occasionally note is made of associated hyperintense edema at the site the hernia.

Following diagnosis, most patients are treated conservatively, with or without support stockings. Occasionally fasciotomy is undertaken in patients with persistent discomfort.

Compartment Syndrome

Compartment syndrome most frequently affects the anterior and lateral compartments of the leg and the anterior compartment of the arm. Hemorrhage and edema complicating either muscle or osseous injury confined by fascial boundaries results in dramatically increased intracompartmental pressures, compressing and impairing capillary flow. Induced ischemia presents as acute pain and often sensory deficit in the calf, often incorrectly attributed to deep vein thrombosis or rupture of a popliteal cyst.

There are four discrete compartments in the calf: the anteromedial compartment containing the tibialis anterior, the extensor hallucis, and the extensor digitorum longus muscles; the peroneal compartment containing the peroneus longus and brevis muscles; and the deep and superficial posterior compartments, the deep containing the flexor hallucis and digitorum longus muscles and the tibialis posterior muscles, and the superficial containing the two heads of the gastrocnemius and soleus muscles (Figs. 32 and 33).

At MR imaging, involved compartments manifest swelling and signal abnormality, conspicuous on fat-suppressed T2 or STIR images, guiding surgical fasciotomy. Angiographic sequences are routinely employed in affected patients to determine vascular patency (88).

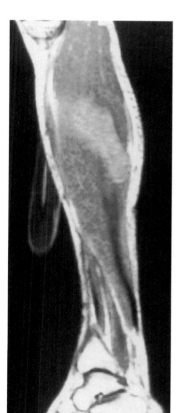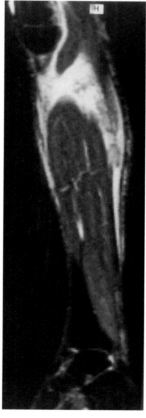

A,B

FIG. 31. (A) Sagittal proton-density- and **(B)** T2-weighted images show local hemorrhage and edema most marked at the junction of the medial head of the gastrocnemius secondary to tear.

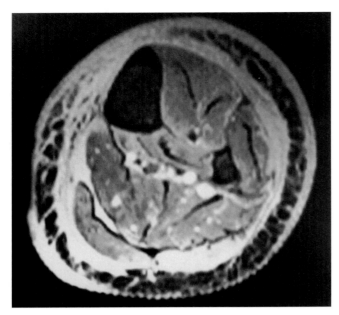

FIG. 32. Axial IR TSE image shows diffuse soft tissue edema with thickening of septae interdigitating through the deep compartments of the calf secondary to fasciitis.

MAGNETIC RESONANCE IMAGING OF ACUTE OSSEOUS (AND CHONDRAL) INJURY

Chondral Injury

As has been discussed in Chapter 4, cartilage is composed of chondrocyte cells (only 5% of total tissue volume) in an extracellular matrix composed of water (70% of total volume) and organized macromolecules—fibrillary collagen and nonfibrillary glycoproteins.

These components combine in different quantities and patterns of organization to form four layers covering subchondral bone. The superficial zone is the thinnest zone but contains most collagen; it affords greatest resistance to shear

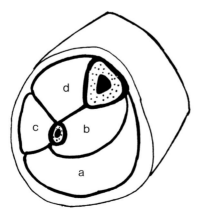

FIG. 33. Axial diagram showing the four compartments of the calf: **(A)** superficial posterior compartment; **(B)** deep posterior compartment; **(C)** lateral compartment; **(D)** anterior compartment.

forces. The transitional zone is composed predominantly of proteoglycans and functions to transmit compression forces to the deeper radial zone. The radial zone is the thickest layer and functions to resist compression forces. The zone of calcified cartilage gives rise to subchondral bone.

In the absence of vascular, lymphatic, or neural contributions to maintenance, cartilage healing following trauma is limited. Intrinsic repair depends on functioning chondrocytes to synthesize new matrix (limited *in vivo*). Extrinsic repair relies on generation of scar, fibrosis, or fibrocartilage at the site of injury triggered by traumatic synovitis or vascular response within deep subchondral bone. Repair following either mechanism is limited (89).

At arthroscopy damage to articular cartilage is defined as linear, stellate, flap, crater, fibrillary, or as thinned and degenerate (90). Improved resolution at MRI, yielded by more powerful gradients, greater image matrix, and improved receiver coils, now allows use of a similar MR-based grading system. Nevertheless, it seems likely that because each form of injury results in disruption of the superficial zone, each will ultimately progress to significant cartilage loss.

There has been extensive interest in the association between subchondral bone bruises and the development of abnormality in overlying cartilage. Although both entities often coexist, particularly following disruption of the anterior cruciate ligament (in which a split-thickness linear crack in cartilage accompanies an extensive subchondral bruise), the association is less common when bruises are identified in non-weight-bearing surfaces. In effect, extensive subchondral bruising is a reflection of extensive subchondral microtrabecular trauma (bruising results from concertina compression of supporting trabeculae). Secondary loss of subchondral structural integrity is transmitted to overlying cartilage, which eventually collapses under the imposed pressure of continued weight bearing. A similar loss of subchondral bone is identified in the femoral head following avascular necrosis, accounting for the crescent sign, which gives rise to articular margin collapse on persistent weight bearing.

Recognizing such a mechanism, a non-weight-bearing regimen advised by most physicians following identification of a bone bruise is appropriate. It might seem prudent to extend this practice to include repeat MR imaging in order to confirm resolution of bone bruise before recommending further weight bearing in affected patients. Graf and colleagues have previously documented resolution of bone buises in up to 90% of patients 6 weeks following anterior cruciate ligament injury (91).

Tibial Plateau Fractures

Tibial plateau fractures are reported to account for 1% of fractures in total, accounting for up to 8% in the elderly. Originally described as being the "bumper or fender" fracture, it is now recognized that tibial plateau fracture may follow acute valgus, acute varus, axial loading, or a combination of these forces most frequently encountered following either a motor vehicle accident or a fall from a height (89,90). It is the combination of both varus or valgus stress accompanying axial loading of up to 8,000 lb, producing both shearing and compression that accounts for the incidence of soft tissue disruption accompanying this injury.

Reflecting the prevalence of valgus injury, up to 70% of tibial plateau fractures involve the lateral articular surface; the medial is involved in 20% of cases, and bilateral plateau involvement occurs in 10%. Based on anatomic location, Schatzker (91) recognizes six patterns of tibial plateau fracture (Fig. 34). Types 1 to 3 fractures are of the lateral tibial plateau: type 1 fracture is a vertical split, type 2 is a vertical split with depression, and type 3 is a depressed fracture of the plateau without a vertical component; type 4 fractures are fractures of the medial tibial plateau (either wedge, split, depressed, or comminuted); type 5 fractures are bicondylar; and type 6 fractures are characterized by a transverse or oblique fracture of the proximal tibia separating the tibial metaphysis from the diaphysis in combination with fractures of either the medial or lateral tibial plateaus.

According to the Schatzker classification, type 1 fractures, splits of the lateral tibial plateau without depression, invariably occur in young adults with strong cancellous bone and are often associated with lateral meniscal tear, either detached peripherally or displaced into the fracture site, and in the setting of valgus strain are often accompanied by injury to the medial collateral and anterior cruciate ligaments (Fig. 35). Because of the prevalence of lateral meniscal injury, either MR imaging or arthroscopy is undertaken in these patients before surgical intervention. Type 2 fractures, where there is both depression and vertical split, occur in older patients above 40 years (Figs. 36 and 37). Depression of the tibial plateau decreases valgus strain and appears to decrease the prevalence of collateral ligament disruption. Many investigators believe that an intact collateral ligament on one side of the knee is necessary for a depressed fracture to occur in the contralateral plateau (Fig. 38). In these patients, preoperative MR imaging facilitates the evaluation of accompanying soft tissue injury but also allows evaluation of articular surface depression. Type 3 fractures are isolated depressions in the articular surface of the lateral tibial plateau. Meniscal injury is common, although this is dictated by the site of the depression. Posterior depressions are more unstable than central depressions and are more likely to require surgical intervention, particularly in young patients. Linear tomography, computed tomography, or MRI may be used to determine the site and extent of the articular depression (see Fig. 38). Type 4 fractures of the medial tibial plateau are uncommon, but when they occur, they are associated with high-energy varus trauma and dislocation and hence are frequently associated with extensive soft tissue injury to the cruciates, menisci, lateral collateral ligament, and to both the peroneal nerve and popliteal artery. Nonoperative treatment of these fractures is undertaken only in patients in whom there is complete restoration of anatomic alignment by closed techniques (Fig. 39). A Schatzker type 5 fracture is a bicondylar fracture, most frequently with split and depression of the lateral plateau. Reflecting the complex nature of the applied trauma, soft tissue injury may be extensive and bilateral. Type 6 fractures, like type 5 fractures, reflect complex trauma and are therefore associated with complex soft tissue injury. The accompanying metaphyseal dissociation accounts for the higher incidence of popliteal arterial injury and compartment syndrome that accompanies this injury (91).

Conventional management of fractures involves restoration of anatomic alignment and immobilization of the affected bone to allow early healing. In this regard, cast immobilization is undertaken in undisplaced tibial plateau fractures in the absence of soft tissue injury, while surgical intervention, screw-and-plate fixation, or buttressing is undertaken in plateau fractures with displacement or distraction of fracture fragment or significant articular margin step-off (greater than 5 mm) (92). Because tibial plateau fractures are commonly associated with intra-articular soft tissue injury, meniscal tear, cruciate or collateral ligament injury, surgical management may be required even in undisplaced fractures. Similarly, a knowledge of the presence or absence of soft tissue injury prior to surgical intervention is helpful even in displaced fractures, triaging patients into those in whom simple extra-articular buttressing can be undertaken (those without meniscal or cruciate ligament disruption) and those in whom a combined intra-articular repair of soft tissue injury must be undertaken in conjunction with extra-articular buttressing.

In order to facilitate operative planning, preoperative imaging must allow multiplanar visualization, allow evaluation

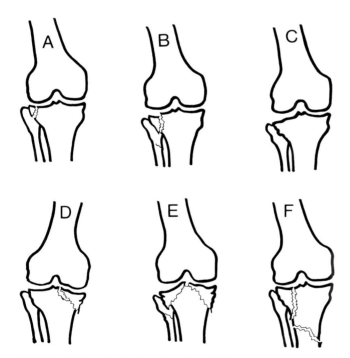

FIG. 34. Schatzker's classification of tibial plateau fractures: **(A)** type 1, **(B)** type 2, **(C)** type 3, **(D)** type 4, **(E)** type 5, **(F)** type 6.

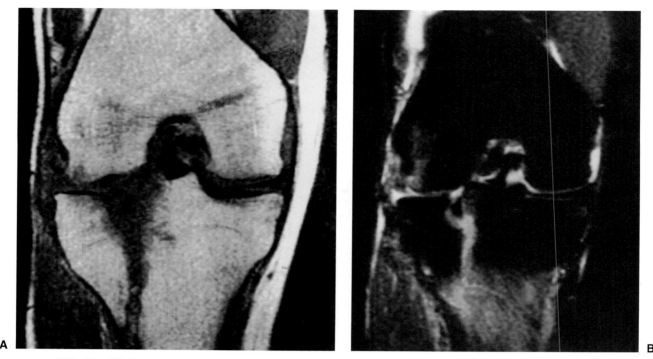

FIG. 35. (A) Coronal TSE T1 and **(B)** IR TSE images show a vertical split (Schatzker type 1) fracture of the lateral tibial plateau with interposition of the meniscus within the fracture margin.

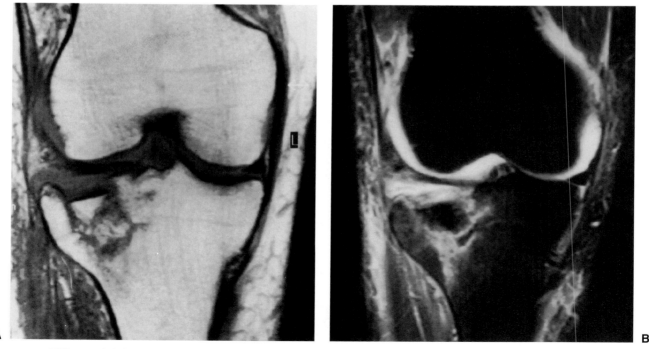

FIG. 36. (A) Coronal TSE T1 and **(B)** IR TSE images show a type 2 fracture with depression and split.

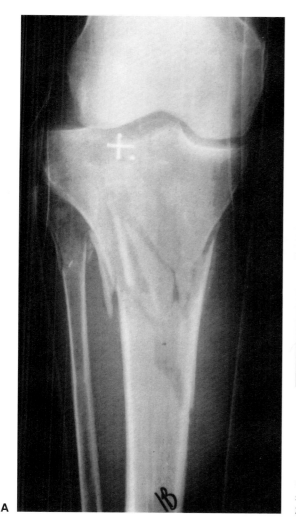

A

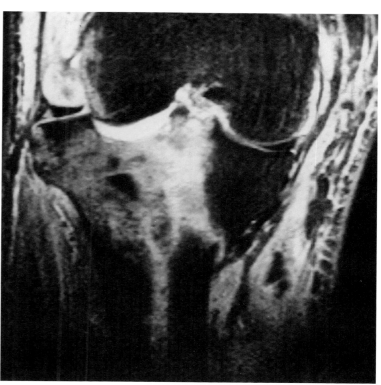

B

FIG. 37. (A) Radiograph shows a lateral tibial plateau fracture with splaying of fragment. **(B)** Coronal IR TSE confirms presence of a type 2 fracture with lateral splaying and preservation of the meniscus.

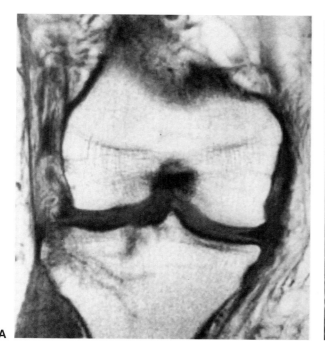

A

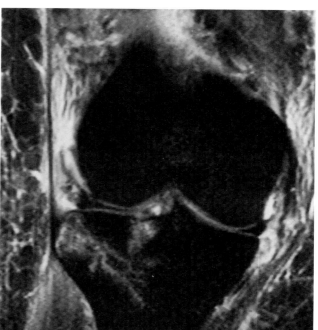

B

FIG. 38. Lateral tibial plateau fracture without depression or displacement of fragment. Impaction forces dissipated by associated disruption of the medial collateral ligament.

123

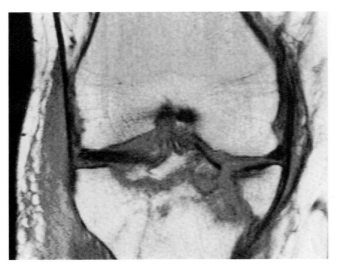

FIG. 39. Coronal TSE T1-weighted image showing medial tibial plateau fracture complicating acute varus (Schatzker type 4 fracture).

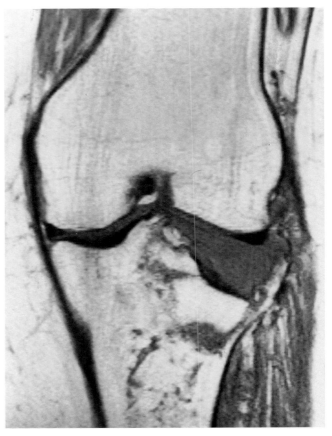

FIG. 40. Coronal TSE T1-weighted image shows gross depression of the lateral tibial plateau, with associated disruption of the lateral collateral ligament but preservation of the meniscus.

of the amount of displacement and distraction of fragment, accurately determine the amount of articular margin step-off (more than 5 mm requires operative fixation), and allow visualization of adjacent soft tissues (93–95). Computed tomography with multiplanar reconstruction has been shown to be more accurate than either plain film radiographs or linear tomography in determining the fracture extent and has been shown to be accurate in determining the amount of articular margin step-off (96). Nevertheless, neither plain film radiography, conventional tomography (95), nor CT gives accurate information concerning concomitant meniscal and ligament injuries (96,97).

Magnetic resonance imaging has recently been shown to allow accurate evaluation of fracture extent, fracture displacement, articular margin step-off, and also associated soft tissue injury (98). Magnetic resonance imaging is well recognized as an accurate technique for defining ligament and meniscal injuries of the knee in elective cases. Because meniscal tears commonly accompany tibial plateau fractures, occurring in 40% to 82% of tibial plateau fractures in surgical series (99) and in 47% (17 of 36 cases) in an arthroscopic series (100), preoperative evaluation by MR imaging is likely to be rewarding. Because wedging of meniscus at the fracture site can prevent reduction, preoperative identification may avoid this drastic complication.

Although the impact of collateral ligament injury on postoperative stability is unclear, it is clear that residual instability following tibial plateau fractures is associated with poor outcome (Fig. 40) (101). Delamarter et al., in a review of 39 patients with collateral ligament injury, 19 of whom were treated surgically, concluded that primary repair of collateral ligaments with open reduction and fixation of the plateau was indicated (102). Persistent morbidity was observed in five patients with unrepaired medial collateral, two patients with unrepaired lateral collateral, and three patients with

unrepaired cruciate ligaments. Bennet and Brower, in a series of 30, observed medial collateral ligament injury in 20%, lateral collateral ligament injury in 3%, meniscal injury in 20%, anterior cruciate ligament injury in 10%, and injury to the peroneal nerve in 3% (Fig. 41) (103).

In a recent study, Kode et al. (104) compared CT and MR imaging in the preoperative evaluation of 22 patients with tibial plateau fractures. They concluded that MR imaging was equivalent or superior to computed tomography for depiction of fracture configuration in all except three patients with complex, markedly comminuted fractures (Fig. 42). In addition, in the same study, MR imaging allowed the visualization of associated ligamentous injury in 68% (15 of 22 patients) and meniscal tears in 55% of cases not visualized at computed tomography. In another study comparing MRI and linear tomography, Barrow et al. (98) concluded that MRI allowed evaluation of depression equivalent to that by tomography but improved on the evaluation of comminution. In their study, MRI allowed detection of soft tissue injury in patients with Schatzker 2, 4, and 6 fractures.

Because of the prevalence of compartment syndromes and popliteal arterial injury in patients with types 4, 5, and 6 fractures, many now perform routine MR angiography in these patients at initial presentation.

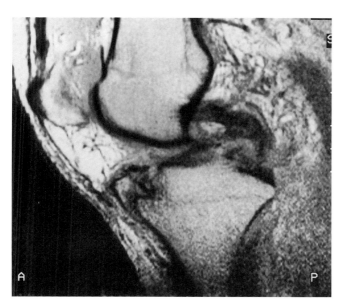

FIG. 41. Sagittal proton-density-weighted image in a patient following hyperextension injury with a compression fracture of the anterior margin of the tibial plateau and posterior avulsion at the insertion of the posterior cruciate ligament.

Arthroscopy or MRI in Tibial Plateau Fractures

Traditionally arthroscopy has been used as an alternative to MRI to evaluate suspected internal derangement in patients with tibial plateau fractures and, to a lesser extent, as a therapeutic tool, enhancing repair of both soft tissue and osseous components of the fracture (105–107).

Advantages of Arthroscopy

Direct Visualization of Internal Structures
Allows Articular Washout of Hemarthrosis
Allows Meniscal Repair
Assists Reduction of Low-Energy Lateral Tibial Plateau Fractures, Schatzker 1–3

Disadvantages

Almost 50% of Patients Have No Internal Derangement
Does Not Evaluate Collateral Ligaments
Increased Incidence of DVTs
Increased Incidence of Infection
Extravasation of Fluid to Soft Tissues—Compartment Syndrome

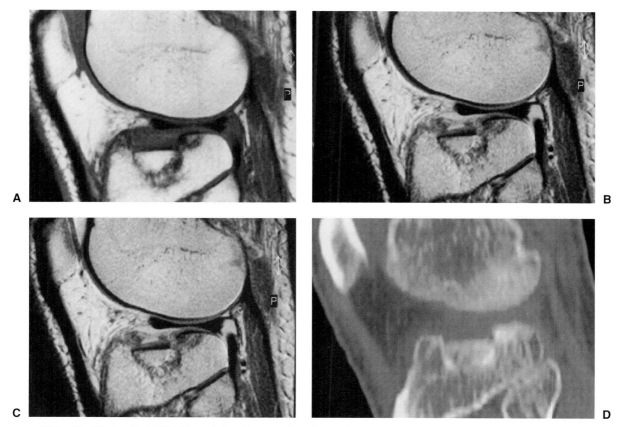

FIG. 42. (A) Sagittal TSE T1-weighted image showing a depressed central fragment complicating tibial plateau fracture, with **(B)** improved contrast and edge enhancement on the proton-density-weighted TSE image. **(C)** Sagittal proton-density-weighted TSE image affords equivalent evaluation of bone injury to sagittal reformatted CT image **(D)**.

Avulsions

Avulsion injuries around the knee are relatively common. As a result of acute stressors at the musculotendinous insertion secondary to acute tensile or rotational forces, avulsions may be identified at the insertions of the medial and lateral collateral and cruciate ligaments and at the insertions of the extensor mechanism.

In general, avulsions occur more frequently before growth plate closure, after which time, tears in either muscle or tendon occur rather than in bone (108).

Lateral Collateral Ligament Avulsions

The Segond Fracture or Lateral Capsular Sign. The Segond fracture is a cortical avulsion of the meniscotibial portion of the middle third of the lateral capsular ligament, originally described by Segond in 1879 (109).

The lateral capsular ligament runs from the patella and patella tendon to the posterior cruciate ligament (PCL) and is divided into three sections. The middle section, defined anteriorly by the iliotibial band and posteriorly by the fibular collateral ligament, which has strong femoral and tibial attachments, is the site of this injury. Acute strain imposed by rotation and varus angulation results in tear or avulsion of the ligament from its meniscotibial insertion, similar to the rotational torque mechanism recognized to induce ACL disruption. In such a way, although a Segond fracture may appear innocuous, it is frequently accompanied by internal joint derangement, with rupture of the ACL in up to 90% of cases and tear of menisci in up to 70% (110).

Although apparent on a conventional AP radiograph as avulsed fragments originating 2 to 10 mm below the cortex of the tibial plateau, posterior and superior to Gerdy's tubercle, small fragments are often visualized only at MRI. Primary fragment size is variable, ranging from 4 to 27 mm, although the injury is commonly accompanied by avulsions at other sites including the fibular head, Gerdy's tubercle, and the tibial eminences (Fig. 43) (111).

Arcuate Complex Avulsions. The arcuate complex is the posterolateral ligamentous complex of the knee and includes the fibular collateral ligament and the tendon of the biceps femoris, which merge to form the conjoint tendon that inserts on the fibular head, the popliteus tendon and the arcuate ligament itself. Injury is usually a sequel to anteromedial impaction to an extended knee with induced posterolateral subluxation. Following such an injury, radiographs are often either apparently normal or reveal the presence of an innocuous small ossific fragment adjacent to the fibular head. In such a way, when MR imaging is undertaken, the extent of soft tissue disruption may be surprising (Fig. 44). Because of the impact of posterolateral knee instability, most patients with this injury are referred for surgical repair.

Medial Collateral Avulsions (Steida Fracture)

Medial collateral ligament avulsions following acute valgus strain are uncommon, from either femoral or tibial insertions. In most cases, valgus strain induces intrasubstance rupture; occasionally in patients in whom a torque injury

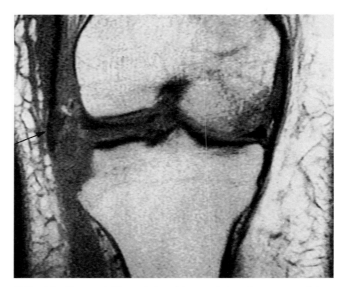

FIG. 43. Coronal T1-weighted image showing an avulsion from the middle portion of the lateral capsule and collateral ligament, typical of a Segond injury.

accompanies valgus, avulsions occur at the femoral attachment of the ligament (Steida fracture) (112).

Intercondylar Notch Avulsions of the Tibial Spines

Isolated injuries to the tibial spines are uncommon in adulthood and, when they occur, usually accompany high-energy plateau fractures, particularly Schatzker 4, 5, and 6 patterns.

In children, isolated avulsions may occur following rotational torque injury or may follow dashboard impaction in

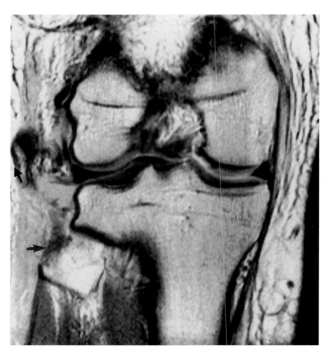

FIG. 44. Coronal TSE T1-weighted image showing avulsion from the fibula head with retraction of the posterolateral stabilizers of the knee *(arrows)*.

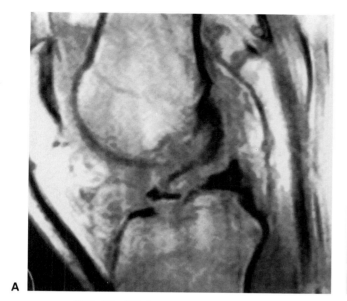
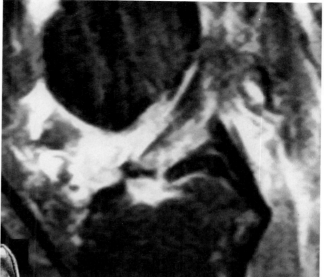

FIG. 45. (A) Sagittal T1 and (B) inversion recovery images of an intercondylar notch avulsion acquired with a dedicated extremity magnet. (Courtesy of Lunar Artoscan.)

a motor vehicle accident and clinically manifest with knee joint pain and swelling functionally mirroring an acute intra-substance ACL disruption.

Meyers and McKeever (113) initially classified intercondylar notch avulsions in 1959 based on the degree of fracture displacement. In a type 1 fracture, only the anterior edge of the eminence is elevated; in a type 2 fracture, more than half of the avulsed fragment is elevated; in a type 3 fracture, the entire avulsed fragment is displaced; and in a type 3b fracture, the fragment is avulsed and rotated (Fig. 45).

Affected patients hold the knee in flexion, attempted extension inducing excruciating pain. Surgical correction is undertaken to restore alignment and ACL function and to repair commonly associated meniscal tears.

Anterior Collateral Ligament Avulsions from the Intercondylar Notch

Although they have been unreported and previously undetected on conventional radiographs, we have identified several adult patients with small avulsions from the inner aspect of the lateral femoral condyle at the insertion of the ACL. Most frequently avulsions are localized to involve either the insertion of the anteromedial or posterolateral bundles of the

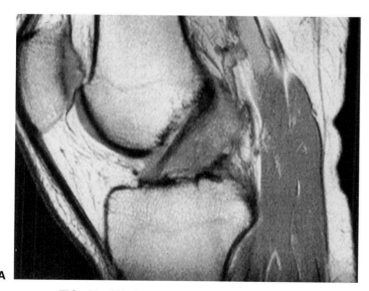
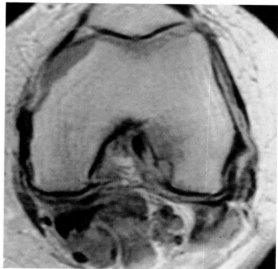

FIG. 46. (A) Sagittal and (B) axial images show swelling of ACL despite preservation of orientation. Axial images show an osteochondral abnormality at the insertion of the posterolateral bundle at site of avulsion injury. Anteromedial fiber bundle maintains orientation.

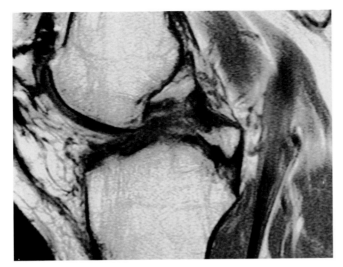

FIG. 47. Sagittal image showing large avulsion fragment at the insertion of the posterior cruciate ligament.

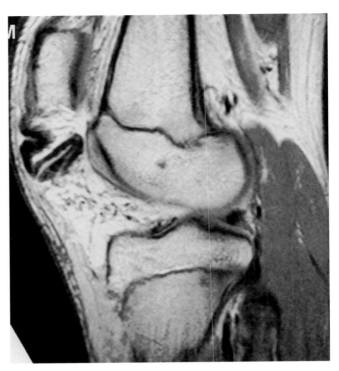

FIG. 48. Sagittal proton-density-weighted TSE image shows avulsion of the patella tendon from the tibial tuberosity with marked retraction.

ligament and, although radiographically occult, are clearly visualized at MRI. In each case, observations at MRI have subsequently been confirmed at surgical intervention (Fig. 46).

Posterior Cruciate Ligament Avulsions

Injury to the PCL is uncommon, most frequently following motor vehicle accident with forced posterior displacement of the tibia, and therefore is commonly accompanied by fractures of the patella and of the posterior column of the acetabulum. When it occurs, injury most frequently results in intrasubstance rupture; avulsion at the insertion of the PCL may occasionally occur, and it is usually associated with avulsion of a bulky fragment and is therefore usually readily apparent on conventional radiographs (Fig. 47) (65–67).

Extensor Mechanism Avulsions

Tibial Tuberosity Avulsions

This injury, usually occurring in young adults, results from forced flexion against a contracted extensor complex. Watson-Jones has identified three patterns of injury: type 1 injury is characterized by avulsion of a separate center for ossification at the tibial tuberosity, most frequently between 12 and 14 years; type 2 injury is characterized by a tongue-like avulsion of bone from the tibial epiphysis, also between 12 and 14 years; whereas type 3 injury is characterized by avulsion of a tongue-like extension directly into joint in a slightly older group, usually between 15 and 17 years (Fig. 48) (114).

Osgood-Schlatter disease represents a specific entity characterized by repeated microavulsions from the tibial tuberosity. It is most frequently identified in adolescent, athletic boys and is bilateral in 40%. Although it is classified along with Keinboch's disease, Kohler's disease, Freiberg's dis-

ease, and other osteochondroses, trauma or avulsions appear more important than ischemia (115).

Inferior Pole of Patella Avulsions—Sinding Larson

Avulsion from the inferior pole of the patella is unusual without preexisting inflammatory change at that site. Sinding Larson describes inflammatory change at the tendon insertion on the inferior pole of the patella secondary to microavulsions and ischemia (Fig. 49) (116).

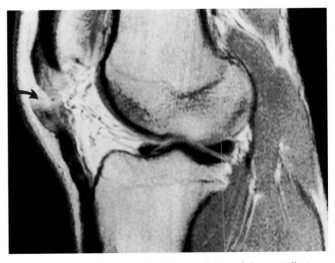

FIG. 49. Sagittal image showing avulsion of the patella tendon from the inferior pole of the patella (arrow).

Avulsions from Proximal Pole of Patella

Although quadriceps tendon injury usually occurs in adulthood, and avulsions at this age are generally uncommon, small superior pole patella avulsions frequently accompany quadriceps tendon injury (117,118).

Patella Fractures

Patella fractures are uncommon and, when they occur, most frequently accompany direct trauma. Fractures are classified as transverse, stellate, or comminuted, longitudinal, proximal pole, distal pole, or osteochondral in type. Transverse fractures are the most common, constituting 50% to 80%, and most frequently involving the lower pole; stellate fractures account for most of the remainder (119).

Surgical approaches to patella fractures have radically altered with time, the earliest surgeons believing that patellectomy improved quadriceps function. It is now recognized that the patella, acting as a fulcrum, is an important functional component, and attempts are now made at salvage at all costs. Surgery is now undertaken in only a third of cases (120).

Surgical approaches include simple open screw fixation of transverse fractures, tension band wiring of complex stellate fractures through to patellectomy in severely comminuted cases. Although complete evaluation may be yielded on conventional radiographs, MRI is occasionally undertaken in severely comminuted cases, the presence of intact articular cartilage prompting salvage rather than excision (Fig. 50). The likelihood of developing patellofemoral osteoarthritis by salvage (reported to occur in up to 50% of cases) is weighed against the likelihood of developing impaired extensor function and rupture at the surgical site following patellectomy (reported to occur in up to 20% of cases). In this regard, intact articular cartilage readily identified at MRI usually prompts attempt at patella salvage (121–123). Nonunion in patella fractures is uncommon and occurs in fewer than 3% of cases.

Supracondylar and Condylar Fractures

The supracondylar area is defined as the zone between the femoral condyles and the metaphysis of the distal femur, comprising 9 cm of the distal femur.

In younger patients, fractures of the distal femur are most frequently observed following complex injury; in older patients, the fractures often follow a minor slip, in which fractures are superimposed on osteoporotic bone.

Deformities following these fractures reflect the initial direction of displacement and the pull of the thigh muscles: the gastrocnemius muscles pull the distal fragment posteriorly, the adductors pull the proximal fragments medially, and the hamstrings and quadriceps result in shortening and overlap (124,125).

In practice, fractures are divided into intra-articular, extra-articular, supracondylar, and condylar types. Factors influencing management and outcome include the amount of displacement, the degree of comminution, the extent of soft tissue injury, amount of osteoporosis, intra-articular extension, and the presence or absence of accompanying soft tissue injury (126,127).

Although diagnosis, with the exception of undisplaced insufficiency fractures in the elderly, can usually be made with a conventional radiograph, MRI is of value in patients with intra-articular fractures, which are often associated with internal derangement, and in patients in whom fractures are accompanied by fractures of the tibial plateau, fractures through the fibular head (associated with peroneal nerve injury and complex lateral collateral ligament injury), by suspected patella subluxation (see next section), in patients in whom popliteal arterial injury is suspected (distal fragment markedly displaced), and in those in whom there is concern about integrity of underlying bone (suspected metastatic disease) (Fig. 51).

Management of supracondylar fractures varies, although frequently, in the absence of intra-articular extension, nonoperative management is undertaken, which includes closed reduction, skeletal traction, and prolonged immobilization. The goal in this setting is not anatomic reduction but restoration of length and axial alignment. Operative reduction, when undertaken, is frequently based on the use of the blade plate and screw fixation device. Condylar fractures are occasionally fixed using solitary lag screws (125,126).

DISLOCATIONS

Knee

Traumatic dislocation of the knee is rare: only 14 knee dislocations were recorded in 2 million admissions to the

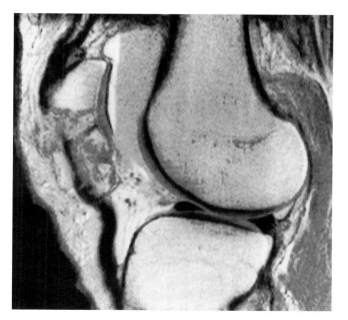

FIG. 50. Sagittal proton-density TSE image shows a comminuted fracture of the patella, with preservation of patellofemoral articular cartilage. Note lipohemarthrosis.

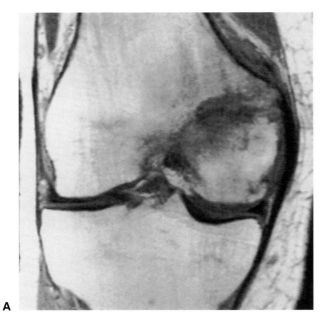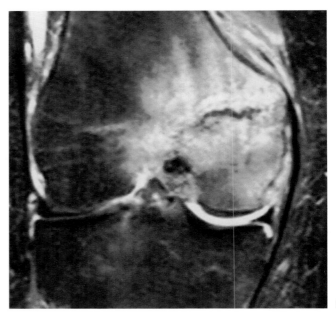

A   B

FIG. 51. (A) Coronal TSE T1 and **(B)** IR TSE images showing an undisplaced occult fracture of the medial femoral condyle.

Mayo Clinic, and when it occurs, it is the sequel of complex high-energy trauma (127).

Knee dislocations are classified as anterior, posterior, medial, lateral, rotatory, and occult and, reflecting the complexity of the injury, are always associated with injury to collateral and cruciate ligaments. An MRI is frequently undertaken in our institution in patients in whom occult dislocation is suspected. Although we do not have absolute criteria for diagnosis, we suggest major injury in patients in whom there is disruption of both collateral and cruciate ligaments (particularly the posterior cruciate ligament). When these are suspected, our routine imaging is accompanied by time-of-flight images to evaluate the popliteal vessels (128,129).

Patella: Transient Subluxation

As a result of mild physiological valgus at the knee, a minor change in biomechanics results in a tendency to laterally sublux the patella on flexion-extension.

Normal function or patellofemoral tracking is maintained by a deep intercondylar notch with an angle not greater than 140° with which the patella articulates. In such a way, the medial articular surface or facet articulates with the medial condyle, and the lateral facet articulates with the lateral condyle within a deep groove (131,132).

Wiberg has previously described three patella configurations: type 1, in which the medial and lateral facets of the patella are equal; type 2, in which the lateral facet is larger than the medial facet; and type 3, in which the medial facet is almost nonexistent, being replaced by a dominant lateral facet. Patients with a deep intercondylar notch and a Wiberg type 1 patella are least likely either to dislocate or to sublux;

patients with a shallow intercondylar notch and a flat dominant lateral patella facet are most likely to both dislocate and sublux, either chronically (tracking disorder) or acutely following trauma (Fig. 52) (133).

As a result of physiological valgus at the knee and the physiological tendency to sublux laterally, minor additional valgus strain, particularly to a flexed knee, which accompanies most knee injuries may result in acute patella dislocation or subluxation, with or without disruption of the medial collateral ligament. On extension, relocation commonly occurs spontaneously with minimal residual local soft tissue swelling (134–138).

Radiographic diagnosis of transient patella dislocation or subluxation is not possible. At MRI, the injury is manifest by *contre-coup* bone bruises high on the lateral femoral con-

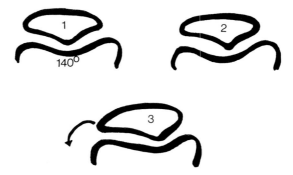

FIG. 52. Diagrammatic representation of patellar shapes (Wiberg types 1–3). Normal intercondylar notch is less than 140° in order to confer stability.

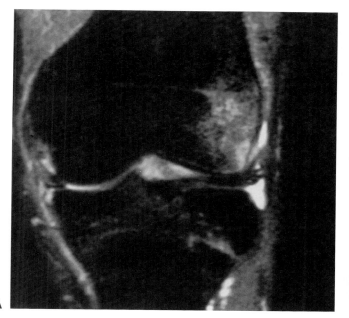

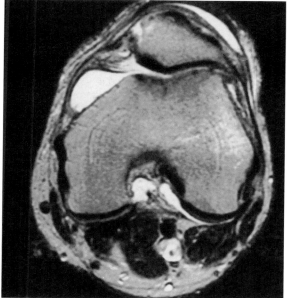

A

B

FIG. 53. **(A)** Coronal IR TSE image of a patient with disruption of the medial collateral ligament complicating an acute valgus injury. Image shows a high lateral bone bruise secondary to patella impaction complicating transient patella subluxation. **(B)** Axial image shows laxity of the disrupted medial retinaculum.

dyle at the site of impaction and deep to the medial patella facet, often accompanied by a local osteochondral fracture most conspicuous on fat-suppressed images (Fig. 53) (134,135). In adults, cartilage often tears at the junction of the calcified and uncalcified cartilage zones to produce chondral injury. In adolescents, lacking the calcified zone in cartilage, shearing forces are transmitted directly to underlying bone, resulting in osteochondral fractures. Dedicated cartilage sequences are used in this setting to enhance evaluation of cartilage injury (see Chapter 3).

As in chondromalacia, acute cartilage injury may manifest as local fibrillation and swelling (grade 1), a rent or defect in cartilage (grade 2), or as a rent or defect in cartilage and underlying bone (grade 3) (Fig. 54) (139–142).

Following patella subluxation or dislocation, it is important to evaluate the fibers of the medial retinaculum, integrity of which dictates the likelihood of persistent tracking anomalies and of need for surgical repair. Injury is manifest by local swelling, hemorrhage, and edema or discontinuity readily identified in the axial plane. The patellar retinacular ligaments are a composite of multiple fascial elements originating from the medial and lateral collateral ligaments extending anteriorly to insert on the margins of the patella. The retinaculae are normally well defined hypointense bands; following injury, they become indistinct and retracted or thickened and irregular with local hemorrhage and edema.

As a result of valgus strain, patella subluxation is commonly associated with injury to the medial collateral ligament, which extends anteriorly into the medial retinaculum, and may be accompanied by injury to the anterior cruciate ligament, complicating interpretation of bone bruises.

Tibiofibular Dislocation

Although described by Nelation in 1874 (143), dislocation at the superior tibiofibular articulation is extremely rare. Reflecting the anatomy of the joint, the conjoint tendon must be relaxed by a flexed knee to allow fibular motion. In such

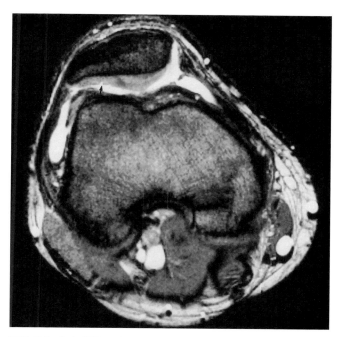

FIG. 54. Axial T2-weighted fast field-echo image with off-resonance magnetization transfer saturation shows a discrete rent in the cartilage overlying the lateral patellar facet *(arrow)*.

a way, marked acute inversion at the tibiotalar articulation may be transmitted superiorly to result in anterior subluxation rather than fibular neck fracture (which may occur with acute inversion and an extended knee (Maisonneuve fracture). The injury may present as pain, local swelling, or result in peroneal nerve palsy. Reduction, achieved in most cases without surgical intervention, results in complete restoration of function in most cases (144,145).

REFERENCES

1. Buckwalter KA, Pennas DR. Anterior cruciate ligament: oblique sagittal MR imaging. *Radiology* 1990;175:276.
2. Escobedo EM, Hunter JC, Zink-Brody GC, et al. Usefulness of turbo spin echo MR imaging in the evaluation of meniscal tears: comparison with a conventional spin echo sequence. *Am J Roentgenol* 1996;167:1223.
3. Santyr GE, Mulkern RV. Magnetization transfer in MR imaging. *J Mag Res Imag* 1995;5:121.
4. Wolff SD, Balaban RS. Magnetization transfer imaging: practical aspects and clinical applications. *Radiology* 1994;192:593.
5. Mirowitz SA. Fast scanning and fat-suppression MR imaging of musculoskeletal disorders. *Am J Roentgenol* 1993;161:1147.
6. Crues JV, Mink J, Levy TL, Loytsch M, Stoller DW. Meniscal tears of the knee, accuracy of MR imaging. *Radiology* 1987;164:445.
7. Semelka RC, Kelekis NL, Thomasson D, et al. HASTE MR imaging: description of technique and preliminary results in the abdomen. *J Mag Res Imag* 1996;6:698.
8. Feinberg DA, Kiefer B, Johnson G. GraSE improves spatial resolution in single shot imaging. *Mag Res Med* 1995;33:529.
9. Jung G, Krahe T, Kugel H, et al. Prospective comparison of fast SE and GraSE sequences and echo planar imaging with conventional SE sequences in the detection of focal liver lesions at 1.0 T. *J Comput Assist Tomog* 1997;21:341.
10. Stoller DW, Genant HK. Magnetic resonance imaging of the knee and hip. *Arthritis Rheum* 1990;33:441.
11. Kursunoglu-Brahme S, Resnick D. Magnetic resonance imaging of the knee. *Orthop Clin North Am* 1990;21:561.
12. Mink JH, Deutsch AL. Magnetic resonance imaging of the knee. *Clin Orthop* 1989;244:29.
13. Burk DL Jr, Mitchell DG, Rifkin MD, Vinitski S. Recent advances in magnetic resonance imaging of the knee. *Radiol Clin North Am* 1990;28:379.
14. Reicher MA, Rauschning W, Gold RH, et al. High-resolution magnetic resonance imaging of the knee joint: normal anatomy. *Am J Roentgenol* 1985;145:895.
15. Arnoczky SP, et al. Microvasculature of the human meniscus. *Am J Sports Med* 1982;10:90.
16. Arnoczky SP, et al. The microvasculature of the meniscus and its response to injury. *Am J Sports Med* 1983;11:31.
17. Mandelbaum BR, et al. Magnetic resonance imaging as a tool for evaluation of traumatic knee injuries: anatomical and pathoanatomical correlations. *Am J Sports Med* 1986;14:361.
18. Mesgarzadeh M, Moyer R, Leder D, Revesz G. MR imaging of the knee: expanded classification and pitfalls to interpretation of meniscal tears. *Radiographics* 1993;13:489.
19. DeSmet AA, Norris MA, Yandow DR, Quintana FA. MR diagnosis of meniscal tears of the knee: importance of high signal in the meniscus that extends to the surface. *Am J Roentgenol* 1993;161:101.
20. Crues JV, Mink J, Levy TL, Lotysch M, Stoller DW. Meniscal tears of the knee: accuracy of magnetic resonance imaging. *Radiology* 1987;164:445-448.
21. Lotysch M, Mink J, Crues JV, Schwartz A. Magnetic resonance imaging in the detection of meniscal injuries. *Mag Res Imag* 1986;4:94.
22. Lotysch M, Mink J, Levy T, Schwartz A, Crues JV. Detection of meniscal injuries using magnetic resonance imaging. *Radiology* 1986;161:238.
23. Mink JH, et al. MR imaging of the knee: pitfalls in interpretation. *Radiology* 1987;165(P):239.
24. Stoller DW, et al. Meniscal tears: pathological correlation with MR imaging. *Radiology* 1987;163:452.
25. Watanabe AT, et al. Normal variations in MR imaging of the knee: appearance and frequency. *Am J Roentgenol* 1987;153:341.
26. DeSmet AA, Norris MA, Yandow DR, Graf BK. Diagnosis of meniscal tears of the knee with MR imaging: effect of observer variation and sample size on sensitivity and specificity. *Am J Roentgenol* 1993;160:555.
27. Mink JH, et al. MR imaging of the knee: technical factors, diagnostic accuracy, and further pitfalls. *Radiology* 1987;165:175.
28. Fischer SP, et al. Accuracy of diagnosis from magnetic resonance imaging of the knee. *J Bone Joint Surg [Am]* 1991;73:2.
29. Tyrrell R, et al. Fast three-dimensional MR imaging of the knee: A comparison with arthroscopy. *Radiology* 1987;166:865.
30. Reicher MA, et al. MR imaging of the knee: I. traumatic disorders. *Radiology* 1987;162:547.
31. Hartzman MD, et al. MR imaging of the knee: II. chronic disorders. *Radiology* 1987;162:553.
32. Tuckman GA, Miller WJ, Remo JW, Fritts HM. Radial tears of the menisci. MR findings. *Am J Roentgenol* 1994;163:395.
33. Singson RD, et al. MR imaging of displaced bucket handle tear of the medial meniscus. *Am J Roentgenol* 1991;156:121.
34. Wright DH, DeSmet AA, Norris M. Bucket handle tears of medial and lateral menisci of the knee, value of MR imaging in detection of displaced fragments. *Am J Roentgenol* 1995;165:621.
35. Kaplan EB. Discoid lateral meniscus of the knee joint. *J Bone Joint Surg [Am]* 1957;39:77.
36. Burk DL, et al. Meniscal and ganglion cysts of the knee. MR evaluation. *Am J Roentgenol* 1988;150:331.
37. Kaplan PA, et al. MR of the knee: the significance of high signal in the meniscus that does not clearly extend to the surface. *Am J Roentgenol* 1991;156:333.
38. Herman LJ, et al. Pitfalls in MR imaging of the knee. *Radiology* 1988;167:775.
39. Vahey TN, et al. MR imaging of the knee: pseudotear of the lateral meniscus caused by the meniscofemoral ligament. *Am J Roentgenol* 1990;154:1237.
40. Turner DA, Rapoport MI, Erwin WD, et al. Truncation artifact: a potential pitfall in MR imaging of the menisci of the knee. *Radiology* 1991;179:629.
41. Peterfy CG, Janzen DL, Tirman PF, VanDijke CF. Magic angle phenomenon: A cause of increased signal in the normal lateral meniscus on short-TE MR images of the knee. *Am J Roentgenol* 1994;163:149.
42. Li DKB, et al. Magnetic resonance imaging of the ligaments and menisci of the knee. *Radiol Clin North Am* 1986;24:209.
43. Yu JS, Salonen DC, Hodler J, Haghighi O, Trudell D, et al. Posterolateral aspect of the knee: improved MR imaging with a coronal oblique technique. *Radiology* 1996;198:199.
44. Ekman EF, Pope T, Martin DF, Cuel WW. Magnetic resonance imaging of iliotibial band syndrome. *Am J Sports Med* 1994;22:851.
45. Schweitzer MS, Tran D, Deely DM, Hume EL. Medial collateral ligament injuries: evaluation of multiple signs, prevalence and location of associated bone bruises and assessment with MR imaging. *Radiology* 1995;194:825.
46. Forbes JR, Helms JA, Janzen DL. Acute pes anserine bursitis: MR imaging. *Radiology* 1995;194:525.
47. Hodler J, Highy P, Trudell D, et al. The cruciate ligament of the knee: correlation between MR appearance and gross and histologic findings in cadaveric specimens. *Am J Roentgenol* 1992;159:357.
48. Robertson PL, Schweitzer ME, Bartolozzi AR, Ligoni A. Anterior cruciate ligament tears: evaluation of multiple signs with MR imaging. *Radiology* 1994;193:829.
49. Tung GA, Davis LM, Wiggins ME, Fadale PD. Tears of the anterior cruciate ligament: primary and secondary signs at MR imaging. *Radiology* 1993;188:661.
50. McCauley TR, Moses M, Kier R, Lynch JK, et al. MR diagnosis of tears of anterior cruciate ligament of the knee: importance of ancillary findings. *Am J Roentgenol* 1994;162:115.
51. Brandser EA, Riley MA, Berbaum KS, et al. MR imaging of anterior cruciate ligament injury: independant value of primary and secondary signs. *Am J Roentgenol* 1996;167:121.
52. Fitzgerald SW, Remer EM, Friedman H, Rogers LF, et al. MR evaluation of the anterior cruciate ligament: value of supplementing sagittal images with coronal and axial images. *Am J Roentgenol* 1993;160:1223.
53. Vahey TN, Junt JE, Shelbourne KD. Anterior translocation of the

tibia at MR imaging: a secondary sign of anterior cruciate ligament tear. *Radiology* 1993;187:817.

54. Murphy BJ, Smith RL, et al. Bone signal abnormalities in the posterolateral tibia and lateral femoral condyle in complete tears of the anterior cruciate ligament: a specific sign? *Radiology* 1992;182:221.

55. Speer KP, Warren RF, Wickiewicz TL, Horowitz L. Observations on the injury mechanism of anterior cruciate ligament tears in skiers. *Am J Sports Med* 1995;23:77.

56. Fowler PJ. Bone injuries associated with anterior cruciate ligament disruption. *Arthroscopy* 1994;10:453.

57. Mink JH, et al. Tears of the anterior cruciate ligament and menisci of the knee: MR imaging evaluation. *Radiology* 1988;167:769.

58. Lee JK, et al. Anterior cruciate ligament tears: MR imaging compared with arthroscopy and clinical tests. *Radiology* 1988;166:861.

59. Kezdi-Rogus PC, Lomasney LM. Plain film manifestations of ACL injury. *Orthopedics* 1994;17:969.

60. Kennedy JC. The posterior cruciate ligament. *J Trauma* 1967;7:367.

61. Covery DC, Sapega AA. Anatomy and function of the posterior cruciate ligament. *Clin Sports Med* 1994;13:509.

62. Turner, et al. Acute injury of the ligaments of the knee: magnetic resonance evaluation. *Radiology* 1985;154:717.

63. Loos WC, et al. Acute posterior cruciate ligament injuries. *Am J Sports Med* 1981;9:86.

64. Miller MD, Harner CD. Posterior cruciate ligament injuries, Current concepts in diagnosis and treatment. *Physician Sports Med* 1993;21: 38.

65. Covey DC, Sapega AA. Current concepts review. Injuries of the posterior cruciate ligament. *J Bone Joint Surg* 1993;75(A):1376.

66. Fanelli GC. Posterior cruciate ligament injuries in trauma patients. *Arthroscopy* 1993;9:291.

67. Giessler WB, Whipple TL. Intraarticular abnormalities in association with posterior cruciate ligament injuries. *Am J Sports Med* 1993;21: 846.

68. Andrews JR, Edwards JC, Satterwhite YE. Isolated posterior cruciate ligament injuries: History, mechanism of injury, physical findings, and ancillary tests. *Clin Sports Med* 1994;13:519–530.

69. Grover JS, et al. Posterior cruciate ligament: MR imaging. *Radiology* 1990;174:527.

70. Sonin AH, Fitzgerald SW, Hoff FL, Friedman H, et al. MR imaging of the posterior cruciate ligament: Normal, abnormal, and associated injury patterns. *Radiographics* 1995;15:552.

71. Larsen L, Lund PM. Ruptures of the extensor mechanism of the knee joint. *Clin Orthop* 1986;213:150.

72. Yu JS, Popp JE, Kaeding CC, Lucas J. Correlation of MR imaging and pathologic findings in athletes undergoing surgery for chronic patellar tendinitis. *Am J Roentgenol* 1995;165:115.

73. McLoughlin RF, Raber EL, Vellet AD, Wiley JP, et al. Patellar tendinitis, MR imaging features with suggested pathogenesis and proposed classification. *Radiology* 1995;197:843.

74. Daffner RH, Riemer BL, Lupetin AR, et al. Magnetic resonance imaging of acute tendon ruptures. *Skel Radiol* 1986;15:619–621.

75. Barasch E, Lombardi L, Arena L, et al. MRI visualization of bilateral quadriceps tendon rupture in a patient with secondary hyperthyroidism: Implications for diagnosis and therapy. *Comput Med Imag Graph* 1989;5:407.

76. Seebacher JR, et al. The structures of the postero-lateral aspect of the knee. *J Bone Joint Surg [Am]* 1982;64:536.

77. Westrich GH, Hannafin JA, Potter HG. Isolated rupture and repair of the popliteus tendon. *Arthroscopy* 1995;22:628.

78. Veltri DM, Warren RF. Operative treatment of posterolateral instability of the knee. *Clin Sports Med* 1994;13:615.

79. Helms CA, Fritz RC, Garvin GJ. Plantaris muscle injury: evaluation with MR imaging. *Radiology* 1995;195:201.

80. El Khoury GY, Brandser EA, Kathol MH, et al. Imaging of muscle injuries. *Skel Radiol* 1996;25:3.

81. Anzel SH, Covey KW, Weiner AD, et al. Disruption of muscles and tendons: An analysis of 1014 cases. *Surgery* 1959;45:406.

82. Baker BE. Current concepts in the diagnosis and treatment of musculotendinous injuries. *Med Sci Sports Exerc* 1984;16:323.

83. Rubin SJ, Feldman F, Staron RB, et al. Magnetic resonance imaging of muscle injury. *Clin Imag* 1995;19:263.

84. Fleckenstein JL, Weatherall PT, Parkey PW, et al. Sports related muscle injuries. Evaluation with MR imaging. *Radiology* 1989;172:793.

85. Dooms GC, Fisher MR, Hricak H, et al. MR imaging of intramuscular hemorrhage. *J Comput Assist Tomogr* 1985;9:908.

86. Armstrong RB. Mechanisms of exercise induced delayed onset muscle soreness: A brief review. *Med Sci Sports Exerc* 1984;16:529.

87. Fleckenstein JL, Shellock FG. Exertional muscle injuries. Magnetic resonance evaluation. *Top Mag Res Imag* 1991;3:50.

88. Gulli B, Templeman D. Compartment syndrome of the lower extremity. *Orthop Clin North Am* 1994;25:677.

89. Scuderi GR, Scott WN, Insall JN. Injuries of the knee. In: Rockwood CA, Green DP, Bucholz RW, Heckman JD, eds. *Fractures in Adults*. Philadelphia: Lippincott–Raven 1996;2049–2052.

90. Bauer M, Jackson RW. Chondral lesions of the femoral condyles: a system of arthroscopic classification. *J Arthrosc Rel Surg* 1988;4: 97–102.

91. Graf BK, Cook DA, De Smet AA, et al. Bone bruises on magnetic resonance imaging evaluation of anterior cruciate ligament injuries. *Am J Sports Med* 1993;21:220–223.

92. Palmer I. Fractures of the upper end of the tibia. *J Bone Joint Surg [Br]* 1951;33-B:160–166.

93. Watson JT. High energy fractures of the tibial plateau. *Orthop Clin North Am* 1994;4:723–752.

94. Schatzker J, McBroom R, Bruce D. The tibial fracture: the Toronto experience 1968–1975. *Clin Orthop Rel Res* 1979;138:94–104.

95. Schulak DJ, Gunn DR. Fractures of the tibial plateaus: a review of the literature. *Clin Orthop Rel Res* 1975;109:166–177.

96. Tscherne H, Lobenhoffer P. Tibial plateau fractures: Management and expected results. *Clin Orthop Rel Res* 1993;292:87–100.

97. Moore T, Harvey P. Roentgenographic measurement of tibial plateau depression due to fracture. *J Bone Joint Surg [Am]* 1974;56:155–160.

98. Newburg AH, Greenstein R. Radiographic evaluation of tibial plateau fractures. *Radiology* 1978;126:319–323.

99. Elstrom J, Pankovich AM, Sassoon H, et al. The use of tomography in the assessment of tibial plateau fractures. *J Bone Joint Surg [Am]* 1976;58:551–555.

100. Rafii M, Firoozia H, Golimbu C, et al. Computed tomography of tibial plateau fractures. *Am J Roentgenol* 1984;142:1181–1186.

101. Barrow BA, Fajman WA, Parker LM, et al. Tibial plateau fractures: evaluation with MR imaging. *Radiographics* 1994;14:553–559.

102. Hohl M, Luck JV. Fractures of the tibial condyle. *J Bone Joint Surg* 1956;38A:1001.

103. Vangsness CT, Ghaderi B, Hohl M, et al. Arthroscopy of meniscal injuries with tibial plateau fractures. *J Bone Joint Surg [Br]* 1994; 76B:488–490.

104. Moore TM, Meyers MH, Harvey JP Jr. Collateral ligament laxity of the knee. Long term comparison between plateau fractures and normal. *J Bone Joint Surg* 1976;58A:594.

105. Delamarter RB, Hohl M, Hopp E. Ligament injuries associated with tibial plateau fractures. *Clin Orthop Rel Res* 1990;250:226–233.

106. Bennet WF, Browner B. Tibial plateau fractures: A study of associated soft tissue injuries. *J Orthop Trauma* 1994;8:183.

107. Kode L, Lieberman JM, Motta AO, et al. Evaluation of tibial plateau fractures: Efficacy of MR imaging compared with CT. *Am J Roentgenol* 1994;163:141–147.

108. Rowe PA, Wright J, Randall RL, Lynch JK, et al. Can MR imaging effectively replace diagnostic arthroscopy? *Radiology* 1992;183:335.

109. Itokazu M, Matsunaga T. Arthroscopic restoration of depressed tibial plateau fractures using bone and hydroxyapatite grafts. *Arthroscopy* 1993;9:103.

110. Jennings JE. Arthroscopic management of tibial plateau fractures. *Arthroscopy* 1985;1:160.

111. El Khoury GY, Daniel WW, Kathol M. Acute and chronic avulsive injuries. *Radiol Clin North Am* 1997;35:747–766.

112. Dietz GW, Wilcox DM, Montgomery JB. Segond tibial condyle fracture: Lateral capsular ligament avulsion. *Radiology* 1986;159: 467–469.

113. Goldman A, Pavlov H, Rubenstein D. The Segond fracture of the proximal tibia. A small avulsion that reflects major ligamentous damage. *Am J Roentgenol* 1988;151:1163.

114. Weber WN, Nuemann CH, Barakos JA, et al. Lateral tibial rim (Segond) fractures: MR imaging characteristics. *Radiology* 1991;180:731.

115. Steida A. Medial femoral condylar avulsion. *Arch Klin Chir* 1908; 85:815.

116. Meyers MH, McKeever FM. Fractures of the intercondylar eminence of the tibia. *J Bone Joint Surg* 1970;52A:1677.

117. Watson-Jones R. Injuries of the knee. In: Wilson JN, ed. *Fractures and Joint Injuries, ed 5, vol 2*. Baltimore: Williams & Wilkins, 1976; 1048.

118. Kujala UM, Kvist M, Heinonen O. Osgood Schlatter's disease in adolescent athletes. Retrospective study of incidence and duration. *Am J Sports Med* 1985;13:236–241.
119. Sinding-Larson C. A hitherto unknown application of the patella in children. *Acta Radiol* 1921;1:171.
120. Kelly DW, Carter VS, Jobe FW, Kerlane RK. Patella and quadriceps tendon ruptures. Jumper's knee. *Am J Sports Med* 1984;12:375–380.
121. Kelly DW, Godfrey KD, Johnson PH, Whiting M. Quadriceps rupture in association with roentgenographic tooth sign. A case report. *Orthopedics* 1980;3:1206–1208.
122. Carpenter JE, Kasman R, Matthews LS. Fractures of the patella. *J Bone Joint Surg* 1993;75A:1550–1561.
123. Haxton H. The function of the patella and effects of its excision. *Surg Gynecol Obstet* 1945;80:389–395.
124. Curtis MJ. Internal fixation of fracture of the patella. A comparison of two methods. *J Bone Joint Surg* 1990;72B:280–282.
125. Haajanen J, Karaharju K. Fractures of the patella. One hundred consecutive cases. *Ann Chir Gynaecol* 1981;70:32–35.
126. Cargill AO. The long term effect of the tibiofemoral compartment of the knee joint of comminuted fractures of the patella. *Injury* 1975;6:309–312.
127. Neer CS II, Grantham SA, Shelton ML. Supracondylar fracture of the adult femur. *J Bone Joint Surg* 1967;49A:591–613.
128. Stewart MJ, Sisk TD, Wallace SL Jr. Fractures of the distal third of the femur. *J Bone Joint Surg* 1966;48A:784–807.
129. Siliski JM, Mahring M, Hofer HP. Supracondylar–intercondylar fractures of the femur. *J Bone Joint Surg* 1989;71A:95–104.
130. Schatzker J, Lambert DC. Supracondylar fractures of the femur. *Clin Orthop* 1979;138:77–83.
131. Moore TM. Fracture dislocation of the knee. *Clin Orthop* 1981;156:128.
132. Green NE, Allen BL. Vascular injuries associated with dislocation of the knee. *J Bone Joint Surg* 1977;59A:236–239.
133. Jones RE. Vascular and orthopedic complications of knee dislocation. *Surg Gynecol Obstet* 1979;149:554.
134. Aichroth PM, Al-Duri Z. Dislocation and subluxation of the patella: an overview. In: Aichroth PM, Cannon WD, Disnitz M, eds. *Knee Surgery: Current Practice.* London: Martin Dunitz, 1992;354.
135. Merchant AC. Patellofemoral disorders. In: Chapman MW, ed. *Operative Orthopaedics, 2nd ed.* Philadelphia: JB Lippincott, 1993;2063.
136. Merchant AC. Radiologic evaluation of the patellofemoral joint. In: Aichroth PM, Cannon WD, Disnitz M, eds. *Knee Surgery: Current Practice.* London: Martin Dunitz, 1992;380.
137. Virolainen H, Visuri T, Kuusela T. Acute dislocation of the patella: MR findings. *Radiology* 1993;189:243.
138. Lance E, Deutsch AL, Mink JH. Prior lateral patellar dislocation. MR imaging findings. *Radiology* 1993;189:905.
139. Freiberger RH, Kotzen LM. Fracture of the medial margin of the patella: A finding diagnostic of lateral dislocation. *Radiology* 1967;88:902–904.
140. Hughston JC. Subluxation of the patella. *J Bone Joint Surg* 1968;50A:1003–1026.
141. Ahstrom JP. Osteochondral fracture in the knee joint associated with hypermobility and dislocation of the patella. *J Bone Joint Surg* 1965;47A:1491–1502.
142. Yulish BS, et al. Chondromalacia patellae: assessment with MR imaging. *Radiology* 1987;164:763.
143. Nelation A. *Elements de Pathologie Chirurgicale, vol. 2.* Paris: Librairie Germer Balliere, 1874;282.
144. Sijbeardij S. Instability of the proximal tibiofibular joint. *Acta Orthop Scand* 1978;49:621–626.
145. Burman MS. Subluxation of the head of the fibula. *Am J Surg* 1931;11:108.

CHAPTER 7

The Pelvis and Hip

Stephen J. Eustace

Conventional radiographs yield an accurate diagnosis in most patients with trauma to the pelvis and hip. In a minority, additional evaluation is undertaken, either to evaluate subtle abnormality or to provide a detailed roadmap before surgical intervention. Traditionally, additional imaging has involved the integrated use of computed tomography, arthrography, and scintigraphy.

Axially acquired images at CT improve evaluation of the posterior pelvis and acetabulum and enhance the detection of complicating genitourinary and vascular injury. Scintigraphy has traditionally been employed to supplement radiographic examination of patients with suspected fractures occult to radiographic detection. Arthrography is less frequently employed to detect either labral injury or intra-articular loose bodies.

This chapter outlines techniques, applications, and evolving uses of MR imaging as an alternative or supplement to established techniques employed to evaluate patients with acute pelvic injury.

S. J. Eustace: Department of Radiology, Section of Musculoskeletal Radiology, Boston University School of Medicine and Boston Medical Center, Boston, Massachusetts 02118.

PATIENT POSITIONING AND IMAGING PROTOCOLS

Positioning

Effective MR imaging of the pelvis is usually performed supine, although hip or flank hematoma may necessitate imaging in an oblique or decubitus plane.

Receiver Coil

In most patients, the pelvis is successfully imaged using the body coil. With the body coil and large field of view, signal-rich images allowing simultaneous evaluation of both hips may be obtained with a single excitation, and the large field of view permits the image matrix to be increased to 512 by 512, allowing improved resolution without discernible alteration in image signal to noise. Although a smaller field of view would further improve spatial resolution, images acquired in this way with the body coil are noisy and lack signal.

With locally applied surface coils, high-resolution, signal-rich images may be obtained; however, coverage is often limited. Dedicated phased-array surface coils facilitate the acquisition of signal-rich, high-resolution images with extended coverage.

Imaging Plane

Routine imaging of pelvic trauma is achieved in direct coronal, sagittal, and axial planes; coronal and sagittal images are prescribed off an axial localizer, and axial images are prescribed off a coronal localizer.

When occult hip fracture is suspected, diagnosis is usually made from a single coronal acquisition. Fragment position and number may be determined by additional axial and sagittal acquisitions.

Evaluation of the acetabulum using a localized surface coil is achieved by imaging in sagittal oblique (parallel to a line drawn between the free margins of the anterior and posterior columns), coronal oblique (perpendicular to the sagittal images), and axial planes.

Field of View

Simultaneous evaluation of both hips is usually achieved using a 30- to 35-cm field of view. High-resolution images of individual hips, using a phased-array surface coil, are obtained using a 14-cm field of view. (Recently developed extended phased-array coils now allow simultaneous evaluation of both hips.)

Slice Thickness

Contiguous 3-mm slices allow detailed evaluation of both bony and soft tissue abnormalities in the coronal plane. In the sagittal plane, extended coverage is yielded by increasing slice thickness to 5 mm and incorporating an interslice gap up to 5 mm. Axial images are acquired in 3-mm contiguous slices.

Motion Suppression

Motion is generally not a source of image degradation in the pelvis, particularly when images are acquired in the standard supine plane.

In infants referred with suspected slipped capital femoral epiphyses, imaging is achieved using chloral hydrate sedation (75 mg/kg up to 10 kg weight, 50 mg/kg for weight above 10 kg).

Imaging Protocol

Patients referred following pelvic trauma are routinely imaged with a 35-cm field of view.

Initial imaging is performed in the coronal plane using a fat-suppressed sequence, using either frequency-selective fat saturation or T1-based inversion recovery. With inversion recovery, fat suppression is obtained with an inversion time of 160 msec (at 1.5 T). In such a way, a 90° excitatory pulse (with a 180° refocusing pulse) is applied 160 msec following an initial 180° inverting pulse. Signal is obtained with a repetition time of 2,000 msec and an echo time of 20 msec, an echo train length of six, and a low-high k-space mapping profile. When extended coverage is required, repetition time may be increased incrementally, increasing the number of excited slices, although this results in a slight increase in the total acquisition time. In patients referred with suspected occult fracture, imaging is limited to a coronal inversion recovery and TSE T1 sequences.

Turbo spin-echo T1 imaging, similar to that in all other joints, is achieved using a repetition time of 500 msec, an echo time of 15 msec, a short echo train of up to six, and a low-high echo to view the k-space mapping profile. Use of a short echo train facilitates the use of a short repetition time, enhancing T1 weighting and further decreasing acquisition time.

If a fracture is identified, manifest as a hypointense line, additional sagittal and axial images are acquired using the turbo TSE T1 sequence.

Following pelvic trauma, hip fracture, or surgery, two-dimensional (2D) time-of-flight venographic images are occasionally acquired in order to exclude deep pelvic vein thrombosis. These images are acquired following the placement of an arterial saturation band above the pelvis. Venographic images are acquired in the axial plane using a short TR of approximately 30 msec, a short out-of-phase TE of 6.9 msec, and a T1-weighted flip angle of 50°. Individual source images are reconstructed to generate a diagnostic venogram using a MIP reconstruction algorithm. It is important to review individual axial source images rather than the reconstructed data before formulating a diagnosis.

To avoid in-plane saturation effects, time-of-flight arterial images may be enhanced by using an intravenous bolus of gadolinium (40 cc of gadolinium dimeglumine), a short TR of 7 msec, an out-of-phase TE of 2.3 msec, and a flip angle of 60° following the placement of an inferior saturation band to eliminate signal from venous flow. Gadolinium-enhanced images are acquired in the coronal plane, unlike axially acquired unenhanced images.

When a child is referred with suspected slipped capital femoral epiphysis, images are generated using a coronal turbo inversion recovery sequence and a T2-weighted fast field- or gradient-echo sequence with off-resonance magnetization transfer saturation. $T2^*$ weighting is achieved with a low flip angle of 30°, a long repetition time of 500 msec, and an echo time of 15 msec. With this technique, articular cartilage becomes hypointense relative to adjacent synovial fluid, partially saturated by the off-resonance pulse, allowing improved visualization of the unossified growth plate.

In most patients, images are acquired with a matrix of 256 phase-encoded steps (although 512 may be employed when both hips are imaged with a large field of view). Adequate image signal is obtained with two excitations.

Magnetic resonance arthrography with a single contrast injection to the hip joint space improves visibility of articular

TABLE 1. *Imaging protocol following trauma to the hip*

Sequence	Image plane	FOV	TR	TE	ETL	Mapping scheme
Occult or documented fracture evaluation						
IR TSE	Cor direct	14	2000	20	6	Linear
TSE T-1	Cor direct	14	500	15	4	Low-High
+ or − additional planes						
Pediatric growth plate injury						
T-2 FFE	Multiple planes	14	500	15		With off resonance MT

cartilage and may improve the evaluation of patients with suspected labral tears. When this is done, 4 to 5 cc of a gadolinium, 1% lidocaine, and renografin solution is injected directly into the hip joint space using a 22-gauge needle (0.1 ml of gadolinium DTPA to 5 ml of 1% lidocaine and 15 cc of renografin 60). T1-weighted images are subsequently drained in three planes with fat saturation (Table 1).

MAGNETIC RESONANCE IMAGING OF SOFT TISSUE INJURY FOLLOWING ACUTE TRAUMA

Labral Tears

The acetabular labrum represents a discontinuous semilunar ring of fibrocartilage marginating the anterior, superolateral, and posterior columns of the acetabulum. The inferior margins of the acetabulum are bridged by the transverse acetabular ligament. The fibrocartilaginous labrum is triangular in cross section, is most frequently inverted in orientation, and is usually thicker posterosuperiorly than anteroinferiorly reflecting its function to provide stability and prevent subluxation (Fig. 1). The synovial lined capsule of the hip joint arises from bone adjacent to the outer attachment of the labrum. In such a way, a sulcus, termed the paralabral sulcus, is created between the labrum and capsule, lined by synovium, from which vascularity to the labrum is derived.

Articular hyaline cartilage extends to the inner or medial margin of the labrum but does not extend between the labrum and underlying bone (1,2). The junction of the articular cartilage and the fibrocartilage may be mistaken for a partial tear.

Following injury, in most cases posterior hip subluxation or dislocation, the labrum becomes torn or detached. Affected patients present with pain, impaired motion, and clicking, accentuated by hip flexion and rotation (3). Although complete detachment of the labrum may be identified at computed tomography (particularly when associated with posterior column avulsed fractures) (4), reproducible evaluation of the labrum can only be undertaken at MRI (5) (Fig. 2).

With MRI, imaging may be performed with or without intra-articular contrast. Under ideal circumstances, imaging is performed with a dedicated phased-array flexible surface coil allowing signal-rich high-resolution images with a 14- to 18-cm field of view (6). Following trauma, examination is usually with a larger field of view, as injury to the hip is often accompanied by further injuries to the pelvis.

Without intra-articular contrast, optimum imaging and detection of labral tears is achieved with T2* weighting. In such a way, any joint fluid is hyperintense, articular cartilage is isointense, and labrum is dark or hypointense. Tears are diagnosed on the basis of signal abnormality, linear signal hyperintensity, or on the basis of altered morphology, an absent labrum, or an abnormal labral configuration. The presence of subchondral cystic change adjacent to or below the labrum is often associated with labral abnormality and should trigger additional scrutiny (6).

When employed, MR arthrography is performed using a 4 to 5 cc of a gadolinium, 1% lidocaine, and renografin solution introduced into the hip joint space using a 22-gauge needle (0.1 ml of gadolinium DTPA to 5 ml of 1% lidocaine and 15 cc of renografin 60). Intra-articular contrast improves visualization of the labrum, the appearance of which is enhanced by distension of the sublabral sulcus. In such a way, the position, morphology (including the presence of surface irregularities), and signal characteristics of the labrum may be identified.

Magnetic resonance arthrography also facilitates the detection of loose bodies following hip trauma, although CT is often favored when this diagnosis is suspected (7).

Pitfalls

Morphologic variants in the configuration of the labrum (like the glenoid labrum) may lead to diagnostic error. In a study of 200 asymptomatic volunteers, the labrum was triangular in shape in two-thirds of patients, round in 10%, flat in 10%, and absent in 14%, and variations increased with age (2).

Variations in intralabral signal correlate poorly with histologic evidence of degeneration. Although some authors conclude that cartilage does not extend beneath the labrum and that linear signal at this site indicates a tear, Petersilge and colleagues report that cartilage may extend beneath the labrum and that discrimination between sublabral cartilage and tear can be made accurately only by using intra-articular gadolinium-enhanced arthrography (5).

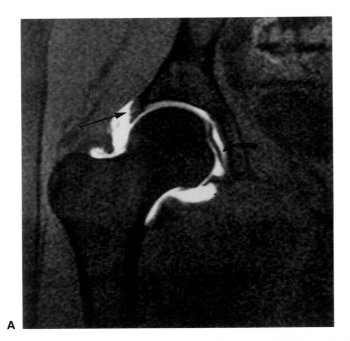

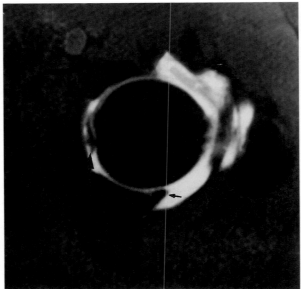

FIG. 1. (A) Coronal conventional T1-weighted spin-echo image with frequency-selective fat suppression following direct gadolinium arthrography shows normal triangular-shaped labrum with contrast outlining the paralabral sulcus *(straight arrow)* and demonstrating the ligamentum teres extending to the fovea centralis *(curved arrow).* **(B)** Sagittal image shows triangular-shaped anterior and posterior *(arrows)* labral margins. **(C)** Axial image shows ligamentum teres in the cotyloid fossa *(arrow),* with dominant posterior labrum *(small arrow).*

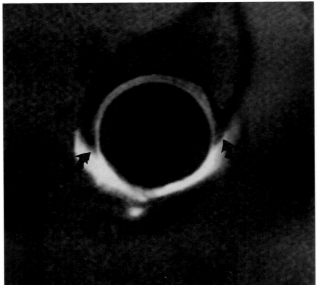

Muscle Injury

Muscle injury around the hip joint is relatively common and is frequently identified in athletes, usually as part of an overuse syndrome. Injury usually involves one of three muscle groups, the quadriceps, the adductors, or the hamstrings.

The Quadriceps

Injury or tear of the rectus femoris is frequently seen in kicking sports, less frequently in sprinters. Although the ex-

tent of injury is variable, injury is usually manifest by the presence of local edema on T2-weighted or fat-suppressed images. In most cases, injury follows minor trauma and is characterized by local edema corresponding to a site of focal tenderness (8). Less frequently, injury is more severe and is characterized by partial or complete disruption of muscle fibers. Grade 1 injury is characterized by local muscle edema and hemorrhage without a significant change in morphology. Grade 2 injury is characterized by partial tear of up to 50% of tendon fibers. Grade 3 injury is characterized by near-complete rupture with or without retraction (9). Following injury, hemorrhage and edema may become localized with

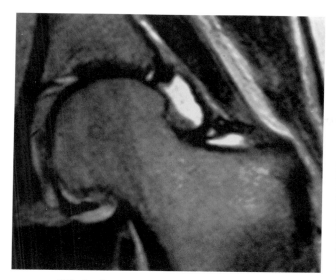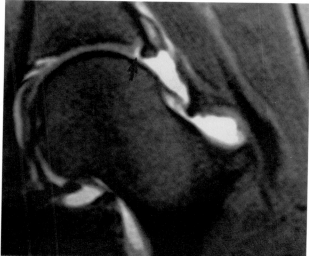

FIG. 2. Coronal fat-suppressed images show truncation of and signal abnormality within the posterosuperior labrum, with contrast interdigitating between it and the underlying acetabular margin *(arrow)* at a site of tear, proven at arthroscopy. (Courtesy of Arthur Newberg, M.D., New England Baptist Hospital, MA.)

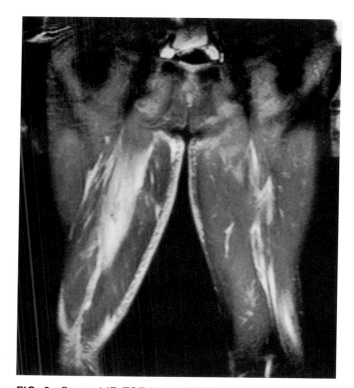

FIG. 3. Coronal IR TSE image (TI 160 msec, TE 20 msec, TR 2,000 msec) shows diffuse hemorrhage and edema within the muscle belly of the semimembranosus or hamstring in a young athlete.

capsular or pseudocyst formation. Hypointense fibrous encasement may occur in chronicity, resulting in a pseudotumor appearance. Susceptibility blooming on gradient-echo sequences (within the hematoma) and lack of internal enhancement allow differentiation from a true tumor (10).

Hamstring Muscle Injuries

Hamstring injuries are common in professional athletes and are characterized by tear, most frequently at the proximal musculotendinous junction (11) (Fig. 3). Partial tear results in local hemorrhage and edema, which are acutely hyperintense on T2-weighted scans but become hyperintense on both T1- and T2-weighted scans when subacute.

Intramuscular Hematoma

Intramuscular hematomas may be spontaneous, complicate trauma (secondary to insulin injections in diabetics), or complicate iatrogenic administration of anticoagulants.

Following a fall or following reduction of posterior hip dislocation, hematomas are frequently identified in the buttocks. Poorly monitored anticoagulant therapy may result in spontaneous retroperitoneal hemorrhage, usually sited in the psoas but occasionally sited in the iliacus tracking to the thigh (12).

Magnetic Resonance Imaging of Repetitive Hip Trauma

Snapping Hip Syndrome

Snapping hip syndrome is the term used to describe a snapping sensation encountered in the region of the hip as the

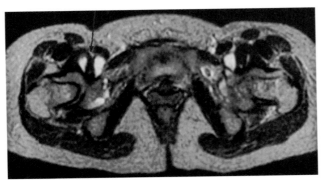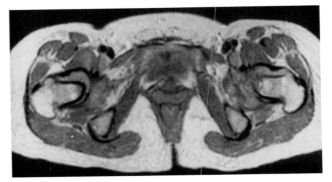

FIG. 4. Axial proton density (right) and T2-weighted images of the hips in a patient with snapping hip syndrome with bilateral iliopsoas bursae bridged by the iliopsoas tendons (more marked on the left) (arrow).

iliopsoas tendon passes over and catches on the ileopectineal eminence of the pubis, usually associated with iliopsoas bursal inflammation (Fig. 4). Infrequently, the snapping hip syndrome is attributed to a catching of the iliofemoral ligaments as they slide over the femoral head in flexion-extension or to a snapping of the long head of the biceps as it slides over the ischial tuberosity on flexion-extension (13).

Trochanteric Bursitis

Occasionally the trochanteric bursa becomes inflamed by friction and trauma imposed by the repetitive motion of the iliotibial band or tensor fascia latae sliding over the greater trochanter during active sports. In chronicity, induced bursal inflammation may result in marked bursal distension (14).

MAGNETIC RESONANCE IMAGING OF OSSEOUS INJURY FOLLOWING ACUTE TRAUMA

Pelvic Ring Fractures

The pelvis is a ring structure composed of integrated osseous and ligamentous structures. The osseous ring is composed of the sacrum, the ilium, the ischium, and the pubis. A ring configuration affords stability disrupted only following acutely applied forces in the vertical, lateral or anteroposterior planes, or a combination of all three (15–17) (Fig. 5). Fractures of the pelvis are classified as stable, in which the ring structure is not disrupted (avulsion injuries), or unstable, in which the inner ring is disrupted and injury is aggravated by persistent weight bearing.

Unstable Pelvic Ring Injuries

Lateral compression results in acute pelvic implosion with injury to the pelvis both anteriorly and posteriorly, typically transverse pubic rami fractures and sacral compression fractures (concertina in configuration) (see Fig. 5B). Anteroposterior compression occurs as a result of forces applied anteriorly or as a result of compression

applied through impacting lower extremities. Such forces result in symphyseal diastasis with dislocations in the posterior pelvis (see Fig. 5C,D). Vertical forces result in shear to the pelvis with vertical rami fractures, vertical symphyseal diastasis, sacroiliac joint disruption, and malgaigre fracture (see Fig. 5A). Vertical shear injuries are often associated with soft tissue injuries including arterial lacerations of the internal iliac vessels (18–20). Conventional radiographs facilitate routine evaluation of osseous injury, although evaluation of sacrum and sacroiliac joints is often limited. Computed tomography is routinely employed to supplement evaluation in the axial plane, particularly to improve evaluation of the sacroiliac joints (21). Magnetic resonance imaging in the axial plane affords similar evaluation of the sacrum and sacroiliac joints, although it is currently rarely employed for this purpose. Sensitivity to marrow edema may improve detection of undisplaced fractures (Fig. 6) and may allow concomi-

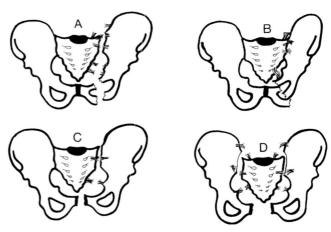

FIG. 5. Diagrammatic representation of pelvic fractures by mechanism: (A) ipsilateral Malgaigne fracture secondary to vertical shear; (B) horizontal rami fractures with impaction secondary to lateral compression; (C) symphyseal diastasis secondary to anteroposterior compression; (D) symphyseal and bilateral sacroiliac joint diastasis (open book type) secondary to anteroposterior compression.

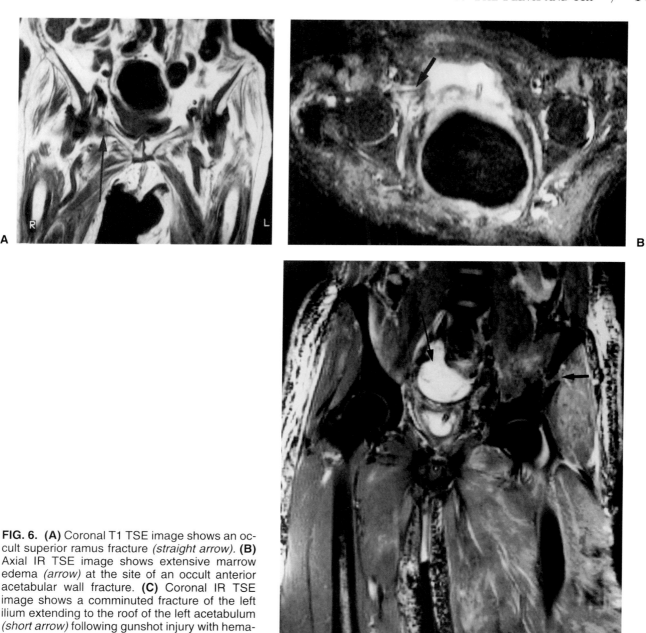

FIG. 6. (A) Coronal T1 TSE image shows an occult superior ramus fracture *(straight arrow)*. **(B)** Axial IR TSE image shows extensive marrow edema *(arrow)* at the site of an occult anterior acetabular wall fracture. **(C)** Coronal IR TSE image shows a comminuted fracture of the left ilium extending to the roof of the left acetabulum *(short arrow)* following gunshot injury with hematoma deep to the left iliacus and free fluid in the pouch of Douglas (straight arrow).

tant evaluation of soft tissue (bladder) and vascular structures.

Stable Pelvic Ring Injuries: Avulsions and Coccygeal Injuries

The musculotendinous unit is composed of a muscle belly that attaches either directly to bone or indirectly through an inelastic tendon. Trauma may induce injury to any part of the unit, compression resulting in contusion, tension resulting in eccentric contraction, muscle strain or tear in tendon rupture or avulsion from bone.

Before growth plate closure, the apophysis, the site of attachment of tendon to bone, is the weakest point in the musculotendinous unit and is the most frequent site of injury following acutely applied tensile forces (22). In maturity, following growth plate closure, tensile forces result in tear either at the musculotendinous junction (usually a site of poor vascular perfusion) or in the muscle belly itself. Injury to or weakening of the tendon following intratendinous steroid injection or as a result of peritendinous inflammation (bursitis) may lead to intrasubstance tendon rupture. Following long-term anabolic steroid therapy, abnormal muscle bulk places intolerable strain on the tendon during contraction of the muscle belly, producing a similar outcome, tendon rupture (23).

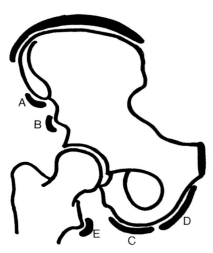

FIG. 7. Diagrammatic representation of sites of pelvic avulsion fractures: **(A)** sartorius; **(B)** rectus femoris; **(C)** hamstrings; **(D)** adductors; **(E)** Iliopsoas muscles. Adapted from El-Khoury et al. (63).

In the pelvis, apophyses appear later than epiphyseal centers in long bones, and so avulsions tend to occur after adolescence (Fig. 7).

Ischial Avulsions

The ischial tuberosity is the site of insertion of the conjoined tendon of the hamstrings and is the most common site of pelvic avulsion fracture. Repeated rapid contraction of the muscle belly in athletes (hurdlers) or an acute contraction as an athlete attempts to maintain stability as he or she slides or hyperflexes at the hip is transmitted to the ischial apophysis, resulting in avulsion. Acute undisplaced injury usually heals over 6 weeks to 3 months if immobilized. Displaced acute avulsions are usually treated by surgical internal fixation with excellent results. Injury as a result of chronic or repetitive trauma may produce local remodeling or osseous overgrowth as repeated attempts at healing are thwarted by further trauma. Callus superimposed on callus may lead to gross bony spur formation at the site of trauma in maturity, occasionally resulting in sciatic nerve compression (24).

Displaced avulsion fractures are easily recognized on conventional radiographs. Magnetic resonance imaging is of value in undisplaced avulsions: the sensitivity of fat-suppressed sequences to marrow edema allows ready identification in the coronal, sagittal, and axial planes (25).

Occasionally, chronic avulsions are associated with bone and soft tissue edema and irregularity and may mimic osteomyelitis. Chronic ischial hamstring avulsions are frequently identified in patients with spastic paraparesis, in whom chronic flexion contractures at the hips result in persistent hamstring traction (26) (Figs. 8 and 9).

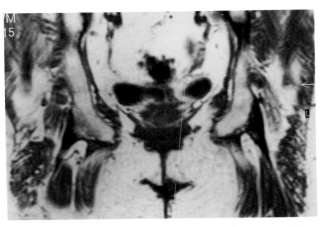

FIG. 8. Coronal T1-weighted image showing normal hamstring insertions bilaterally.

Pubic Ramus Avulsions

The adductor longus, magnus, and brevis insert on the pubic rami, at the junction of the inferior ramus and the symphysis. Repeated or acute traction may result in avulsion with osseous irregularity at this site (Fig. 10). Although it is usually self-evident, osseous irregularity may be misinterpreted as being caused by a malignant tumor, most frequently Ewing's sarcoma (27). Biopsy should not be undertaken without a detailed review, as biopsy of marginal callus, secondary to attempted healing, may present tissue indistinguishable from a malignant osseous sarcoma. Scintigraphy typically reveals focal accumulation of radiotracer at the site of avulsions, a focal hot spot. In this setting, MR imaging may be misleading, revealing extensive edema within both

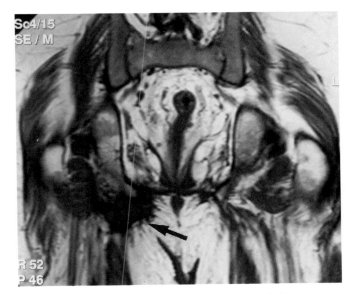

FIG. 9. Coronal T1-weighted image showing inflammatory change at the insertion of the hamstring on the right *(arrow)* in a patient with spastic quadriparesis and chronic hamstring avulsion injury.

bone and soft tissues. Avulsion should be suspected when edema or enhancement tracks along the adductors (28). Although acute avulsions are associated with minimal focal edema in the ramus, repetitive trauma may produce more marked or diffuse bone bruising or edema (see Fig. 10).

The presence of multiple avulsions in the same patient is uncommon although well described, presumably because athletes cease activity as a result of the incurred pain (29). Nevertheless, societal emphasis on exercise may lead to more frequent recognition of avulsions, such as occurs following the use of stairmaster exercise equipment.

Iliac Spine Avulsions

Iliac spine avulsions occur more commonly superiorly at the insertion of the sartorius and tensor fascia lata (ASIS) than inferiorly at the insertion of the rectus femoris (AIIS), which tends to be less symptomatic (Fig. 11). Unlike avulsions in the ischial tuberosity, reflecting vascularity (red marrow), avulsions of the iliac spine usually heal without intervention (30).

Lesser and Greater Trochanteric Avulsions

Avulsions are occasionally identified at the insertion of the iliopsoas on the lesser trochanter and at the insertion of the glutei, particularly in athletes involved in jumping or kicking (Fig. 12).

Coccygeal Injuries

The coccyx usually consists of four fused vertebral bodies, rudimentary in nature without laminae and with few processes. The most cephalad segment articulates via a small disk with the caudad portion of the sacrum and has articulating processes projecting upward to unite with the sacral cornua via ligaments (31).

As a result of position and delicacy, the coccyx is com-

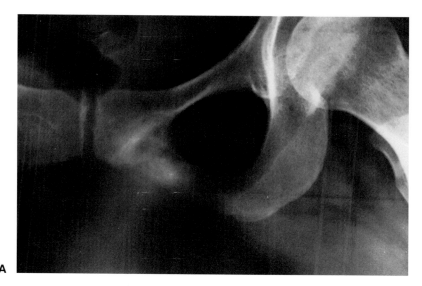

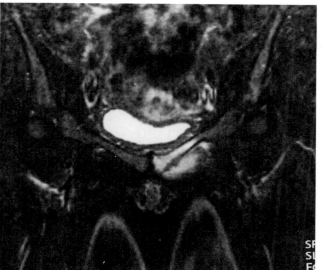

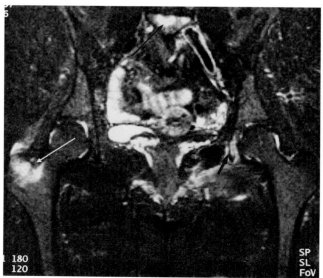

FIG. 10. (A) Radiograph shows lytic destruction at the insertion of the adductor muscle, mimicking aggressive tumor. (B) This IR TSE image shows extensive marrow edema through the superior pubic ramus and extending to the adductor compartment, suggesting avulsion injury. (C) Another IR TSE image in the same patient showing additional marrow edema in the right greater trochanter extending to the glutei, with trace edema in the left acetabulum and in the superior end plate of L5. History revealed daily exercise regimen on a Stairmaster machine. (Courtesy of S. Valentine, M.D., Calgary, Alberta.)

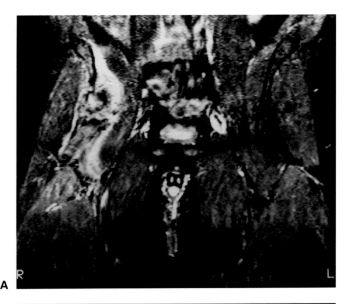

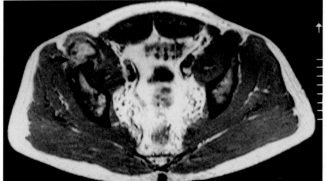

FIG. 11. (A) Coronal IR TSE image of a patient referred with a suspected tumor shows edema tracking to the muscle belly of the rectus femoris muscle on the right. (B,C) Axial proton density and fast field-echo images show avulsion of bony fragments from the anterior inferior iliac spine by the rectus femoris muscle, mimicking soft tissue mass (arrows).

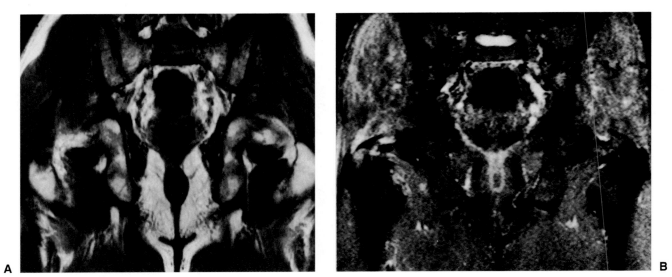

FIG. 12. Coronal TSE T1 (A) and IR TSE (B) images show edema in the right greater trochanter extending to the glutei secondary to avulsion injury.

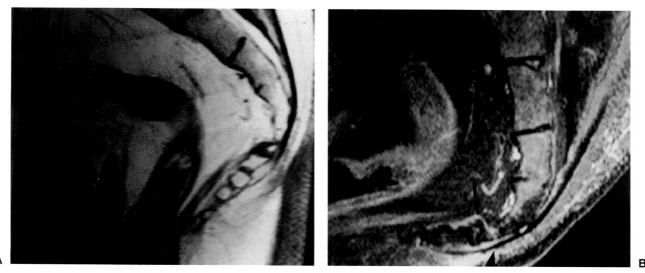

FIG. 13. Sagittal TSE T1 **(A)** and IR TSE **(B)** images show an occult fracture of the coccyx manifest by marrow edema and step-off *(arrow)* in a patient presenting with posttraumatic coccydynia.

monly injured following a direct blow as occurs following a fall on the buttocks. The coccyx is poorly visualized on both anteroposterior and lateral conventional radiographs as a result of overlying soft tissues. At scintigraphy, focal accumulation of radiotracer may be identified in the region of the coccyx, but anatomic resolution is poor. Despite tomographic imaging at computed tomography, injuries to the coccyx are poorly evaluated in this way, as images are acquired in the axial plane, and the orientation of the coccyx is variable.

Direct sagittal imaging and sensitivity of MR images to edema allow optimal evaluation and detection of coccygeal injury, ranging from contusion through fracture to dislocation (Fig. 13). Although management of coccygeal injury is usually conservative, accurate diagnosis is often important

in the trauma setting, as the injury may have medicolegal implications.

Acetabular Fractures

The acetabulum is composed of an anterior column, superior column, posterior column, and roof (quadrilateral plate). Injury to the acetabulum, most frequently secondary to femoral head impaction, usually involves the posterior column, less frequently the roof. Injury to the anterior column is less common but usually occurs complicating extension of a ramus fracture (32) (Fig. 14). Fractures are generally identified on conventional radiographs, supplemented by oblique Judet views, on the basis of integrity of six acetabular lines (Fig. 15). Computed tomography is undertaken in these inju-

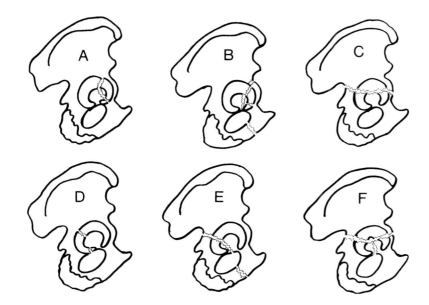

FIG. 14. Diagrammatic representation of acetabular fractures: **(A)** anterior wall fracture; **(B)** anterior column fracture; **(C)** horizontal fracture; **(D)** posterior wall fracture; **(E)** posterior column fracture; **(F)** T-shaped acetabular fracture.

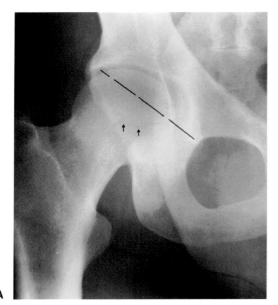

A

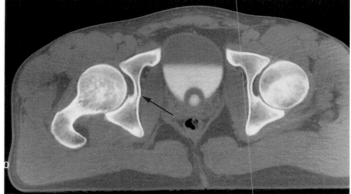

B

FIG. 15. (A) Oblique view of the right acetabulum (Judet view) to improve visualization of the posterior column shows a transverse fracture *(arrows)* extending through the posterior column. *Interrupted line* indicates the anterior margin of the anterior column. **(B)** Axial CT scan of the same patient: 2-mm slice thickness shows subtle step-off in the quadrilateral plate *(arrow)*. **(C)** Coronal TSE T1 image (1 min 5 sec acquisition) shows a transverse fracture extending through the posterior wall of the acetabulum *(arrow)*. Coronal oblique **(D)** and axial **(E)** T1-weighted images in another patient show oblique fracture through the roof of the acetabulum **(D,** *arrow)* and through the posterior wall **(E,** *arrow)*.

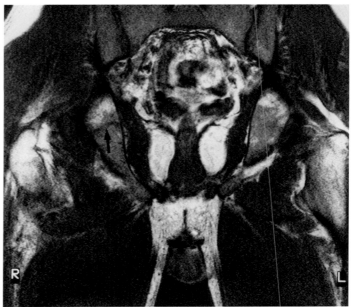

C

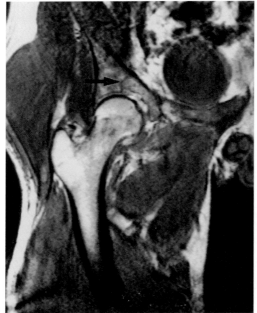

D

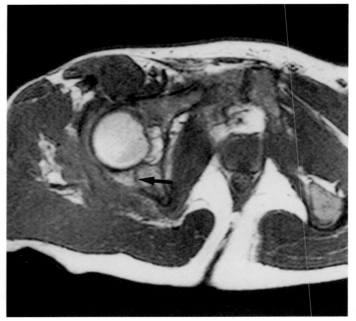

E

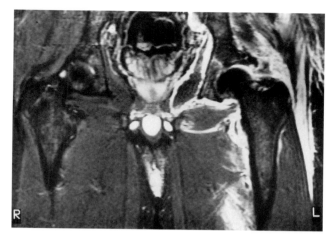

FIG. 16. Coronal IR TSE image shows an occult acetabular fracture (left hip) with extensive hemorrhage and edema in a patient referred with a suspected subcapital fracture of the proximal femur.

ries to provide tomographic evaluation of fracture position, to accurately detect amount of articular margin step-off (more than 2 mm is generally treated surgically) and to evaluate for associated loose intra-articular fragments (33). When fractures are in the axial plane, computed tomography may be misleading. In-plane fracture phenomena may lead to fractures actually being obscured (see Fig. 15A,B). Because they are not visualized in the source data, they are therefore not identified in subsequent reconstructions popularized by referring orthopedists. The ability to image in multiple planes using MRI reduces the likelihood of in-plane fracture obscuration, and sensitivity to edema allows detection of undisplaced injuries (Figs. 16 and 17).

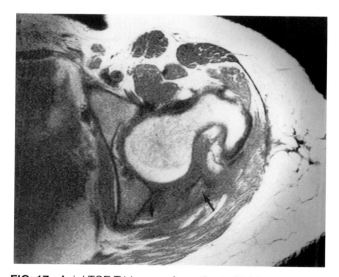

FIG. 17. Axial TSE T1 image of a patient with hip pain following motor vehicle accident shows a displaced fracture of the posterior wall with truncation of the osseous margins of the posterior acetabulum (arrows).

Trauma to the Proximal Femur

Posttraumatic Bone Marrow Edema Syndrome

Occasionally, following trauma, patients present with hip pain in the absence of a discernible fracture on conventional radiographs. When MR imaging is undertaken, images show diffuse femoral head and neck edema without a hypointense line, as is seen in occult fractures (34) (Fig. 18). Affected patients may develop radiographic demineralization before spontaneous resolution. It is unclear whether the observed bone marrow edema represents simple femoral head contusion and microtrabecular trauma or whether it represents a variant of reflex sympathetic dystrophy, with hyperemia-induced demineralization and neurogenic pain (35).

Similar marrow edema may be seen in patients with early avascular necrosis secondary to impaired venous drainage or in patients with transient migratory osteoporosis. Transient migratory osteoporosis was originally described in women in the third trimester, in whom it invariably involved the left hip, but is now more commonly identified in men, in whom it may be bilateral.

Magnetic resonance images are nonspecific and are characterized by extensive poorly marginated edema in each circumstance, hypointense on T1 and hyperintense on T2 and STIR images (36).

Fractures of the Proximal Femur

Fractures of the proximal femur are classified as intra- or extra-articular. Intra-articular fractures involve the femoral head and neck, typically at the head–neck junction, termed subcapital, or midneck, termed transcervical. Intra-articular fractures may disrupt vascular supply to the femoral head via the circumflex vessels. Extra-articular fractures are classified as intertrochanteric or subtrochanteric. Stability of these fractures is dictated by the obliquity or axis of the fracture (37).

Garden's classification is widely employed to grade femoral neck fractures. It describes the relative displacement of

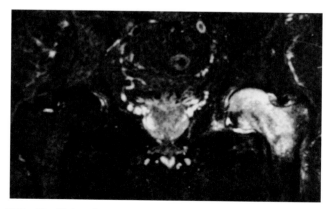

FIG. 18. Extensive posttraumatic edema in the left femoral head without a fracture, 8 weeks following injury, secondary to transient osteoporosis complicating hip trauma.

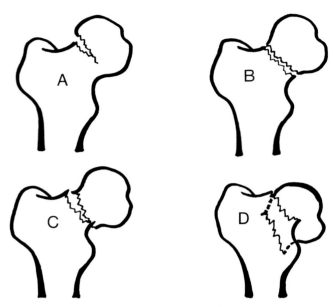

FIG. 19. Diagrammatic representation of Garden's classification of fractures of the femoral neck: **(A)** incomplete subcapital fracture; **(B)** complete undisplaced subcapital fracture; **(C)** minimally displaced complete subcapital fracture; **(D)** markedly displaced complete subcapital fracture.

fracture fragment and hence the relative risk of subsequent development of avascular necrosis of the femoral head (38) (Fig. 19).

Occult Fracture Detection

The multiplanar imaging capability and improved contrast afforded by MR imaging facilitates its use in the detection of fractures undetected by conventional radiographs. Fractures in the region of the hip are reported to account for 30% of all fractures requiring hospitalization in the United States and almost half of the bed occupancy attributed to a fracture (39). Although femoral neck fractures are usually identified following review of plain film radiographs, undisplaced (Garden type 1 and 2) fractures may remain occult without further imaging. Undisplaced fractures may be particularly difficult to detect in elderly osteopenic patients in whom minor alterations in trabecular alignment resulting from fracture may be harder to perceive and hence remain undetected. Patients with recognized undisplaced femoral neck fractures require acute admission from the emergency room and early screw fixation in most cases. Patients with unrecognized fractures continue to bear weight as much as is tolerable following discharge until finally fracture fragments displace with drastic consequence. In one study of 38 patients with delayed diagnosis, seven of nine patients with displaced fractures developed either avascular necrosis or nonunion following delayed operative intervention (40).

In the past, authors have advocated the use of nuclear scintigraphy to detect these fractures on the premise that early osteoblastic reaction at fracture margins results in focal linear accumulation of radiopharmaceuticals at that site (41). Although computed tomography, by allowing multiplanar evaluation, improves the detection of these fractures, MR imaging is both more sensitive and specific.

Magnetic resonance imaging facilitates immediate detection of undisplaced fractures, manifest as a hypointense fracture line surrounded by adjacent edema (Fig. 20). In contrast, uptake of a radiopharmaceutical (^{99m}Tc-MDP) at nuclear scintigraphy mirrors osteoblastic response at fracture margins, which may be delayed in the elderly and only begin to occur as late as 72 hr following injury. Poor accumulation of radiotracer has previously been reported in patients with congestive heart failure, chronic renal failure (impaired excretion decreasing the soft tissue to target bone ratio), and in the elderly, in whom blood supply to the femoral head is markedly reduced even in health (42). The improved contrast resolution afforded by MR imaging improves the detection of marrow edema at the site of fracture, which is not radiographically detectable at computed tomography.

Although marrow edema accompanying a fracture has been observed to clear within months, bone scintiscans may remain positive for up to 2 years as a result of posttraumatic vascular recruitment (43).

Magnetic resonance imaging is favored in preference to scintigraphy, as it is equally sensitive, more specific, and because it allows immediate diagnosis. An MRI of a patient with a suspected fracture facilitates either early intervention or discharge from the emergency room, limiting not only patient morbidity but also the costs of a protracted hospital stay. In contrast to scintigraphy, MR imaging not only allows specific characterization of the fracture type but also the axis of the fracture, allowing optimal surgical planning. Although the American College of Radiology recommends a single coronal T1-weighted scan to evaluate patients with suspected femoral neck fractures (44), most combine evaluation using both a coronal T1 and fat-suppressed image, such as achieved using STIR. Additional sequences contribute little to the overall time of study, which is predominantly dictated by the time taken to get the patient on and off the scan table.

Bogost et al. have emphasized the prevalence of additional unsuspected fractures of the pelvis in patients referred with suspected femoral neck fractures, additional unsuspected fractures being identified in 27% in their study (45) (see Fig. 16).

Pathologic Fractures

Pathologic fractures are suspected when fracture occurs through bone either in the absence of or following minor trauma (secondary to either tumor infiltration or abnormal bone mineralization, termed *insufficiency fracture*), or when fracture union is delayed despite appropriate fixation.

When pathologic fracture is suspected, MR imaging allows definitive evaluation, either confirming or excluding the presence of tumor deposit, allowing evaluation of tumor extent before surgical resection or fixation, and occasionally can be used to evaluate the total body and search for the presence of an unknown primary tumor (Figs. 21 and 22).

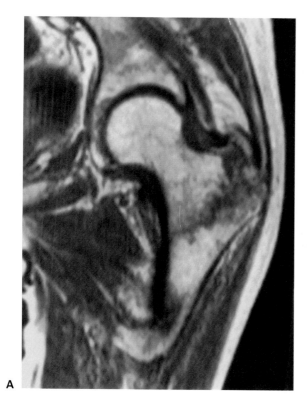

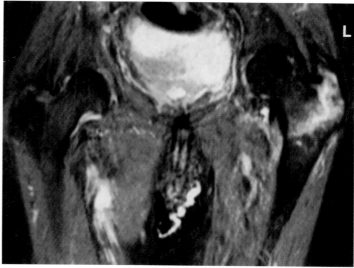

A

FIG. 20. **(A)** This TSE T1 image shows an oblique intertrochanteric fracture through the proximal shaft of the left femur (1 min acquisition). **(B)** The IR TSE image shows extensive marrow edema at the site of fracture (2 min acquisition).

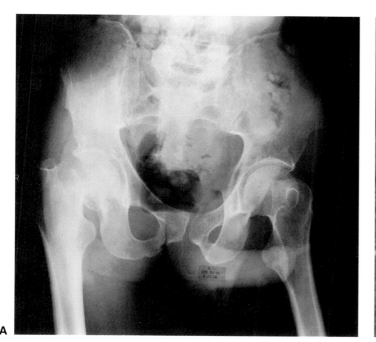

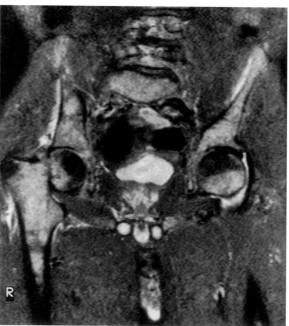

A

B

FIG. 21. **(A)** Frontal radiograph shows a fracture of the right proximal femur. **(B)** Coronal IR TSE image in the same patient shows diffuse marrow replacement secondary to multiple myeloma.

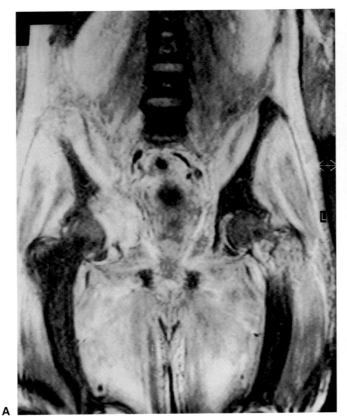

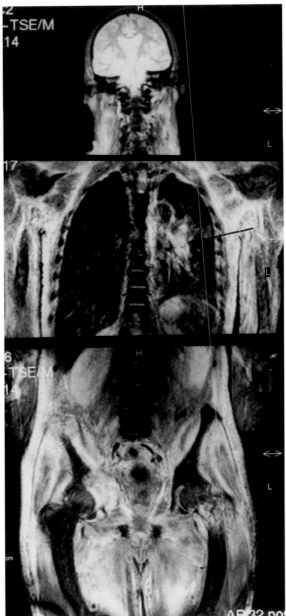

FIG. 22. (A) Coronal IR TSE image shows a pathologic fracture through metastatic deposit in the left hip, with further deposits in the right acetabulum and ilium. **(B)** Whole-body IR TSE image shows an occult lung tumor in the apical segment of the left lower lobe *(arrow)*.

Magnetic Resonance Imaging of Pathologic Fractures

Confirms Presence or Absence of Tumor
Determines the Extent of Tumor Infiltration
Allows Total Body Imaging and Search for Unknown Primary Tumor

---

Stress Fractures: Fatigue Versus Insufficiency

Stress fractures result from either fatigue, in which they occur as a result of abnormal stress on normal bone, or insufficiency, in which they occur as a result of stress on abnormal bone (46). In general, the term stress fracture is used to describe fatigue fractures rather than insufficiency, and although they occur as a result of chronic stress, they often present as a result of acute fracture to a site weakened over time.

Fatigue Fractures

Femoral neck stress fractures are not uncommon and occur in long-distance athletes and military recruits, who present with persistent groin pain exacerbated by exercise. Although suspected, stress fractures at this site are radiographically occult on radiographs in up to 50% of cases but in chronicity are manifest by a focal periosteal reaction, a

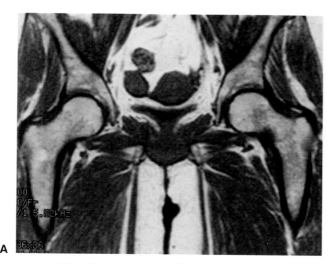 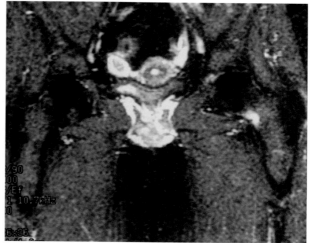

FIG. 23. Coronal T1 **(A)** and IR **(B)** images show a fatigue fracture in the left femoral neck. Note marked sclerosis or signal hypointensity.

cortical break, and a band of sclerosis. Reflecting induced osteoblastic activity, they are usually readily detected at scintigraphy manifest as a linear band of uptake perpendicular to the long axis of the shaft. A normal bone scan essentially excludes the diagnosis of stress fracture (47).

At MR imaging, a low-signal band perpendicular to and continuous with the cortex of the medial femoral neck is seen on all pulse sequences, secondary to osteoblast activity and bony sclerosis (Fig. 23). Within 3 weeks of the onset of symptoms, note is often made of adjacent edema and hemorrhage manifest as signal hyperintensity on T2 and fat-saturated sequences (STIR) (48). After 3 weeks, following resolution of edema, hypointense sclerosis at sites of fractures may be obscured adjacent to hypointense fat on both inversion recovery and frequency selective sequences. Evaluation of suspected stress fracture is therefore best achieved using a T1-weighted spin-echo sequence in which the hypointense line is contrasted against hyperintense marrow fat.

Insufficiency Fractures

Pelvic insufficiency fractures occurring in osteoporotic or osteomalacic bone are seen in pubic rami, the femoral necks, and the sacrum, where they occur parallel to the sacroiliac joints. Sacral insufficiency fractures are most frequently identified in patients who have undergone previous pelvic radiation therapy, most frequently for cervical cancer, in whom the sacrum is within the therapeutic field of view (49,50) (Fig. 24).

In contrast to fatigue fractures, where margins are grossly sclerotic and hypointense, impaired healing response in abnormal bone produces minimal sclerosis at the site of injury. Lack of sclerosis minimizes signal hypointensity at MRI. In contrast to fatigue fractures, insufficiency fractures are manifest by marked marrow edema at the site of injury and

are therefore best visualized on fat-suppressed sequences such as STIR. Sacral insufficiency fractures are best visualized in the coronal plane oblique to the axis of the sacrum off a sagittal localizer (51).

Slipped Capital Femoral Epiphysis

During adolescence and rapid growth, the unfused epiphysis represents a site of biomechanical weakness during weight bearing. In such a way, abnormal weight bearing, particularly in obese adolescents (earlier in girls), is manifest

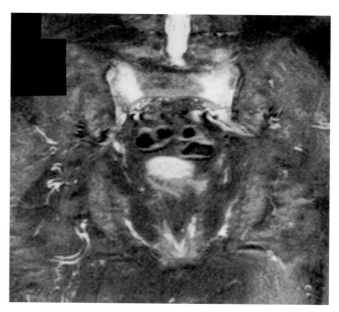

FIG. 24. Coronal IR TSE image shows linear marrow edema paralleling the sacroiliac joints bilaterally at sites of radiation induced insufficiency fractures.

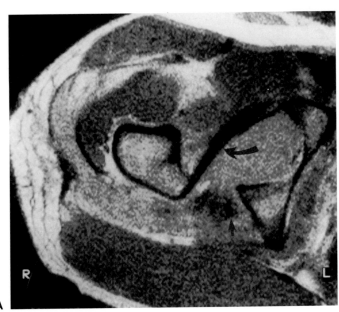
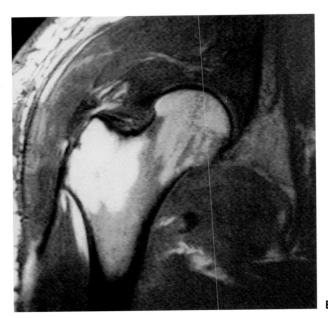

FIG. 25. (A) Axial image shows a posterior hip dislocation, with displaced posterior labral fragment (arrow) and iliopsoas tendon (curved arrow). **(B)** Coronal TSE T1 weighted image shows fixed dislocation of the femoral head above the acetabulum.

as posteroinferior displacement of the proximal femoral epiphysis relative to the femoral neck. Although readily identified on conventional radiographs, multiplanar tomographic imaging afforded by MR imaging improves detection in subtle cases.

Dislocations

Hip dislocation is a severe injury accompanying high-velocity trauma (52). It commonly accompanies motor vehicle accidents as part of a dashboard injury. Impaction against the dashboard is transmitted through patella and femur to the posterior column of the acetabulum. In severe injury, the femoral head either subluxes or dislocates posteriorly, with or without fracture of the posterior column of the acetabulum, with or without fracture of the femoral head. Dislocation is readily evaluated on conventional radiographs and infrequently requires additional imaging. The incidence of avascular necrosis (AVN) complicating posterior dislocation is high, as both circumflex vessels and the ligamentum teres are disrupted, and AVN occurs in almost 100% of cases if reduction is delayed over 24 hr (Fig. 25).

COMPLICATIONS OF PELVIC TRAUMA

Acute Hemorrhage Following Pelvic Trauma

Acute hemorrhage complicating pelvic trauma is most frequently secondary to venous hemorrhage from bone (19). Such bleeding is therefore readily controlled by external tamponade achieved through an external pelvic clamp, which, following realignment, reapposes the fracture sur-

faces. Occasionally bleeding is continuous and occurs secondary to arterial laceration, most frequently derived from the internal iliac vessels adjacent to the anterior sacroiliac joint and the sacrotuberous and sacrospinous ligaments. Traditionally, this diagnosis of arterial injury was made at contrast angiography, now employed because it offers the therapeutic option of coil embolization if a bleeder is identified. Now, many centers perform contrast-enhanced CT of the pelvis before angiography, as it offers the ability to confirm or exclude arterial bleed and therefore triage patients into those who do and do not require conventional angiography. Extravasation of contrast to local soft tissues anterior to the sacroiliac joint is used as a marker of arterial hemorrhage. When practical, MR angiography may be employed rather than CT. When used in this setting, MR imaging affords evaluation of osseous, soft tissue, and vascular structures. Magnetic resonance angiography is generally performed following the administration of 40 ml of gadolinium DTPA (20) (Fig. 26).

Pelvic Deep Vein Thrombosis

Pulmonary embolus complicating pelvic trauma is not uncommon and in most cases occurs secondary to pelvic vein thrombosis rather than thrombosis in veins of the lower extremity (53).

Doppler examination has essentially replaced the use of contrast venography to evaluate patients with suspected extremity deep vein thrombosis, but its ability to detect pelvic thrombosis is poor. Although contrast venography allows evaluation of pelvic veins, MR venography is now frequently used as an alternative, as it requires no contrast injec-

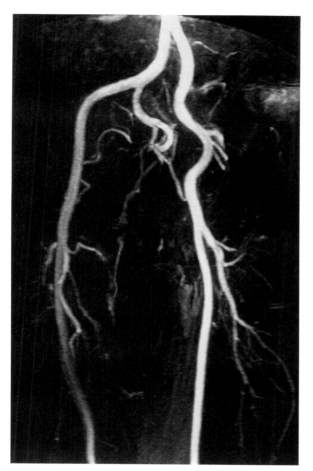

FIG. 26. Coronal MIP reconstruction from gadolinium enhanced source data shows normal pelvic arterial supply without hemorrhage or laceration following pelvic trauma.

tion and allows simultaneous evaluation of suspected osseous injury (Fig. 27).

In general, despite in-plane saturation effects, venous patency is evaluated using 2D time-of-flight technique without

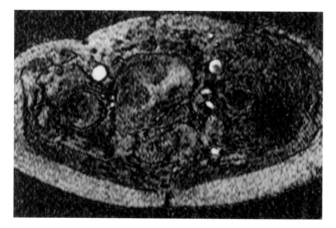

FIG. 27. Axial 2D time-of-flight image shows thrombus within the left common femoral vein.

gadolinium enhancement, with individual axial images acquired perpendicular to common iliac, internal iliac, and femoral veins. In such a way images are acquired of vessels on the right side of pelvis and then of vessels on the left side of pelvis.

AVASCULAR NECROSIS OF THE FEMORAL HEAD

The vascular supply to the femoral head is predominantly through perforating branches (superior retinacular artery) of the circumflex femoris artery, although additional perfusion is yielded through the ligamentum teres (54).

Fractures of the femoral neck result in disruption of retinacular and sinusoidal vessels, markedly reducing perfusion following injury. In undisplaced fractures, vascular recanalization or healing frequently occurs, and the subsequent development of bone necrosis is uncommon. Studies of resected specimens show foci of ischemic necrosis in 60% to 75% of cases, although revascularization through the artery of the ligamentum teres is identified in over 50% of these cases (55). In practice, evidence of osteonecrosis is identified in 10% of undisplaced fractures and in up to 35% of displaced fractures. Because both the retinacular vessels and the artery of the ligamentum teres are injured following posterior dislocation of the hip, the incidence of avascular necrosis in this group is even higher at up to 50%, particularly patients with fracture dislocation. Delayed reduction following hip dislocation over 24 hr increases the rate of avascular necrosis to almost 100%.

Magnetic resonance imaging allows the earliest detection of avascular necrosis. Posttraumatic ischemia generates less marrow edema than other causes in which impaired vascular drainage (secondary to raised intramedullary pressure) leads to congestion and edema. In contrast, disruption of vascular supply as occurs following fracture reduces overall femoral head fluid content (56).

Dynamic gadolinium-enhanced techniques allow the earliest evaluation of vascular integrity. By use of a fat-saturated T1-weighted fast field-echo sequence with sequential keyhole acquisitions, relative enhancement of the femoral head may be determined. At the time of this writing, the actual significance of observed ischemia is unclear, as it is recognized that in almost 50% of cases, reperfusion occurs. It is thought that the early identification of ischemia might promote prolonged immobilization and hence even greater vascular reperfusion (57).

As ischemic necrosis progresses, the zone of ischemia becomes marginated by a serpiginous dark outer and a bright inner band, the so-called double-line sign, evident up to 3 months before detection of abnormality on conventional radiographs (58) (Fig. 28). This sign is thought to reflect vascular ingrowth from the viable margins to the infarcted segment, hypointense sclerosis or new bone being laid down behind the hyperintense fluid-rich tissue as vascular ingrowth occurs.

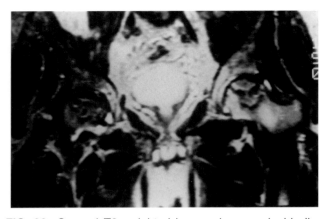

FIG. 28. Coronal T2 weighted image shows a double line sign in the left femoral head secondary to avascular necrosis. Chronic avascular necrosis is identified in the right femoral head.

In established ischemia, subchondral bone becomes necrotic and collapses to produce the radiographic crescent sign. Loss of subchondral biomechanical integrity is followed by articular margin collapse and eventually joint space osteoarthritis (59).

MYOSITIS OSSIFICANS

Heterotopic bone formation within para-articular soft tissues is a well-recognized complication of hip trauma. Although it is occasionally identified in the absence of trauma, there is a history of isolated or repeated hip trauma in two-thirds of cases. Following muscle trauma, mesenchymal cells proliferate at the site of tissue damage, and become mineralized as they differentiate into osteoblastic components and subsequently into mature bone (60).

Mineralization may be seen in the damaged soft tissues as early as 11 days, characterized by focal accumulation of radiotracer (^{99m}Tc-MDP) at scintigraphy or edema and signal hyperintensity at MR imaging.

The complication is most frequently identified in patients with preexisting hyperparathyroidism, Paget's disease, seronegative arthritis, or paralysis. Progressive mineralization may be limited by immediate radiation therapy in patients following its identification. Nevertheless, in most patients, surgical resection is the definitive therapy. Therefore, once identified, imaging is used both to determine the true extent and also the maturity of the process. Surgery before completed ossification may result in incomplete resection and recurrence. No change in the extent on three serial radiographs, markedly reduced concentration of radiotracer at scintigraphy (similar uptake to adjacent mature bone), and absence of edema surrounding heterotopic bone at MR imaging are used as markers of mature heterotopic bone (61,62).

REFERENCES

1. Keane GS, Villa RN. Arthroscopic anatomy of the hip: an *in vivo* study. *Arthroscopy* 1994;10:392.
2. Hodler J, Yu JS, Goodwin D, Haghigh P. MR arthrography of the hip: improved imaging of the acetabular labrum with histologic correlation in cadavers. *Am J Roentgenol* 1995;165:887.
3. Lecouvert FE, Vande Berg BC, Malghem J, et al. MR imaging of the acetabular labrum. Variations in 200 asymptomatic volunteers. *Am J Roentgenol* 1996;167:1025–1028.
4. Adam P, Labbe JL, Alberge Y, et al. The role of computed tomography in the assessment and treatment of acetabular fractures. *Clin Radiol* 1985;36:13–18.
5. Petersilge CA, Haque MA, Petersilge WJ, et al. Acetabular labral tears: evaluation with MR arthrography. *Radiology* 1996;200:231–235.
6. Czerny C, Hoffman S, Neuhold A, et al. Lesions of the acetabular labrum: accuracy of MR imaging and MR arthrography in detection and staging. *Radiology* 1996;200:225.
7. Guy RL, Butler-Manuel PA, Holder P, et al. The role of three dimensional CT in the assessment of acetabular fractures. *Br J Radiol* 1992;65:384–389.
8. Fischer MR, Dooms GC, Hricak H, et al. MRI of normal and pathological musculoskeletal system. *Mag Res Imag* 1986;4:491.
9. Fleckenstein JL, Shellock FG. Exertional muscle injuries: MRI evaluation. *Top Mag Res Imag* 1991;3:50–70.
10. DeSmet AA, Fisher DR, Heiner JP, Keane JS. Magnetic resonance imaging of muscle tears. *Skel Radiol* 1990;19:283–286.
11. Brandser EA, El-Khoury GY, Kathol MH, Callaghan JJ. Hamstring injuries: radiographic, conventional tomographic, CT and MR imaging characteristics. *Radiology* 1995;197:257.
12. Dooms GC, Fisher MF, Hricak H, et al. MR imaging of intramuscular hemorrhage. *J Comput Assist Tomogr* 1985;9:908.
13. Vaccaro JP, Sauser DD, Beals RK. Iliopsoas bursa imaging: efficacy in depicting abnormal iliopsoas tendon motion in patients with internal snapping hip syndrome. *Radiology* 1995;197:853.
14. Garret WE. Muscle strain injuries: Clinical and basic aspects. *Med Sci Sports Exerc* 1990;22:436–443.
15. Dunn EL, Berry PH, Connally JD. Computed tomography of the pelvis in patients with multiple injuries. *J Trauma* 1983;23:378–382.
16. Pennal GF, Tile M, Waddell JP, et al. Pelvic disruption. Assessment and classification. *Clin Orthop* 1980;151:12–21.
17. Tile M. *Fractures of the Pelvis and Acetabulum.* Baltimore: Williams & Wilkins, 1984.
18. Evers MB, Cryer HM, Miller FB. Pelvic fracture haemorrhage. *Arch Surg* 1989;124:422–424.
19. Cryer HM, Miller FB, Evers BM, et al. Pelvic fracture classification: correlation with hemorrhage. *J Trauma* 1988;28:973–980.
20. Ben-Menachem Y, Coldwell DM, Young JWR, et al. Hemorrhage associated with pelvic fractures: causes, diagnosis and emergent management. *Am J Roentgenol* 1991;157:1005–1014.
21. Gill K, Bucholz RW. The role of computerized tomographic scanning in the evaluation of major pelvic fractures. *J Bone Joint Surg* 1984;66:34–39.
22. Zarins B, Ciullo JV. Acute muscle and tendon injuries in athletes. *Clin Sports Med* 1983;2:167–182.
23. Fernbach SK, Wilkinson RH. Avulsion injuries of the pelvis and proximal femur. *Am J Roentgenol* 1981;137:581–584.
24. Brandser EA, El-Khoury GY, Kathol MH. Adolescent hamstring avulsions that simulate tumors. *Emerg Radiol* 1995;2:273–278.
25. Tehranzadeh J. The spectrum of avulsion and avulsion like injuries of the musculoskeletal system. *Radiographics* 1987;7:945–974.
26. Wooten JR, Cross MJ, Holt KWG. Avulsion of the ischial apophysis. *J Bone Joint Surg [Br]* 1990;72-B:625–627.
27. Schneider R, Kaye JJ, Ghelman B. Adductor avulsive injuries near the symphysis pubis. *Radiology* 1976;129:567–569.
28. Metzmaker JN, Pappas Am. Avulsion fractures of the pelvis. *Am J Sports Med* 1985;13:349–358.
29. Sundar M, Carty H. Avulsion fractures of the pelvis in children: A report of 32 fractures and their outcome. *Skel Radiol* 1994;23:85–90.
30. Cleaves EN. Fracture avulsion of the anterior superior iliac spine of the ilium. *J Bone Joint Surg [Am]* 1938;20:490.
31. Williams PL, Warwick R, Dyson M, et al. *Gray's Anatomy, 37th ed.* New York: Churchill Livingstone, 1989.
32. Saks BJ. Normal acetabular anatomy for acetabular fracture assessment. CT and plain film correlation. *Radiology* 1986;159:139–145.
33. Harley JD, Mack LA, Winquist RA. CT of acetabular fractures. Comparison with conventional radiography. *Am J Roentgenol* 1982;138:413–417.
34. Hofman S, Engel A, Neuhold A, et al. Bone marrow edema syndrome

and transient osteoporosis of the hip. *J Bone Joint Surg [Br]* 1993; 75B:210–216.

35. Junk S, Ostrowski M, Kokoszczynski L. Transient osteoporosis of the hip in pregnancy complicated by femoral neck fracture. *Acta Orthop Scand* 1996;67:69–70.

36. Hayes CW, Conway WF, Daniel WW. MR imaging of bone marrow edema pattern: transient osteoporosis, transient bone marrow edema syndrome, or osteonecrosis. *Radiographics* 1993;13:1001–1011.

37. Kyle RF, Gustilo RB, Premer RF. Analysis of 622 intertrochanteric hip fractures: a retrospective and prospective study. *J Bone Joint Surg* 1979;61A:216–221.

38. Garden RS. Stability and union in subcapital fractures of the femur. *J Bone Joint Surg* 1964;46B:630–647.

39. Blickenstaff LD, Morris JM. Fatigue fracture of the femoral neck. *J Bone Joint Surg* 1966;48A:1031–1047.

40. Asnis SE, Gould ES, Bansal M, et al. Magnetic resonance imaging of the hip after displaced femoral neck fractures. *Clin Orthop* 1994;298:191–198.

41. Deutsch AL, Mink JH, Waxman AD. Occult fractures of the proximal femur. MR imaging. *Radiology* 1989;170:113–116.

42. Ruland LJ, Wang GJ, Teates CD, et al. A comparison of magnetic resonance imaging to bone scintigraphy in early traumatic ischemia of the femoral head. *Clin Orthop* 1992;285:30–34.

43. Lang P, Mauz M, Schorner W, et al. Acute fractures of the femoral neck. Assessment of femoral neck perfusion with gadopentate dimeglumine enhanced MR imaging. *Am J Roentgenol* 1993;160:335–341.

44. Quinn SF, McCarthy JL. Prospective evaluation of patients with suspected hip fracture and indeterminate radiographs: Use of T1 weighted MR images. *Radiology* 1993;187:469–471.

45. Bogost GA, Lizerbram EK, Crues JV. MR imaging in evaluation of suspected hip fracture: frequency of unsuspected bone and soft tissue injury. *Radiology* 1995;197:263–267.

46. Anderson MW, Greenspan A: Stress fractures. *Radiology* 1996;199:1.

47. Davies AM. Stress fractures: current concepts. *Am J Roentgenol* 1992; 159:245–252.

48. Peh WCG, Khong PL, Yin Y, et al. Imaging of pelvic insufficiency fractures. *Radiographics* 1996;16:335–348.

49. Brahme SK, Cervilla V, Vint V, et al. Magnetic resonance imaging appearance of sacral insufficiency fractures. *Skel Radiol* 1990;19:489–493.

50. Blomlie V, Lien HH, Iversen T, et al. Radiation induced insufficiency fractures of the sacrum: evaluation with MR imaging. *Radiology* 1993; 188:214–244.

51. Blomlie V, Rofstad EK, Talle K, et al. Incidence of radiation induced insufficiency fractures of the female pelvis. Evaluation with MR imaging. *Am J Roentgenol* 1996;167:1205–1210.

52. Vas WG, Wolverson MK, Sundaram M, et al. The role of computed tomography in pelvic fractures. *J Comput Tomogr* 1982;6:796–801.

53. Montgomery KD, Potter HG, Helfet DL. *The use of magnetic resonance imaging to evaluate the deep venous system in the pelvis in patients with acetabular fractures.* Paper presented at Surgery of the Pelvis and Acetabulum: The Second International Consensus, Pittsburgh, 1993.

54. Bluemke DA, Petri M, Zerhouni EA. Femoral head perfusion and composition: MR imaging and spectroscopic evaluation of patients with systemic lupis erythematosis and at risk for avascular necrosis. *Radiology* 1995;197:433–438.

55. Bayliss AP, Davidson JK. Traumatic osteonecrosis of the femoral head following intracapsular fracture: incidence and earliest radiological features. *Clin Radiol* 1977;28:407–414.

56. Arnoldi CC, Linderholm H. Intraosseous pressures in patients with fracture of the femoral neck. *Acta Chir Scand* 1969;135:407–411.

57. Nadel SN, Debatin JF, Richardson WJ, et al. Detection of acute avascular necrosis of the femoral head in dogs. Dynamic contrast enhanced MR imaging versus spin echo and STIR sequences. *Am J Roentgenol* 1992;159:1255–1261.

58. Hauzeur JP, Pasteels JL, Schoutens A, et al. The diagnostic value of magnetic resonance imaging in nontraumatic osteonecrosis of the femoral head. *J Bone Joint Surg [Am]* 1989;71A:643–648.

59. Vande Berg BE, Malghem JJ, Labaisse MA, et al. Avascular necrosis of the hip. Comparison of contrast enhanced and nonenhanced MR imaging with histologic correlation. *Radiology* 1992;182:445–450.

60. Goldman AB. Myositis ossificans circumscripta: A benign lesion with malignant differential diagnosis. *Am J Roentgenol* 1976;126:32.

61. Norman A, Dorfman HD. Juxtacortical circumscribed myositis ossificans: evolution and radiological features. *Radiology* 1970;96:301.

62. Ehara S, Nakasato T, Tamakawa Y, et al. MRI of myositis ossificans circumscripta. *Clin Imag* 1991;15:130.

63. El-Khoury GY, Daniel WW, Kathol MH: Acute and chronic avulsive injuries. *Radiol Clin North Am* 1997;35:747.

CHAPTER 8

The Cervical Spine

Elias R. Melhem and Stephen J. Eustace

Under ideal circumstances, conventional radiographs detect up to 93% of cervical spine fractures, including flexion wedge and teardrop fractures, extension teardrop fractures, unilateral and bilateral facet dislocations, and most injuries around the craniocervical junction. Of the 7% missed fractures, odontoid, hangman's, and facet fractures are the most frequent, and these are often better evaluated with axial CT. As a result of availability, cost, and rapid acquisition, many now employ MR imaging as an alternative to CT, immediately following radiographic examination, as it affords concomitant multiplanar evaluation of both bone and soft tissue structures.

PATIENT POSITIONING AND IMAGING PROTOCOLS

Significant progress has been made in the areas of device compatibility, fast MR pulse sequences, and surface coil technology, allowing routine use of MR imaging to evaluate patients immediately following cervical spine trauma.

Compatibility Issues

Continuous hemodynamic monitoring, respiratory support, and external fixation devices are frequently a necessity

E. R. Melhem: Department of Radiology, Section of Neuroradiology, Boston University School of Medicine and Boston Medical Center, Boston, Massachusetts 02118.
S. J. Eustace: Department of Radiology, Section of Musculoskeletal Radiology, Boston University School of Medicine and Boston Medical Center, Boston, Massachusetts 02118.

in acutely traumatized patients. Problems resulting from these devices in the magnetic environment include induction of electric currents, heating, dislodgment, and image-degrading artifacts (1). Cervical spine-stabilizing devices made from MR-compatible materials such as aluminum, graphite, and plastic have significantly reduced the risk of induced patient morbidity and of metal-induced artifacts limiting image interpretation. The introduction of appropriately RF-shielded monitoring devices or those operating at frequencies outside the MR scanner RF spectrum has facilitated the safe imaging of the hemodynamically unstable patient (2).

Image Quality Issues

Turbo spin-echo imaging has revolutionized cervical spine imaging (3,4). Because of the acquisition of multiple data lines in k-space per TR interval (significant improvement in scanning efficiency) and the maintenance of spin-echo contrast, turbo spin echo has replaced conventional spin-echo and to a large extent gradient-echo sequences in routine T2/T2*-weighted imaging. The significant improvement in time resolution offered by turbo spin-echo techniques has allowed timely imaging of the critical patient, improvements in image spatial resolution and signal to noise, and routine implementation of formerly time-consuming inversion recovery MR sequences (STIR and FLAIR) (5). In addition to gross motion-related artifacts, the multiple 180° RF pulses and the relatively short echo spacing implemented in turbo spin-echo techniques play an important role in the reduction of susceptibility-related artifacts originating from paramagnetic or ferromagnetic hardware (6,7). Unfortunately, the latter advantage renders this fast MR technique

TABLE 1. *Magnetic resonance sequences used in imaging cervical spine injury*

Type of MR sequence	Parameters	Utility
Sagittal T1	TR/TE: 500/15 Slice thickness/gap (mm): 3.0/0.3	Epidural hematoma, cord swelling
Sagittal T2 Turbo SE	TR/TE/ETL: 2000/80/8 Slice thickness/gap (mm): 3.0/0.3	Cord edema, spondylosis, cord compression
Sagittal Turbo STIR	TR/TI/TE/ETL: 2000/160/20/5 Slice thickness/gap (mm): 3.0/0.3	Bone marrow edema, ligamentous and soft tissue injury
Sagittal T2* GRE	TR/TE/Flip angle: 480/25/25° Slice thickness/gap (mm): 3.0/0.3	Cord hematoma, disk herniation, bone fragments
Axial T1	TR/TE: 574/17 Slice thickness/gap (mm): 4.0/0.4	Epidural hematoma, posterior element fractures
Axial T2 Turbo SE	TR/TE/ETL: 3,000/100/8 Slice thickness/gap (mm): 4.0/0.4	Cord edema, cord compression

suboptimal for detecting subtle acute hemorrhage in the cord and necessitates the routine implementation of a T2*-weighted gradient-echo sequence in spine trauma imaging. Another disadvantage of this technique in imaging the traumatized spine is related to the bright signal originating from fat within the bone marrow and paraspinal soft tissue. This can lead to difficulty in detecting edema in the bony spine and paraspinal ligaments on T2-weighted imaging. For this reason, fat suppression techniques (frequency- or T1 relaxation-selective) coupled to turbo spin-echo readouts have become routine in imaging the traumatized cervical spine (8).

Recently, circularly polarized (quadrature) phased-array coils functioning in receive mode have become the mainstay for imaging the cervical spine in the setting of trauma. The phased-array coil is a series of small coils linked in a ladder-like configuration that allows examination of a large area while taking advantage of the high signal to noise offered by smaller coils. Although the Helmholtz-like volume coil configuration may provide slightly superior signal to noise in imaging the cervical spine compared to the phased-array coil, the frequent use of fixation and monitoring devices often precludes the use of the former coil in MR imaging of the traumatized patient.

Magnetic Resonance Imaging Protocols

Positioning

All patients with neurologic deficit referrable to the spinal cord or evidence of cervical spine fracture/dislocation are imaged using a set MR protocol (Table 1) under the supervision of an emergency department physician and a radiologist. The need for cardiac and respiratory monitoring during MR imaging is determined by the trauma team and usually dictates patient positioning.

Receiver Coil

All MR imaging of the cervical spine is done using surface coils functioning in receive mode (quadrature phased array).

Imaging Protocol

When patient stability permits, a sagittal T1-weighted spin-echo image is acquired and used to assess alignment of the cervical spine, integrity of the individual vertebral bodies, and the caliber of the spinal cord (focal swelling). A sagittal T2-weighted TSE image (Fig. 1) is then acquired to detect cord edema, cord compression, and spondylotic changes. A sagittal turbo STIR image is then employed to detect subtle paraspinal ligamentous injury (Fig. 2) and bone marrow edema. A sagittal T2*-weighted fast field echo is acquired to facilitate exquisite demonstration of acute cord hemorrhage (Fig. 3) and acute posttraumatic disk herniation. This sequence maintains high signal within the disks even in the presence of severe degeneration, which makes easier the differentiation between a herniated disk and a bone fragment. Finally axial T1-weighted SE and T2-weighted turbo SE images are acquired to detect posterior element fractures and to confirm and localize the abnormalities detected on sagittal imaging.

Fractures within the vertebral body are readily detected as a result of intense edema induced within cancellous bone. Posterior elements lack cancellous bone and therefore generate less edema following injury; posterior element fractures are therefore often localized by the presence of edema in the adjacent soft tissues.

All MR images are systematically analyzed (Table 2) and correlated with other available imaging modalities (plain radiographs and CT) as well as the patient's neurologic exam. An immediate evaluation of the stability of the cervical spine and the status of the spinal cord is made.

Background

Cervical spine trauma is a serious and often catastrophic injury that commonly affects young men at the time of peak productivity. Enormous resources are dedicated to the medical and surgical management as well as rehabilitation of affected individuals. In peacetime, most cervical spine injuries result from motor vehicle accidents, recreational sports, and diving-related accidents (9).

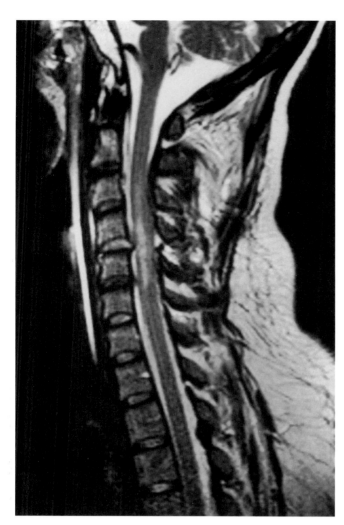

FIG. 1. A 46-year-old woman with hyperflexion injury and anterior cord syndrome. Sagittal T2-weighted TSE (2,000/80: TR/TE) nicely demonstrates a spindle-shaped area of hyperintensity in the cord extending from C2 to C5 representing contusion. A small acute disk herniation at the C4-5 level and mild prevertebral soft tissue edema at the C4 level are also demonstrated.

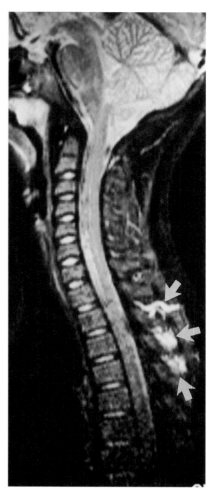

FIG. 2. An 11-year-old girl with hyperflexion injury and persistent pain at the cervicothoracic junction. Sagittal IR TSE (2,000/160/20:TR/TI/TE) demonstrates edema in the interspinous ligaments of the upper thoracic spine (arrows).

Cervical spine and spinal cord injuries have been classified based on neurologic deficits (Table 3), type of injury (blunt versus penetrating trauma), mechanisms of injury (Table 4), and anatomic location of injury (cervicocranial junction versus lower cervical spine). With these various classification schemes as guidelines, there are two fundamental issues unique to the spine that need to be addressed before planning appropriate therapy and judging prognosis. The first relates to characterization of direct injury to the spinal cord, and the second relates to identification of spinal instability and associated spinal cord damage (10).

Plain radiographs and x-ray CT scanning continue to play an instrumental role in the evaluation of the acutely injured cervical spine, in particular with regard to identification of spinal instability. These imaging modalities have been less than optimal in the characterization of direct spinal cord injury and identification of nonosseous causes of cord compression (11).

In the last decade, MR imaging has demonstrated enormous potential for characterizing direct injury to the spinal cord and for identifying osseous instability in a timely and definitive fashion.

Role of MRI in the Characterization of Spinal Cord Injury

The reaction of spinal cord to penetrating and blunt injury covers a wide range. Spinal cord abnormalities are related to site, intensity, and distribution of impact and to biochemical, electrophysiological, and hemodynamic derangements (12).

Spinal cord injuries can be categorized as concussion, contusion, and compression (11). Concussion of the cord is a purely functional and fully reversible derangement that has been attributed to transient deficiencies in the cord's

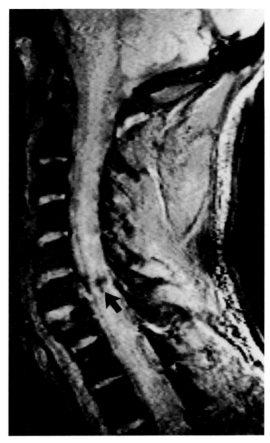

FIG. 3. A 25-year-old man with hyperflexion injury and paraplegia. Sagittal T2*-weighted GRE (480/25/25°:TR/TE/flip angle) demonstrates acute intramedullary hemorrhage at the C6 level as a focus of hypointensity caused by magnetic susceptibility effects *(arrow).*

TABLE 3. *Frankel's functional classification of spinal cord injury*

Grade	Neurologic deficit
A	Complete motor and sensory loss
B	Preserved sensory function
C	Preserved motor activity (nonfunctional)
D	Preserved motor activity (functional)
E	Complete neurologic recovery

microcirculation (13). Demonstration of cord edema on T2-weighted MR images is uncommon and transient. Contusion is an injury of the cord with a spectrum extending from simple edema, petechial hemorrhages, to severe hemorrhagic necrosis and even complete transection (14). Subsequent demyelination, micro- and macrocystic myelomalacia, and arachnoiditis are common. Contusion can result from transient compression or stretching of the cord. Cord compression results from the same spectrum of injury to the cord as contusion with the additional demonstration of the compressive lesion (bone fragment, subluxation/dislocation, disk herniation, epidural hematoma, and spondylotic bar). A 50% or greater reduction in the anterior–posterior dimension of the spinal canal has been suggested as a necessary condition for cord compression. The identification of an acute compressive lesion is of utmost clinical importance because in many trauma centers, its identification mandates immediate surgical intervention (15).

Magnetic resonance imaging is undoubtedly superior to other imaging modalities in demonstrating spinal cord injuries, namely, cord contusion and compression. Kulkarni et al.

TABLE 2. *Systematic inspection of the MR images in cervical spine trauma*

Alignment	Subluxation/dislocation
Spinal cord	Edema
	Swelling
	Hemorrhage
	Compression
Epidural space	Disk herniation
	Bone fragment
	Hematoma
Spinal column	Vertebral body fracture
	Posterior element fracture
	Bony edema
	Spondylosis
Ligaments	Anterior longitudinal ligament
	Posterior longitudinal ligament
	Interlaminar ligaments (Flava)
	Supra-/interspinous ligaments
Vascular	Vertebral artery (Fig. 5)

TABLE 4. *Functional classification of cervical spine fractures and dislocations*

Mechanism of injury	Type
Hyperflexion	Anterior subluxation (sprain)
	Bilateral interfacetal dislocation
	Simple wedge fracture
	Clay shoveler's fracture
	Teardrop fracture
Hyperextension	Dislocation (sprain or strain)
	Avulsion fracture of the anterior arch of C1
	Fracture of the posterior arch of C1
	Teardrop fracture of C2
	Laminar fracture
	Hangman's fracture
	Fracture or dislocation
Vertical compression	Jefferson fracture
	Burst fracture
Hyperflexion and rotation	Unilateral interfacetal dislocation
Hyperextension and rotation	Pillar fracture
Lateral flexion	Uncinate process fracture
Indeterminate	Atlanto-occipital disassociation
	Odontoid fractures

TABLE 5. *Magnetic resonance signal pattern in acute spinal cord injury*

Magnetic resonance pattern	T1-weighted images	T2-weighted images	
		Central	Peripheral
I	Heterogeneous	Large area of hypointensity	Thin rim of hyperintensity
II	Normal	Hyperintensity	Hyperintensity
III	Normal	Small area of hypointensity	Thick rim of hyperintensity

(16) describe three MR imaging patterns of spinal cord injury (Table 5). In the acute phase the first pattern is characterized by an area of hypointensity relative to the normal cord on T2-weighted images with the development of a thin rim of hyperintensity on short-term follow-up (3 to 7 days). On the axial T2-weighted images, the foci of hyperintensity are often seen at the gray–white matter junction. T1-weighted images demonstrate focal cord swelling. The second pattern is characterized by a spindle-shaped area of hyperintensity relative to the normal cord on T2-weighted images (see Fig. 1). Follow-up imaging demonstrates rapid resolution of the hyperintensity. The third pattern is characterized by a small area of hypointensity surrounded by a thick rim of hyperintensity on T2-weighted images (Figs. 4). Follow-up imaging demonstrates partial resolution of the lesion, seen as filling in of the central area by hyperintense signal. More importantly, these patterns correlate well with admission and discharge neurologic functionality of the injured patients. The first pattern is associated with the highest degree of acute neurologic deficit and the least degree of improvement. The second and third patterns are associated with less acute neurologic deficit and most improvement. Also, MR imaging of spinal cord injury has very high positive and negative predictive values for neurologic deficits (14). The well-documented poor correlation between plain radiographic/CT findings and neurologic functionality in patients with cervical spine injury has rendered MR imaging the sole modality for patient stratification and prognostication (17) (Fig. 5).

The importance of distinguishing cord contusion from direct cord compression is based on both experimental and clinical evidence showing improvement or resolution of acute and chronic neurologic deficits following surgical decompression (18). Although the benefit of emergency spine decompression is somewhat controversial, most authorities agree to the need for immediate intervention in patients with acute cord compression regardless of the severity of neurologic deficit (15). Possible explanations for this controversy include inaccurate characterization of cord injury, significant cord compression, or satisfactory decompression; different types and approaches to surgical intervention; or inaccurate assessment of initial neurologic deficits.

Currently, MR imaging is the method of choice for demonstrating and characterizing the causes of cord compression. In particular, nonosseous causes, such as disk herniation (Fig. 6) and epidural hematoma (Fig. 7), are much better demonstrated on MR imaging compared to plain radio-graphs, x-ray CT, and myelography. When MR imaging is used as a standard of reference, CT has approximately 33% and 44% sensitivity for the detection of posttraumatic spinal cord compression and disk herniation, respectively (14). Further, emergency MR imaging is still needed in patients with definite evidence of osseous cord compression on other imaging modalities. This is advocated to prevent worsening

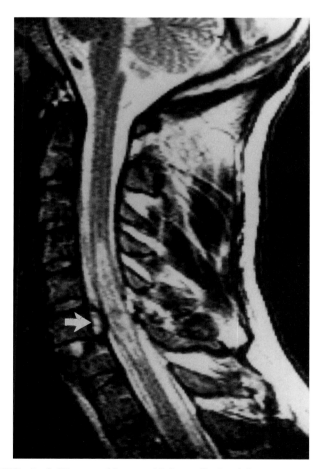

FIG. 4. A 25-year-old man with hyperflexion injury and paraplegia. Sagittal T2-weighted TSE (2,000/80:TR/TE) demonstrates Kulkarni's third pattern, which is characterized by a small area of hypointensity secondary to acute intramedullary hemorrhage at the level of C6 surrounded by a thick rim of hyperintensity representing cord edema. A small epidural hematoma *(arrow)* behind the C6 vertebral body compressing the cord with disruption of the posterior longitudinal ligament is also demonstrated.

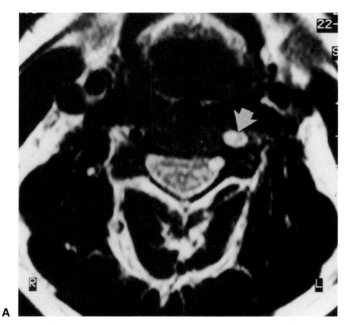
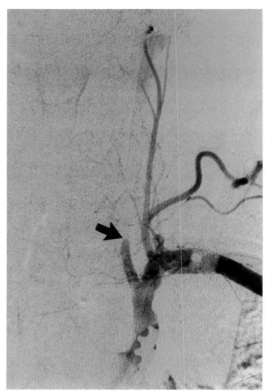

A   **B**

FIG. 5. A 29-year-old man with a burst fracture secondary to axial loading injury. Axial T2-weighted TSE (2,000/80:TR/TE) **(A)** demonstrates hyperintensity in the left transverse foramen *(arrow)*, where a flow void in the vertebral artery is expected. Occlusion of the left vertebral artery *(arrow)* secondary to posttraumatic dissection is confirmed on digital subtraction angiogram **(B)**.

cord compression and neurologic function from an unsuspected extruded disk fragment after cervical reduction (19). Also, patients with severe cervical spine spondylotic changes who experience hyperextension injury may present with neurologic deficits (central cord syndrome) despite the presence of normal conventional radiographs and CT (20). In these patients, MR imaging is invaluable for demonstrating spinal cord injury and compression (Fig. 8). On MR imaging, the neurologic level of injury corresponds precisely to the site of compression.

Role of MR Imaging in the Identification of Spinal Instability

Instability of the cervical spine is defined as the inability to maintain normal association between vertebral segments while under a physiological load (21). Instability, in the setting of trauma, results from the loss of structural integrity of the bony spine and ligaments, which may lead to damage to the spinal cord and nerve roots or to pain and incapacitating deformity of the spinal column. Several clinical criteria have been established to suggest spinal instability. By dividing the spine into three columns (Table 6), Denis (22) defines instability as disruption of at least two of these columns (Fig. 9). Other more objective criteria that are completely reliant

on imaging include the displacement of two adjacent vertebrae more than 3.5 mm and angulation greater than 11° (21).

The role of MR imaging in the evaluation of spinal instability is less well defined. Patients with clear evidence of instability on plain radiographs, without signs of spinal cord injury, or patients in whom reduction of misalignment is not contemplated do not require MR imaging. On the other hand, if the clinical evaluation and plain radiographic/CT findings are inconclusive but suggest instability, then MR may become necessary for confirmation. The superiority of MR imaging in the detection of ligamentous injuries or tears and

TABLE 6. *Components of the three columns of the cervical spine*[a]

Column	Components
Anterior	Anterior longitudinal ligament
	Anterior annulus fibrosis
	Anterior vertebral body
Middle	Posterior vertebral body
	Posterior annulus fibrosis
	Posterior longitudinal ligament
Posterior	Posterior elements
	Facet capsules
	Interlaminar ligaments (Flava)
	Supra-/interspinous ligaments

[a] Instability requires disruption of at least two columns.

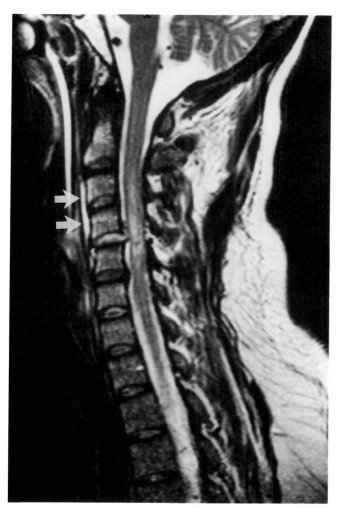

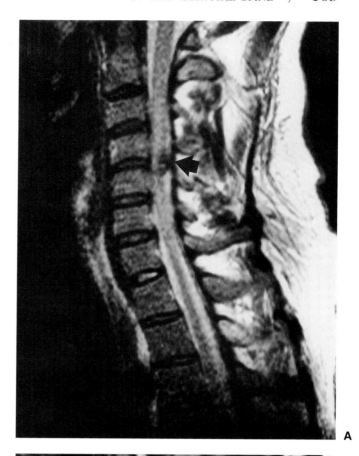

A

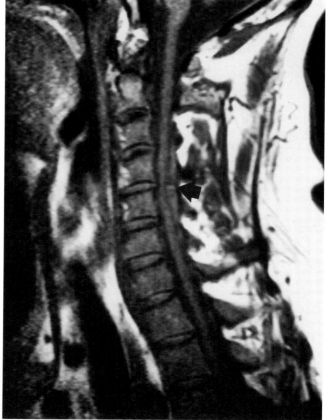

B

FIG. 6. 41 year-old woman with hyperflexion injury and anterior cord syndrome. Sagittal T2-weighted TSE (2,000/80:TR/TE) demonstrates a hyperintense moderate-sized acute disk herniation at the C4-5 level causing cord compression. This is associated with type 3 Kulkarni cord changes, minimal anterior subluxation of C4 on C5, mild prevertebral edema *(arrows),* and disruption of the posterior longitudinal ligament.

FIG. 7. A 40-year-old man with minor hyperextension injury and no abnormality on conventional radiographs of the cervical spine. Sagittal T2-weighted TSE (2,000/80:TR/TE) **(A)** and sagittal T1-weighted SE (500/15: TR/TE) **(B)** demonstrate a spindle-shaped acute posterior epidural hematoma compressing the cord *(arrow).* The epidural hematoma is hypointense on the T2-weighted TSE and isointense to cord on the T1-weighted SE images.

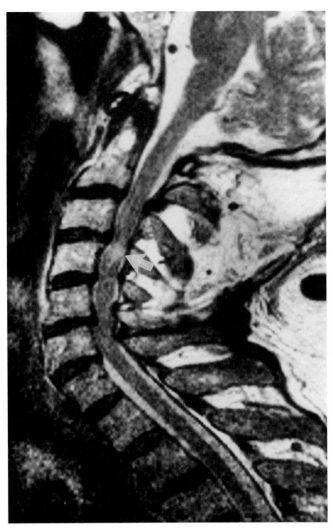

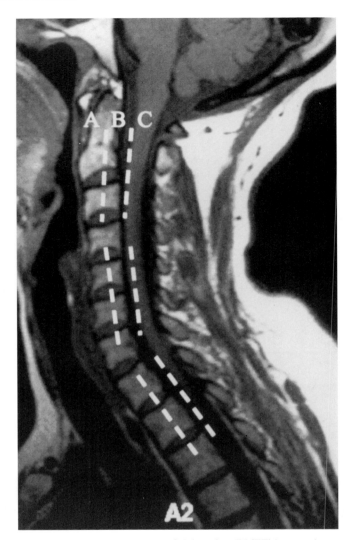

FIG. 8. A 69-year-old man with minor hyperextension injury and moderate spondylotic changes in the cervical spine. Sagittal T2-weighted TSE (2,000/80:TR/TE) images demonstrate moderate spinal stenosis at the C3-4 and C5-6 levels secondary to spondylotic disease. There is cord edema (arrow) at the C4 level resulting from the hyperextension injury.

FIG. 9. Sagittal T1-weighted SE (500/15:TR/TE) image demonstrating three-column structure of the cervical spine: anterior **(A)**, middle **(B)**, and posterior **(C)**.

the questionable reliability of cervical spine flexion-extension radiography in the acute setting have rendered MR the imaging method of choice for the confirmation of instability (23). The reported sensitivity of MR imaging, using high-resolution CT as standard, in the demonstration of cervical spine fractures is variable and ranges from 25% to 100% (14). The wide range reflects significant differences in the ability of MR to demonstrate vertebral body versus posterior element fractures and variability in the MR imaging techniques implemented. Subtle bony fractures of the posterior elements, which may be the only evidence of a second column disruption, can be missed on current MR imaging techniques. For the time being, this limitation secures the role of high resolution CT in the evaluation of cervical spine trauma.

CLASSIFICATIONS OF CERVICAL SPINE INJURIES

Penetrating Trauma

Penetrating trauma to the cervical spine can be further divided into missile injuries and puncture wounds. In peacetime, the most common missile injuries are the result of bullet fragments. Spinal cord damage from missile injuries can result from direct passage of the missile through the cord or, more commonly, from displaced bone fragments and blast effects (24).

On the other hand, puncture wounds are the result of stabbing with a sharp instrument. Because of the protective nature of the bony posterior elements, especially the laminae and spinous processes, most entry sites are off-midline through the interlaminar ligaments, and most injuries involve the dorsolateral aspect of the cord.

Magnetic resonance imaging plays an important role in

the evaluation of penetrating trauma. Victims of puncture wounds, in whom the injury is frequently limited to soft tissues and spinal cord, may have completely negative plain radiographic and CT exams. The MRI can provide critical information regarding location, extent, and type of cord injury as well as precise correlation with the level of neurologic deficit (Fig. 10). In contrast, MR imaging for the evaluation of direct missile injuries may be limited by ferromagnetic susceptibility artifacts.

Blunt Trauma

Blunt trauma to the cervical spine is classified according to anatomic location of injury (cervicocranial junction versus lower cervical spine). Injuries at the cervicocranial junction are further divided into those involving the atlanto-occipital articulation and the atlantoaxial articulation. Lower cervical spine injuries are more common because of increased mobility and are commonly classified according to underlying mechanism (see Table 4) (25).

Atlanto-Occipital Disassociation

This injury is commonly fatal and describes any separation of the atlanto-occipital articulation (26). The separation may be complete (dislocation) or partial (subluxation) with posterior, anterior, or superior (distraction) displacement of the skull. The primary injury is ligamentous with disruption of the ligaments that provide structural support to the cervicocranial junction, namely, atlanto-occipital capsular ligaments, anterior and posterior atlanto-occipital membrane ligaments, paired lateral atlanto-occipital ligaments, longitudinal component of the cruciate ligament, apical ligament, paired alar ligaments, and tectorial membrane.

Multiplanar capability and sensitivity to ligamentous injury render MR the best imaging modality for the demonstration of the relationship between the basion/opisthion and the tip of the dens, between the occipital condyle and the superior facets of the atlas, and the disruption of the supporting ligaments. Also, commonly existing cord injuries are well demonstrated on MR imaging (26).

Atlantoaxial Dissociation

This disassociation can be either secondary to distraction with superior displacement of the atlas and skull (Fig. 11) or secondary to odontoid fractures with resultant anterior or posterior displacement of the atlas. The former is commonly

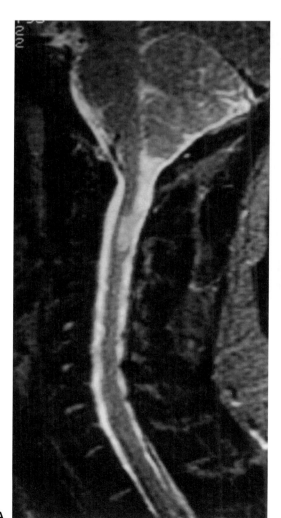

A

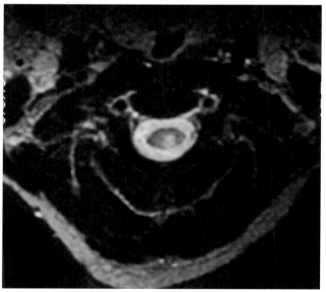

B

FIG. 10. A 26-year-old man who developed Brown-Sequard syndrome after a penetrating injury to the neck. Sagittal **(A)** and axial **(B)** T2-weighted SE (2,000/80:TR/TE) images demonstrate focal swelling and hyperintensity involving the left posterolateral aspect of the cord at the C2-3 level secondary to contusion.

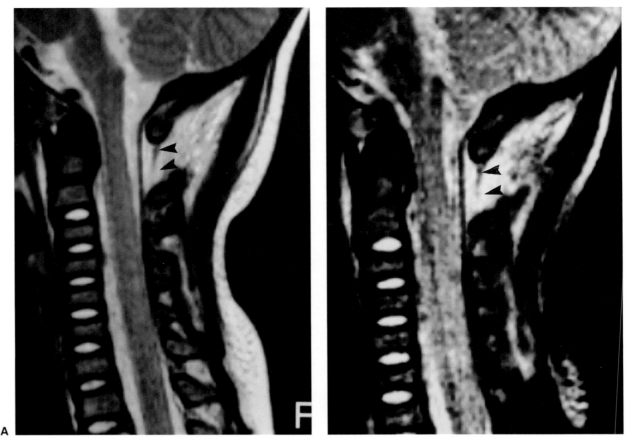

FIG. 11. A 4-year-old boy with a disassociation injury at the cervicocranial junction. Sagittal T2-weighted TSE (2,000/80:TR/TE) **(A)** and sagittal IR TSE (2,000/160/20:TR/TI/TE) **(B)** images demonstrate posterior ligamentous injury *(arrow)* and mild superior displacement of the atlas and skull with respect to C2. There is mild prevertebral edema anterior to C2.

associated with atlanto-occipital disassociation and is primarily the result of ligamentous disruption.

On the other hand, in odontoid fractures, the bony injury predominates. Generally, the mechanism of injury in odontoid fractures is not well understood, although hyperflexion is suspected to represent a dominant component. These fractures are typed by Anderson and D'Alonzo based on the location of the fracture in the axis (Table 7) (Fig. 12) (27).

Again, the disruption of the supporting ligaments and the relationship of the atlas to the axis are well demonstrated

TABLE 7. *Classification of odontoid fractures (Anderson and D'Alonzo)*

Type	Description
I	Avulsion fracture of the tip of the dens
II	Transverse fracture of the dens above the body of C2
III	Fracture of the superior body and the superior articulating facets of C2

on MR imaging. In addition, spinal cord injury and compression are best shown on MR imaging. With respect to odontoid fractures, MR imaging may often demonstrate the fracture lines and associated bone marrow edema (especially when implementing fat saturation techniques). However, high-resolution CT, plain film tomography, or ^{99m}Tc-MDP bone scan may be better than MR imaging for the detection of subtle cortically based fractures (e.g., type I).

Hyperflexion Injuries

Flexion injury of the cervical spine results in the forward rotation or translation of the vertebra in the sagittal plane. This injury is caused by direct trauma to the head and neck in the flexed position or by forces that cause hyperflexion of the neutral cervical spine. There are several subtypes (see Table 4) of flexion injuries with associated different degrees of cord injury and instability depending on the severity of the traumatic force and the position of the neck at the time

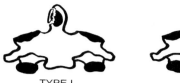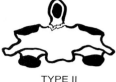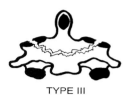

TYPE I   TYPE II   TYPE III

FIG. 12. Schematic representation of fractures of the dens (type I, tip; type II, base; and type III, body).

of impact. The injury tends to be more severe if the cervical spine is flexed at the time of impact (28).

Anterior subluxation of the vertebral body, reversal of cervical lordosis, anterior narrowing and posterior widening of the intervening disk space, anterior displacement of the superior facets, and fanning of the spinous processes are common features of flexion injury. These features are the result of disruption of the posterior ligament complex (inter- and supraspinous ligaments), the interlaminar ligaments, the facet capsules, the posterior longitudinal ligament, and the posterior portion of the annulus fibrosis. The degree of anterior displacement may be minimal (hyperflexion sprain) or obvious (bilateral interfacetal dislocation and teardrop fracture).

The clay shoveler's fracture and the simple wedge fracture tend to be stable, whereas the bilateral interfacetal disloca-

tion and the teardrop fracture (29) are unstable fractures (Figs. 13 and 14). The hyperflexion sprain results in delayed instability. Also, the bilateral interfacetal dislocation and the teardrop fracture frequently result in cord injury and compression.

Most flexion injuries are well demonstrated on MR imaging. In addition to the demonstration of alignment abnormalities and fractures, MR imaging provides unique information regarding ligamentous injury, cord abnormalities, and acute disk herniations commonly associated with hyperflexion injury (30).

The importance of MR imaging is highlighted by its ability to differentiate between anterior subluxation caused by chronic spondylotic changes and that caused by hyperflexion sprain. In the acute setting, because of the questionable reliability of flexion-extension radiography (23), MR imaging

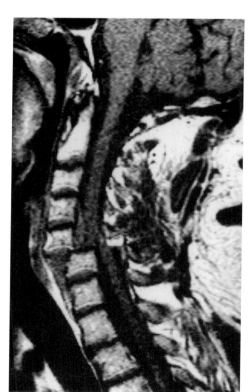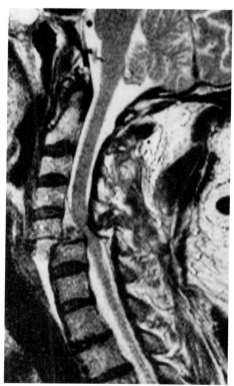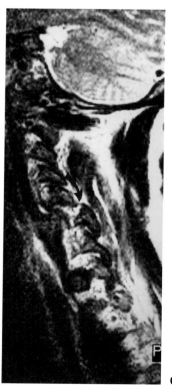

FIG. 13. A 65-year-old man with severe hyperflexion injury resulting in bilateral interfacetal dislocation. Sagittal T1-weighted SE (500/15:TR/TE) **(A)** and sagittal and parasagittal T2-weighted TSE (2,000/80: TR/TE) **(B,C)** demonstrate complete disruption of all three columns with marked anterior translation of the C5 vertebral body on C6 resulting in cord compression and complete interfacetal dislocation *(curved arrow).* There is moderate prevertebral edema from C6 to T1.

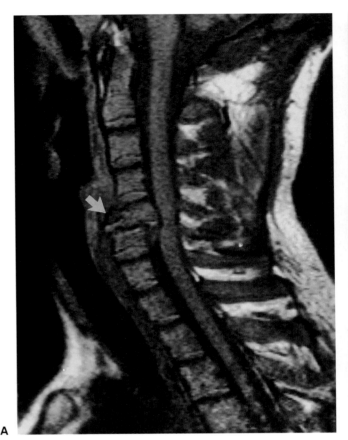
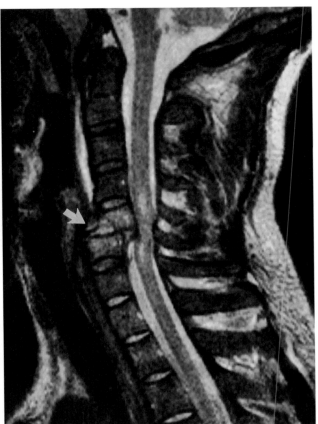

A   B

FIG. 14. A 31-year-old man with severe hyperflexion injury resulting in flexion teardrop fracture. Sagittal T1-weighted SE (500/15:TR/TE) **(A)** and sagittal T2-weighted TSE (2,000/80:TR/TE) **(B)** images demonstrate reverse curvature of the cervical spine with compression fracture of the C5 vertebral body on C6, producing the characteristic triangular fragment that comprises the anteroinferior aspect of the vertebral body *(arrow)*. The retropulsed fragment has caused cord compression and contusion. Note is made of additional disruption of the posterior longitudinal ligament, of moderate prevertebral edema extending from C2 to C4, and of bruising of the C6 vertebral body.

becomes a valuable alternative capable of demonstrating posterior ligamentous injury and hence confirming the presence of hyperflexion sprain.

Hyperextension Injuries

Extension injury of the cervical spine results in the backward rotation or translation of the vertebra in the sagittal plane. It is often the result of an anterior force impacting on the mandible, face, or forehead or of sudden deceleration (28). There are several subtypes of extension injuries (see Table 4) with associated different degrees of cord injury and instability depending on the direction and magnitude of the hyperextensive force.

The different subtypes can be further categorized into stable and unstable fractures. Avulsion fracture of the anterior arch of the atlas and extension teardrop fracture are limited to the anterior column of the cervical spine, whereas isolated fractures of the posterior arch of the atlas and laminar frac-

tures are limited to the posterior column. This limited involvement renders these fractures relatively stable. On the other hand, in more severe types of hyperextension injuries, such as hangman's fracture, hyperextension-dislocation, and hyperextension fracture-dislocation (Fig. 15), at least two columns are disrupted with resultant instability.

Hangman's fracture or C2 traumatic spondylolisthesis is a fracture involving both pars interarticularis or adjacent structures (Fig. 16). This fracture is categorized by Effendi et al. (31) into three types (Fig. 17): type 1 is defined as an isolated hairline fracture of the pars without displacement of the body or facets of C2; type 2 is defined as a fracture of the pars with anterior displacement of the body of C2; and type 3 is defined as a fracture of the pars with anterior displacement of the body of C2 in a position of flexion and associated bilateral facet dislocation. It is felt by some investigators that type 3 hangman's fracture is not a pure hyperextension injury but rather results from a combination of hyperflexion followed by rebound hyperextension.

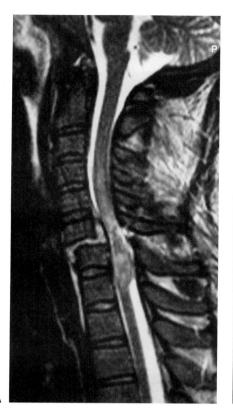

A

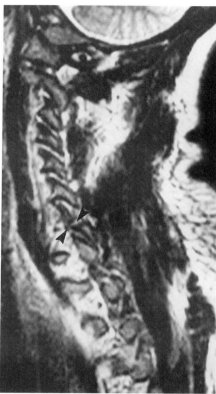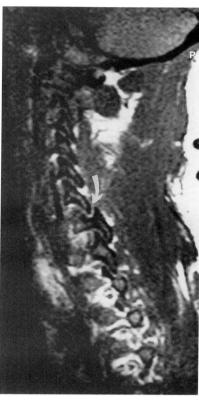

B,C

FIG. 15. A 28-year-old woman involved in a high-speed motor vehicle accident resulting in hyperextension fracture—dislocation injury. Sagittal and parasagittal **(left side)** T2-weighted TSE (2,000/80:TR/TE) **(A,B)** and parasagittal **(right side)** T1-weighted SE (500/15:TR/TE) **(C)** images demonstrate complete disruption of all three columns with mild to moderate paradoxic anterior translation of C6 vertebral body on C7. There is complete interfacetal dislocation of the right C6 on C7 *(curved arrow)* and fracture of the left C7 superior facet *(arrowheads)*. Note the severe cord contusion and posterior buckling of the disrupted C6-7 disk behind C6.

Hyperextension-dislocation injury is a predominantly ligamentous injury resulting in distraction of the anterior column, buckling of the middle column (posterior longitudinal ligament), and transient posterior intervertebral dislocation, which is usually reduced immediately after impact. Plain radiographic findings can be subtle despite commonly associated serious neurologic deficits and include prevertebral soft tissue swelling, avulsion fracture arising from the inferior end plate of the distracted vertebra, widening of the disk space, and a vacuum disk. Magnetic resonance imaging plays a critical role in defining the type of spinal cord injury responsible for the neurologic deficit. It defines the extent of ligamentous injury and it allows identification of an associated acute compressive herniated disk (32).

Vertical Compression Injuries

Axial loading injury of the cervical spine results from forces transmitted through the skull and occipital condyles to a voluntarily straightened spine (28). This type of injury gives rise to the well-described Jefferson fracture of the atlas and the bursting fracture in the lower cervical spine.

The Jefferson fracture consists of simultaneous disruption of the anterior and posterior arches of C1 with or without disruption of the transverse atlantal ligament. Identification of transverse ligament disruption, with resultant atlantoaxial instability, is crucial in the evaluation of this injury. Magnetic resonance imaging, with its superior multiplanar capability and sensitivity to ligamentous injury, nicely demonstrates the lateral displacement of the lateral masses of C1 on the coronal images, the increase in the atlantodental interval on the sagittal images, and disruption of the transverse ligament on the axial images.

As the vertical force is transmitted to the lower cervical spine, it is dissipated by compression of the intervertebral disk. The buildup of pressure within the disk results in either an acute herniated disk or a comminuted fracture in the adjacent vertebral body with associated retropulsion of the posterior body fragments (bursting fracture) (Fig. 18). In either case, MR imaging plays an important role in defining the relationship of the herniated disk or retropulsed fragment to the spinal cord and in demonstrating cord injury.

In summary, continual improvements in MR imaging

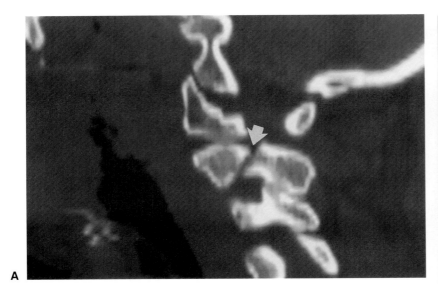

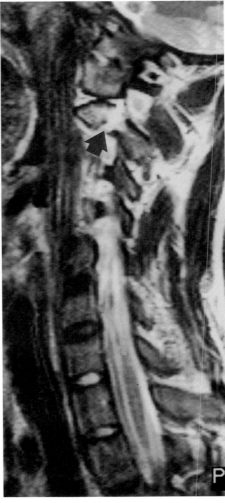

FIG. 16. A 26-year-old woman with hyperextension injury resulting in a type 2 hangman's fracture. Parasagittal reformation from high-resolution axial x-ray CT data **(A)** and parasagittal T2-weighted TSE (2,000/80:TR/TE) **(B)** images demonstrate fracture of the pars interarticularis of C2 *(arrow)* with edema in the superior facet seen only on MR images.

technology and MR-compatible monitoring and fixation devices has allowed the incorporation of this relatively new imaging modality into standard algorithms for cervical spine trauma assessment. The role of MR imaging in defining the type of spinal cord injury, the cause and severity of spinal cord compression, and the stability of the spinal column is unmatched. The heavy reliance of the spine surgeon on MR imaging for decisions regarding the type of therapy, the tim- ing and approach of surgical intervention, and for predicting patient outcome, attests to the critical role played by this modality. Future implementation of fast, high-resolution three-dimensional MR imaging sensitized to bone marrow edema and the application of relatively artifact-free functional MR imaging may enhance our sensitivity for detecting cervical spine instablity and early, possibly reversible, spinal cord injury.

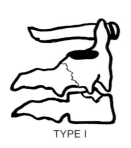

TYPE I

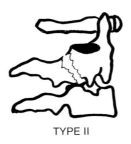

TYPE II

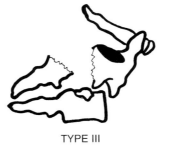

TYPE III

FIG. 17. Schematic representation of the three different types of hangman's fractures: type I, type II, and type III.

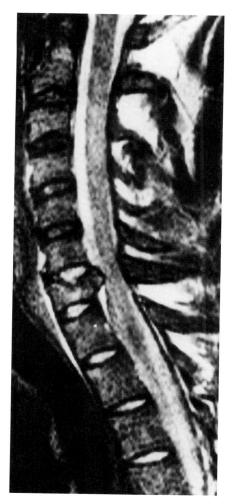

FIG. 18. A 29-year-old man with a burst fracture of C7 secondary to axial loading injury. Sagittal T2-weighted TSE (2,000/80:TR/TE) image demonstrates a burst fracture of the C7 vertebral body with the retropulsed fragment compressing the cord. There is mild prevertebral edema extending from C4 to T2. Note the normal alignment of the cervical spine.

REFERENCES

1. New PF, Rosen BR, Brady TJ, et al. Potential hazards and artifacts of ferromagnetic and nonferromagnetic surgical and dental materials in nuclear magnetic resonance imaging. *Radiology* 1983;147:139–148.
2. Roth JL, Nugent M, Gray JE, et al. Patient monitoring during magnetic resonance imaging. *Anesthesiology* 1985;62:80–83.
3. Melki PS, Jolesz FA, Mulkern RV. Partial RF echo planar imaging with the FAISE method: I. Experimental and theoretical assessment of artifact. *Magn Reson Med* 1992;26:328–341.
4. Melki PS, Jolesz FA, Mulkern RV. Partial RF echo planar imaging with the FAISE method: II. Contrast equivalence with spin-echo sequences. *Magn Reson Med* 1992;26:342–354.
5. Melhem ER, Jara H, Shakir H, Gagliano TA. Fast inversion recovery MR imaging: The effect of hybrid-RARE read-out on the null points of CSF and fat. *Am J Neuroradiol* 1997;18:1627–1633.
6. Eustace S, Goldberg R, Williamson D, et al. MR imaging of soft tissues adjacent to orthopaedic hardware: techniques to minimize susceptibility artifact. *Clin Radiol* 1997;52:589–594.
7. Rockwell D, Melhem ER, Bhatia R: GRASE (gradient- and spin-echo) MR imaging of the brain. *Am J Neuroradiol* 1997;18:1923–1928.
8. Dwyer AJ, Frank JA, Sank VJ, et al. Short T1 inversion-recovery sequence: analysis and initial experience in cancer imaging. *Radiology* 1988;168:827–836.
9. Bracken MB, Freeman DH, Hellenbrand K. Incidence of acute traumatic hospitalized spinal cord injury in the United States, 1970–1977. *Am J Epidemiol* 1981;113:615–622.
10. Masaryk TJ. Spinal trauma. In: Modic MT, Masaryk TJ, Ross JS, eds. *Magnetic Resonance Imaging of the Spine, 2nd ed.* St Louis: Mosby, 1994.
11. Benedetti PF. MR imaging in emergency medicine. *Radiographics* 1996;16:953–962.
12. De La Torre JA. Spinal cord injury: review of basic and applied research. *Spine* 1981;6:315–335.
13. Dohrmann GJ, Wagner FC, Buey PC. The microvasculature in transitory traumatic paraplegia: an electron microscopic study in the monkey. *J Neurosurg* 1971;35:263–271.
14. Flanders AE, Schaefer DM, Doan HT, et al. Acute cervical spine trauma: correlation of MR imaging findings with degree of neurologic deficit. *Radiology* 1990;177:25–33.
15. Quencer RM, Nunez D, Green BA. Controversies in imaging acute cervical spine trauma. *Am J Neuroradiol* 1997;18:1866–1868.
16. Kulkarni MV, McArdle CB, Kopanicky D, et al. Acute spinal cord injury: MR imaging at 1.5 T. *Radiology* 1987;164:837–843.
17. Goldberg AL, Rothfus WE, Deeb ZL, et al. Hyperextension injuries of the cervical spine. *Skeletal Radiol* 1989;18:283–288.
18. Brodkey JS, Miller CF, Harmody RM. The syndrome of acute cervical spinal cord injury revisited. *Surg Neurol* 1980;14:251–257.
19. Robertson PA, Ryan MD. Neurologic deterioration after reduction of cervical subluxation. *J Bone Joint Surg [Br]* 1992;74:224–227.
20. Regenbogen VS, Rogers LF, Atlas SW, et al. Cervical spinal injuries in patients with cervical spondylosis. *Am J Roentgenol* 1986;146:277–284.
21. White AA, Southwick WO, Panjabi MM. Clinical instability in the lower cervical spine: a review of past and current concepts. *Spine* 1976;1:15–27.
22. Denis F. The three column spine and its significance in the classification of acute thoracolumbar spinal injuries. *Spine* 1983;8:817–831.
23. Lewis LM, Docherty M, Ruoff BE, et al. Flexion-extension views in the evaluation of cervical-spine injuries. *Ann Emerg Med* 1991;20:117–121.
24. Yashon D, Jane JA, White RJ. Prognosis and management of spinal cord and cauda equina bullet injury in 65 civilians. *J Neurosurg* 1970;32:163–170.
25. Roaf R. A study of the mechanisms of spinal injuries. *J Bone Joint Surg [Br]* 1960;42:810–823.
26. Goldberg AL, Baron B, Daffner RH. Clinical images. Atlantooccipital dislocation: MR demonstration of cord damage. *J Comput Assist Tomogr* 1991;15:174–178.
27. Anderson LD, D'Alonzo RT. Fractures of the odontoid process of the axis. *J Bone Joint Surg [Am]* 1974;56:1663–1691.
28. Harris JR, Edeiken-Monroe B. *The Radiology of Acute Cervical Spine Trauma, 2nd ed.* Baltimore: Williams & Wilkins, 1987.
29. Kim KS, Chen HH, Russell EJ, et al. Flexion teardrop fracture of the cervical spine: radiographic characteristics. *Am J Roentgenol* 1989;152:319–326.
30. Rizzolo SLJ, Piazza MR, Cotler JM, et al. Intervertebral disc injury complicating cervical spine trauma. *Spine* 1991;16(Suppl 2):187–189.
31. Effendi B, Roy D, Cornish B, et al. Fractures of the ring of the axis: a classification based on the analysis of 131 cases. *J Bone Joint Surg [Br]* 1981;63:319–327.
32. Davis SJ, Teresi LM, Bradley WG, et al. Cervical spine hyperextension injuries: MR findings. *Radiology* 1991;180:245–251.

CHAPTER 9

The Thoracolumbar Spine

Stephen J. Eustace and Elias R. Melhem

Traditional evaluation of trauma to the spine integrates use of conventional radiographs, myelograms and both conventional and computed tomography. Computed tomography is employed when radiographic evaluation is impaired by patient habitus or when surgical intervention is planned. MR imaging offers several advantages, outlined in the following section.

Although utilization of MR imaging in trauma is subject to institutional variation, it should be employed in all patients with neurologic signs accompanying spinal injury, is valuable in the assessment of patients with persistent unexplained symptoms or pain following trauma, and should be undertaken in all patients in whom either closed or open reduction is to be undertaken (even in the absence of neurologic signs). One of the reasons is that disk prolapse may be aggravated by either closed traction or by open reduction.

S. J. Eustace: Department of Radiology, Section of Musculoskeletal Radiology, Boston University School of Medicine and Boston Medical Center, Boston, Massachusetts 02118.

E. R. Melhem: Department of Radiology, Section of Neuroradiology, Boston University School of Medicine and Boston Medical Center, Boston, Massachusetts 02118.

Indications for MR Imaging Following Trauma

Neurologic Signs Complicating Spinal Trauma
Planned Reduction, Either Open or Closed, Following Spinal Trauma
Unexplained Symptoms Following Spinal Trauma

PATIENT POSITIONING AND IMAGING PROTOCOLS

Positioning

Similar to the cervical spine, successful imaging of both the dorsal and lumbar spine is acheived in the supine position, although occasionally images are acquired with the patient either decubitus or prone.

Receiver Coil

Although images of the spine may be obtained with the body coil alone, high-resolution imaging requires dedicated surface coils, often with a rectangular license plate configuration. Phased array coils allow high resolution signal rich imaging with an extended field of view.

Imaging Plane

Images are generally prescribed off a sagittal localizer, with coronals prescribed perpendicular to this axis and axial images prescribed at particular regions of interest.

Field of View

Similar to other sites, a preliminary image, usually a sagittal turbo inversion recovery sequence, is acquired with an extended rectangular field of view to localize sites of acute injury.

Subsequently, images are acquired with a smaller field of view, 25 cm, with a rectangular configuration. In general, turbo TSE T1 and turbo inversion recovery images are acquired in sagittal and axial planes. Coronal images are acquired in complex seat belt injuries. When specific evaluation of the spinal cord is required, imaging is supplemented by the use of FLAIR with and without gadolinium enhancement and T2-weighted turbo spin-echo sequences.

Slice Thickness

Detailed evaluation of bone and cord injury is generally obtained with 3-mm slices. By use of three-dimensional gradient-echo techniques, 1-mm oblique slices may be obtained to evaluate exiting nerves within the intervertebral foramina.

Motion Suppression

Both cardiac and respiratory motion may degrade images. Respiratory motion is limited by imaging the patient in the supine position. Cardiac motion is negated by an elongated saturation band placed adjacent and parallel to the spine. Phase encoding in the superior–inferior plane further limits motion artifact.

Methods of Motion Suppression

1. Gradient motion nulling. Motion suppression is achieved by the application of an additional gradient waveform to compensate for phase changes that occur from moving spins during the application of a bipolar gradient, such as that used in slice selection and readout.
2. Peripheral pulse gating. A peripheral sensor is used to detect peripheral pulse and gate signal acquisition. This approach is routinely employed during T2 signal acquisition.
3. Saturation bands. Bands are placed parallel to the long axis of the spine and saturate signal that would otherwise generate image distortion as a result of either respiratory or cardiac motion (1).

Imaging Protocol

Following trauma, the spine is imaged with an extended rectangular field of view. Initial imaging with an inversion recovery sequence is often undertaken to localize sites of acute injury (1 min). Detailed evaluation is then undertaken integrating a combination of turboSTIR and turbo spin-echo T1-weighted sequences in sagittal and axial planes (1 min 5 sec for each acquisition) using a 25-cm rectangular field of view. Axial T1-weighted images allow accurate evaluation of disk integrity, and configuration which is enhanced by extrathecal fat except in patients with canal stenosis in whom fat planes are lost.

Inversion recovery is often employed in preference to spectrally acquired frequency-selective fat saturation in the spine, as subtle cardiac or respiratory motion may generate local field changes and inhomogeneous fat suppression. Turbo spin-echo T1 imaging, similar to that in all other joints, is achieved using a repetition time of 500 msec, an echo time of 15 msec, a short echo train of up to six, and a low-high echo to view k-space mapping profile. Use of a short echo train facilitates the use of a short repetition time, enhancing T1 weighting and further decreasing acquisition time. Turbo inversion recovery sequences are acquired using an inversion time of 160 msec, a repetition time of 2,000 msec, an echo time of 20 msec, an echo train of six, and a linear echo to view k-space mapping profile.

When disk disease is suspected or an evaluation of cord integrity is required, improved contrast is obtained using either density or T2-weighted fluid-attenuated inversion recovery sequences (FLAIR). Cord edema and contusion may be differentiated from irreversible cord hemorrhage using gadolinium-enhanced proton-density-weighted FLAIR sequences. The former enhances, unlike cord hemorrhage, and is potentially reversible.

A myelographic effect may be achieved using heavily T2-weighted turbo spin-echo sequences with an echo time of 140 msec, imaged in the coronal plane.

Postoperative patients may be successfully imaged using RARE-based Turbo spin-echo and HASTE sequences. Appropriate slice selection, orientation of frequency gradients away from the region of interest (superior-to-inferior orientation of frequency gradients when sagittal images are undertaken to evaluate the spinal cord), and the application of serial refocusing 180° pulses, a part of the RARE sequence, facilitate successful reduction of metal-induced susceptibility artifact.

3D gradient-echo sequences are rarely employed in the lumbar spine, as the need for three-dimensional imaging is limited. Susceptibility effects between fat and trabeculae may generate artifact on gradient-echo sequences, which is magnified in osteoporotic bone (2) (Table 1).

Indications for Gadolinium

Gadolinium enhancement is not routinely employed to evaluate patients with either trauma or disk disease unless

TABLE 1. *Protocol for imaging the lumbar spine following acute trauma*

Imaging Plane	TR	TE	ETL or Flip	Mapping Profile
Sagittal TSE T1	500	15	4	Low-high profile
Sagittal IR TSE	2,000	20	6	Linear profile
Sagittal FFE	500	20	25°	
Axial TSE T1	500	15	4	Low-high profile
Axial FFE	500	20	25°	

concomitant infection is suspected. Gadolinium-enhanced imaging is performed when:

1. No anatomic abnormality is identified in a patient with intractable pain. Normal nerve roots do not enhance. Acutely inflamed nerve sheaths enhance early. Subsequent changes in enhancement (loss of enhancement) are used to predict either nerve recovery or permanent damage.
2. The identified abnormality does not explain clinical mononeuropathy.
3. A lateral disk mirrors the appearance of a schwannoma (diffuse enhancement observed in the schwannoma).
4. Noncontrast images show vertebral body collapse, and metastatic disease is suspected. Benign collapse shows minimal enhancement. Malignant collapse shows diffuse enhancment that persists at 6 weeks.

Gadolinium contrast-enhanced imaging is routinely employed in patients referred with suspected discitis and is routinely employed in the evaluation of postoperative patients with recurrent back pain, allowing differentiation of enhancing scar or fibrous tissue and retained nonenhancing disk fragment (3–6).

Truncation Artifact

Truncation artifact is commonly observed in the spine, mimicking the appearance of the intranuclear cleft (dark band identified in healthy adolescent intervertebral disks). The artifact is commonly observed when phase encoding is in a cephalocaudal direction and a matrix of 256 by 128 is employed. The artifact is minimized by increasing the matrix to 256 by 256.

MAGNETIC RESONANCE IMAGING OF SOFT TISSUE DISORDERS IN THE DORSAL AND LUMBAR SPINE

Intervertebral Disk Degeneration and Herniation

The intervertebral disk is predominantly composed of water and mucopolysaccharide, which accounts for T1 signal hypointensity and T2 signal hyperintensity in health. In adulthood, as disk degeneration develops (thought to be related to biomechanical trauma and changes in vascular supply through lumbar arteries), the disk loses water, resulting in loss of T2 signal hyperintensity, and mucopolysaccharide

content diminishes, resulting in morphologic changes, loss of height, and annular bulging of the disk (Fig. 1) (8).

The precursor to disk degeneration is thought to be tearing of the outer annular fibers either anteriorly, laterally, or posteriorly. In most cases, these annular tears are not identifiable at MR imaging. Occasionally, the tears are conspicuous on heavily T2-weighted scans as foci of hyperintensity (high-intensity zones, HIZs) secondary to the presence of edema and granulation tissue (Fig. 2) (9). Nerve endings are known to exit in the periphery of the annulus and may be irritated by tear, accounting for a documented correlation between HIZs and low back pain. Somatic neurons of the recurrent meningeal nerve of Luschka supply fibers to the posterior longitudinal ligament, the meninges, the blood vessels, the

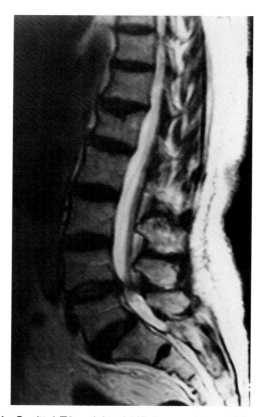

FIG. 1. Sagittal T2-weighted MR image shows diffuse loss of signal throughout the intervertebral disks secondary to degeneration with annular bulge and canal stenosis at L4-5. Incidental note is made of a superior end plate osteoporotic wedge compression at L1.

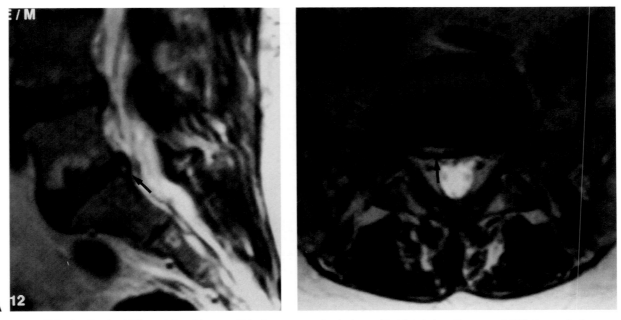

FIG. 2. Sagittal T2-weighted image **(A)** shows annular bulge with high-intensity zone (HIZ) *(arrow)* at the site of a symptomatic annular tear. Incidental note is made of Modic 2 superior end plate marrow change. Axial T2-weighted image **(B)** shows an extensive annular tear.

posterior outer fibers of the annulus, and the vertebral body periosteum (10).

As tears extend, morphology of the disk in both the sagittal and axial planes is lost, with both loss of height and bulging. As annular fibers are stretched, traction effects promote the development of osteophytes at the insertion of the outer annular Sharpey fibers. With MRI, signal abnormalities are noted in the marrow immediately adjacent to the vertebral body end plate adjacent to the degenerating disk, preceding radiographic evidence of end plate sclerosis. Although unexplained, it seems likely that vascular abnormalities contribute to the described signal changes. According to Modic, early in discogenic degeneration (type 1 change), marrow is characterized by end plate T1 signal hypointensity with T2 signal hyperintensity; in chronicity (type 2 change), marrow adjacent to the end plate appears to become fatty with T1 signal hyperintensity and persistent although slightly less marked T2 signal hyperintensity (Figs. 3 and 4). In endstage disease, marrow becomes replaced by dense bone, obvious on radiographs, hypointense on both T1- and T2-weighted scans at MRI. It is important to note that both type 1 and 2 changes enhance following the administration of gadolinium (11).

Modic Marrow Changes

Type 1: Blood-like; T1 Dark, T2 Bright; Enhance with Gd
Type 2: Fat-like; T1 Bright, T2 Bright; Enhance with Gd
Type 3: Fibrous; T1 and T2 Dark; No Enhancement

As the disk degenerates, manifest as loss of T2 signal

hyperintensity at MRI, annular tears, either posterolateral or in the midline, allow herniation of central content, the nucleus pulposus (12).

Loss of both water and mucopolysaccharide from the disk promotes diffuse disk bulging. Superimposed discrete annular tears result in focal extension of the central nucleus pulposus through the defect described as disk protrusion. Disruption of the outer fibers of the annulus, Sharpey's fibers, allows disk extrusion. When extrusion is followed by fragment migration at, above, or below the disk level, the term disk sequestration is applied.

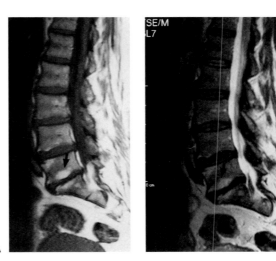

FIG. 3. Sagittal T1 **(A)** and T2 **(B)** images show marked disk degeneration with loss of height at L5-S1 with associated superior end plate marrow hyperintensity on T1 and T2 scans typical of the Modic 2 pattern.

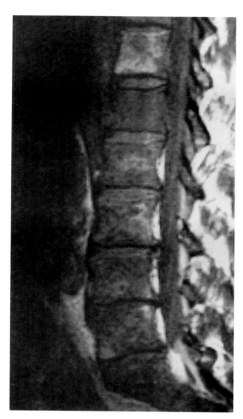

FIG. 4. Sagittal T1-weighted image shows diffuse loss of signal throughout vertebral body marrow (absent yellow marrow), secondary to red marrow conversion or infiltration or, as in this case, secondary to accumulation of marrow iron in anemia of chronic disease, commonly observed in patients with chronic HIV infection.

Global Alteration in Morphology

Disk Bulging; Loss of Water and Polysaccharide
Disk Protrusion; Herniation of Nucleus Through an Annular Tear
Disk Extrusion; Herniation Beyond Disrupted Sharpey's Fibers
Disk Sequestration; Migration of Disk Fragment At, Above, or Below Level

---

Virtually all lumbar and thoracic disk herniations are associated with loss of T2 signal (disk degeneration); nevertheless, only a minority of degenerating disks progress to protrusion or extrusion. The hallmark feature of a herniated disk is a focal contour abnormality (contiguous with the intervertebral portion of the disk by a narrow waist) along the posterior disk margin with a soft tissue mass displacing epidural fat, nerve root, epidural veins, or thecal sac.

Herniations are well visualized on T1-weighted scans, contrasted against epidural fat. On T2-weighted scans, the herniated portion is usually slightly hyperintense relative to the rest of the degenerating disk. The nerve root adjacent to the herniated disk may enhance following the administration of gadolinium (6,12).

Loss in vertebral disk height secondary to degeneration may lead to abnormal facet joint motion with both secondary osteoarthritis and compensatory hypertrophy of the ligamentum flavum (an attempt to resist abnormal motion). The combination of hypertrophic change at the facet joint, ligamentous hypertrophy, and disk prolapse may lead to marked central canal stenosis (anteroposterior diameter less than 11.5 mm, area less than 1.5 cm^2).

In patients with congenital ''short pedicles,'' the effect of these changes is magnified. Asymmetric facet overgrowth (particularly of the superior facet) leads to osseous encroachment of the lateral recesses and the foramina with compression of lateral nerve roots (foraminal stenosis defined as a distance of less than 4 mm between the superior facet and the vertebral body) (13,14).

Spondylolisthesis and Spondylolysis

Spondylolysis is the term used to describe an abnormality of the spine in which a defect or cleft is found in the pars interarticularis. Although the etiology of spondylolysis is unclear, most believe it results from repeated trauma during childhood and that it represents a form of stress fracture. Spondylolysis is not identified in children with neuromuscular diseases who never walk. Although spondylolysis is occasionally identified following local isolated macrotrauma, this is extremely uncommon. Reflecting onset in childhood, the recorded prevalence of between 3% and 10% is noted to be the same in both childhood and adulthood (15).

Although any vertebra can be involved, the L5 posterior element is involved in up to 95% of cases, bilateral involvement occurring in 90%.

In affected individuals, up to 75% of patients remain asymptomatic. Almost 25% of patients develop chronic back pain, usually secondary to complicating facet disease, nerve entrapment, or spondylolisthesis (16,17).

Spondylolisthesis is the term used to describe a forward slip of an upper vertebral body on a lower vertebral body (in contrast to backward slippage described as retrolisthesis). Degree of slippage is graded 1 to 4. Grade 1 represents a slip of between 0% and 25%; grade 2 represents a slip of between 25% and 50%; grade 3 represents a slip of between 50% and 75%; grade 4 represents a slip of greater than 75% (18,19).

Although spondylolisthesis is most commonly secondary to spondylolysis, it is also commonly identified in the elderly secondary to facet joint disease and rarely secondary to a structural deficiency in the vertebral body. Of interest, although unexplained, is the finding that only 50% of patients with spondylolysis develop spondylolisthesis, and only half of these become symptomatic (20).

Pathria has previously demonstrated that almost 70% of patients over 40 years have evidence of significant facet joint osteoarthritis at CT. According to Pathria (21), facet disease is graded 0 to 3: grade 1, mild osteoarthritis; grade 2, moderate osteoarthritis; grade 3, severe osteoarthritis. In contrast

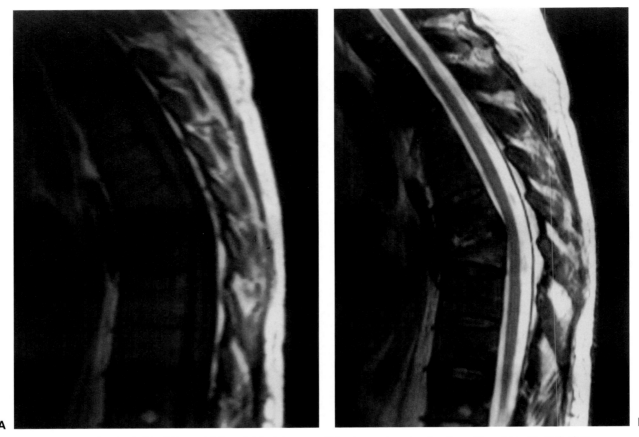

FIG. 5. Sagittal T1- **(A)** and T2-weighted images **(B)** show chronic discitis with adjacent end plate osteomyelitis and wedging in the middorsal spine, secondary to tuberculous infection.

to spondylolysis, spondylolisthesis complicating facet disease is most commonly identified at the L4-5 level (22).

Infection

Spinal infection is generally a sequel to hematogenous spread, either arterial or venous, and rarely complicates medical intervention. Reflecting vascularity, infection in childhood is frequently confined to the vascular disk. In adulthood, infection is initially to vascular red marrow adjacent to the anterior margin of the end plate, with disk infection complicating local osteomyelitis (Fig. 5) (23,24). Occasionally infection spares the disk and spreads via the anterior subligamentous space, particularly in tuberculous or fungal infection. *Staphylococcus* infection accounts for up to 60% of cases, even in immunocompromised patients. In contrast, isolated posterior element infection is invariably secondary to tuberculosis (25,26).

MAGNETIC RESONANCE IMAGING OF ACUTE OSSEOUS INJURY FOLLOWING TRAUMA TO THE DORSAL AND LUMBAR SPINE

Ninety percent of thoracic and lumbar vertebral body fractures occur at the thoracolumbar junction between T11 and L4. Fractures occur at this site because it is the junction of two opposing spinal curvatures, the dorsal kyphosis and the lumbar lordosis, because of a loss of the stabilizing effect of the bony and soft tissue thoracic cage, and because at this point there is change in the orientation of the articular facets from the thoracic coronal to the lumbar sagittal plane (27).

Predisposing Factors in Thoracolumbar Junction Fractures

Loss of Thoracic Cage Support
Fulcrum Between Thoracic Kyphosis and Lumbar Lordosis
Change in Facet Joint Orientation

Reflecting severe trauma, thoracolumbar fractures are often associated with trauma at additional sites; indeed, noncontiguous concomitant fractures are identified in up to 5% of patients. To account for additional sites of trauma, the entire spine should be imaged in all patients with dorsolumbar trauma (28).

Fractures of the Dorsolumbar Spine

Fractures of the thoracolumbar spine are divided into major and minor categories. Injuries involving the vertebral body are considered to be major injuries, whereas injuries involving the posterior elements (the transverse processes, the pars interarticularis, and the spinous processes) are considered to be minor injuries. Minor injuries tend to be stable and not associated with neurologic compromise and do not produce progressive deformity.

Major injuries of the vertebral body may be secondary to anterior wedging (compression fractures), axial loading (burst fractures), or acute hyperflexion (seat belt fractures) with or without rotation.

To classify fractures involving the vertebral body, both Denis and Ferguson divide the spine into three columns (Fig. 6) (29). The anterior column incorporates the anterior longitudinal ligament, the anterior two-thirds of the vertebral body, and the anterior two-thirds of the annulus fibrosis and disk. (It is the site of wedge or compression fractures.) The middle column incorporates the posterior one-third of the vertebral body, the posterior one-third of the annulus fibrosis and disk, and the posterior longitudinal ligament. (Both the anterior and middle columns are involved in burst fractures.) The posterior column incorporates the posterior bony elements (pedicles, articular processes, the lamina, and spinous processes), and the posterior ligamentous complex (ligamentum flavum and the interspinous and supraspinous ligaments). (The middle and posterior columns are involved in lap seat belt injuries.)

All three columns are disrupted in fracture dislocations where rotation is typically superimposed on hyperflexion and distraction forces.

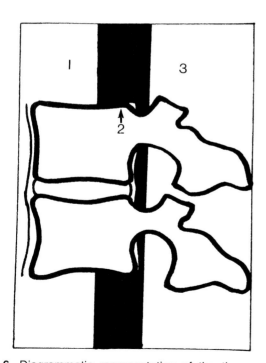

FIG. 6. Diagrammatic representation of the three-column structure described by Dennis: 1, anterior column; 2, middle column; 3, posterior column.

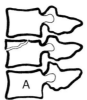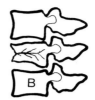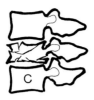

FIG. 7. Diagrammatic representation of spectrum of wedge compression fractures secondary to flexion forces (**A,** mild; **B,** severe) through burst fracture secondary to acute axial loading (**C**).

Three-Column Classification of Dorsolumbar Spine Fractures

Anterior Column: Wedge Compression Fractures
Anterior and Middle Columns: Burst Fractures
Middle and Posterior Columns: Lap Seat Belt Fractures
Three Columns: Fracture Dislocations

Wedge Compression Fractures

Wedge compression fractures follow acute hyperflexion with impaction, accounting for almost 50% of dorsolumbar fractures. Mechanical failure of vertically oriented trabeculae within cancellous bone of the vertebral body, particularly of the anterior column, results in vertebral body wedging with mechanical compression of the superior end plate, which may become comminuted in the presence of bony demineralization (Fig. 7) (30).

Being confined to the anterior column, sparing the middle and posterior columns, wedge compression fractures are generally stable. Instability is conferred by loss of more than 50% of the anterior vertebral body height or compressions at multiple levels (Fig. 8).

Wedge fractures are poorly visualized in the axial plane at CT, as the fracture lines almost parallel the imaging plane, the in plane fracture phenomenon. In contrast, wedging is readily identified at MR imaging in the sagittal plane. Although management is usually conservative, persistent weight bearing and activity in an unrecognized acute wedge may result in progressive compression with the development of instability.

In the presence of severe wedging, MR imaging may be undertaken in order to differentiate an acute stable wedge fracture from an unstable two column burst fracture (Fig. 9) (31,32).

Burst Fractures

Burst fractures are usually the result of acute axial loading such as occurs following a fall from a height. They account for up to 15% of dorsolumbar fractures and are of importance because they are frequently associated with neurologic injury (33).

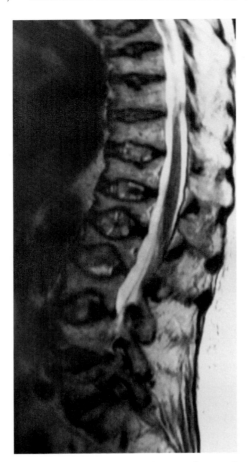

FIG. 8. Sagittal TSE T2-weighted image (fat retains signal secondary to J coupling effect) shows osteoporotic end plate wedging at multiple levels, with loss of height of anterior vertebral body relative to posterior vertebral body margins at multiple levels.

Burst fractures are comminuted fractures involving the anterior and middle columns, the superior or inferior end plates, or both, occasionally in association with vertical fractures through the posterior elements. Frequently comminution is associated with loss of vertebral body height both anteriorly and posteriorly and with retropulsion of bone fragment to the spinal canal (Figs. 10 and 11).

Although burst fractures are readily identified on conventional radiographs, CT is routinely undertaken for this injury because it allows specific evaluation of the degree of vertebral body comminution and localization of retropulsed osseous fragments. Similar information may be obtained with MRI in coronal, sagittal, and axial planes, particularly using the FLAIR sequence. In addition, MR imaging allows improved detection of concomitant disk prolapse and differentiation of acute cord edema and hemorrhage (34,35).

Burst fractures are generally considered to be unstable fractures requiring operative fixation. Associated vertical fracture of the posterior element, particularly the pedicles, is a marker of definite instability (three-column injury).

Lap Seat Belt Fractures: Chance Fractures

Acute hyperflexion over a seat belt, preventing forward propulsion following a motor vehicle accident, may lead to a severe fracture and distraction of the middle and particularly of the posterior columns. Such injuries account for 5% of dorsolumbar spine fractures in adulthood.

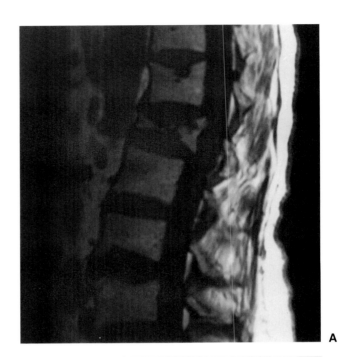

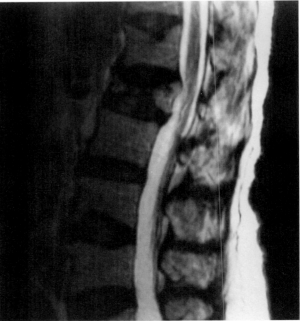

FIG. 9. Sagittal T1 **(A)** and T2 **(B)** images showing a severe wedge compression fracture at the L1 level with retropulsion of bone fragment. There is greater loss of height anteriorly than posteriorly, indicating a flexion mechanism. There is preservation of vertebral body marrow signal, indicating a benign osteoporotic etiology.

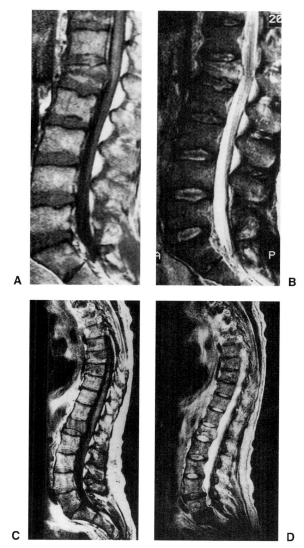

A **B**

C **D**

FIG. 10. Sagittal T1 **(A)** and T2 **(B)** images showing an acute burst fracture at L1 in a patient following a fall from a height. Central concertina effect of trabeculae within cancellous bone accounting for central loss of vertebral body signal on T1- and extensive central signal hyperintensity on T2-weighted scans. Note is made of retropulsion and bowing of the posterior margin of the vertebral body with associated cord hemorrhage and edema. Discrepancy in height of anterior and posterior vertebral body margins makes differentiation of severe flexion and axial load injury difficult although somewhat academic. Sagittal T1- **(C)** and T2-weighted **(D)** images in a patient with similar L1 burst fracture following a fall from a height (lover's leap).

The classic Chance fracture represents a horizontal fracture through the posterior arch, pedicle, and posterior vertebral body; however, many variations in this injury are now recognized, ranging from purely ligamentous disruption through a combination of bone and soft tissue, with disruption of disk rather than vertebral body, with variations often involving more than one vertebral body level (Fig. 12) (36).

Radiographs show widening of the posterior elements fol-

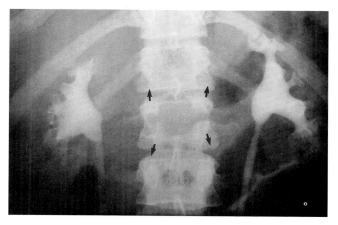

FIG. 11. Frontal radiograph from an intravenous urogram series shows splaying of the posterior elements of the L1 vertebral body *(arrows)* in a patient following a motor vehicle accident.

lowing this injury but may not show extension to the vertebral body or disk (see Fig. 11). Similar to wedge fractures, the plane of this injury often limits its visualization by CT (in plane fracture phenomenon) without sagittal reformatting (Fig. 13). With MRI, sagittal images clearly delineate extension of these fractures through either the vertebral body, disk, or posterior elements. Similar to other injuries, sensitivity to edema facilitates the identification of cord contusion and associated disk disease (Fig. 14).

Lap seat belt fractures are generally considered to be stable because stability is conferred by an intact anterior column and anterior longitudinal ligament. These fractures are unstable in flexion.

Fracture Dislocation

Fracture dislocations of the dorsolumbar spine account for 15% of fractures of the dorsolumbar spine. They are the result of either acute severe hyperflexion (in which dislocation is anterior), acute shear, or acute flexion rotation injury, often following motor vehicle or motorbicycle accident.

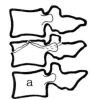 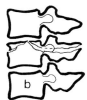 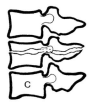

FIG. 12. Diagrammatic representation of variations in lap seat belt injury: **(a)** fracture extension to the pars interarticularis, **(b)** fracture extension to the end plate and spinous process, **(c)** fracture extension through the vertebral body and posterior element.

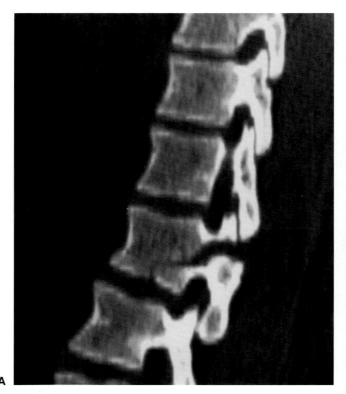
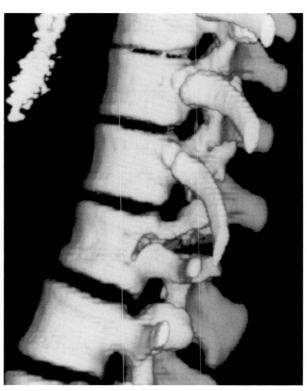

A

B

FIG. 13. (A) Sagittal reformatted CT image acquired from axial source data shows a lap seat belt hyperflexion fracture extending through the inferior vertebral body to the posterior element pars interarticularis. **(B)** Three-dimensional reformatted image in the same patient.

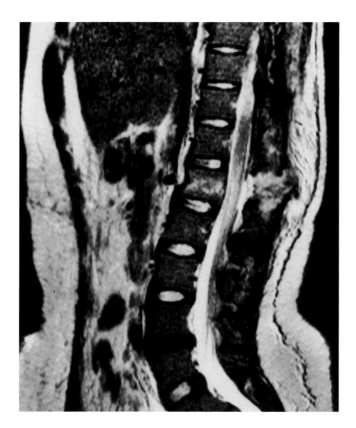

FIG. 14. Sagittal T2-weighted image shows fracture extending posteriorly through the vertebral body to the spinous process in a type c lap seat belt injury (see Fig. 12).

Complete disruption of three columns confers gross instability, usually complicated by acute cord compression or transection.

The injury is readily identified on conventional radiographs, and the degree of osseous injury usually requires no further evaluation. Computed tomography is occasionally undertaken to evaluate position of articular processes and integrity of the spinal canal, although it has now been replaced for this purpose by MRI. In the axial plane, displaced vertebral bodies may be seen in the same plane;

the double-rim sign and unpaired articular processes of the facet joints may be identified, the naked facet sign (Fig. 15) (37).

Injuries Accompanying Fractures of the Dorsolumbar Spine

Reflecting severe trauma, fractures of the dorsolumbar spine are commonly associated with concomitant noncontiguous spinal fractures in 5% of cases. Fractures are often

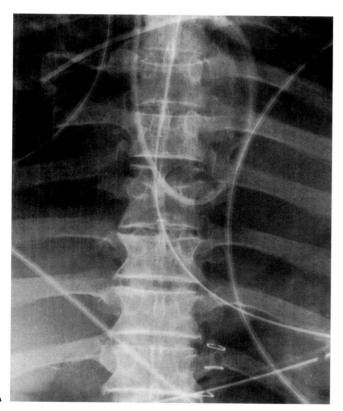
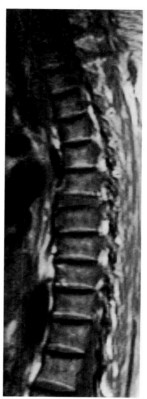
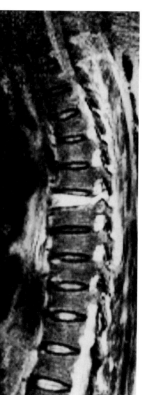

A

C,D

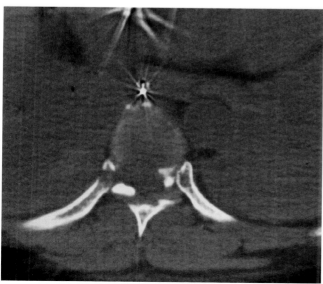

B

FIG. 15. (A) Radiograph shows apparent widening of the T8-9 interspace with associated posterior rib fracture on right in patient with post-MVA paraparesis. (B) Axial CT scan through the T8-9 level shows a naked left facet indicating rotational component or fracture dislocation. (C) Sagittal T1-weighted image and (D) sagittal T2-weighted image show fracture dislocation through the T8-9 disk space and posterior elements with marked distraction at the site of fracture.

accompanied by posterior rib fractures (costovertebral dislocation) and injury to the sternum.

Sternal fractures may be secondary to direct impaction against the steering column, in which case the inferior fragment is displaced posteriorly, or may be secondary to forces applied from above secondary to acute spinal hyperflexion, indirect sternal fracture, in which the superior fragment is displaced posteriorly (38,39).

Isolated dorsal fractures are commonly associated with mediastinal hematoma and hemothorax (mimicking aortic injury) (40), seat belt fractures are associated with traumatic duodenal hematomas (41), and, reflecting a shared mechanism, burst fractures are often associated with compression fractures of the calcaneus.

Pitfalls and Variants

Physiological wedging of the anterior margins of the vertebral bodies is commonly identified at the thoracolumbar junction between T8 and T12. The ratio of the height of the anterior margin of the vertebral body to the posterior margin is 0.8 in men and 0.87 in women (42).

Thinning of the pedicles is commonly identified at the thoracolumbar junction, resulting in apparent widening of the intevetebral foramina (43).

Scheuermann's disease is a self-limiting osteochondrosis of the vertebral body end plate. It is initially manifest as corner apophysitis and subsequently as end plate sclerosis, irregularity, and depression. End plate irregularity may be incorrectly attributed to acute trauma.

Benign Versus Malignant Vertebral Body Collapse

In elderly patients, age-related demineralization of cancellous bone within the vertebral body predisposes to compression fracture, often following minor trauma. In this setting, it may be difficult to exclude the presence of underlying bony metastatic disease (44).

On radiographs, the identification of gas within or between the vertebral body is a reliable indicator of a benign etiology. Similarly, the identification of progressive compression over years on old radiographs is a further marker of benignity (45,46).

Because bony metastatic disease is rarely solitary, a bone scan is often undertaken to localize additional sites of disease. If uptake of radiotracer is identified at multiple sites, the likelihood of metastatic compression fracture is markedly increased, and transpedicular biopsy is undertaken. As an alternative, whole-body MR imaging using a turboSTIR technique may be employed. In a recent study, whole-body MR imaging demonstrated disease in 57 of 175 sites, as compared with bone scan, which identified disease in 42 of 175 sites. Whole-body MR imaging is particularly valuable in patients in whom compression fractures are identified during dedicated MR imaging of the lumbar spine. In these patients, the investigation may be performed while the patient is on the table rather than as an additional study following formal interpretation of the MR study (47).

When compression fractures are identified at MR imaging, complete loss of normal vertebral body marrow signal, inferior end plate fracture, extension of abnormal signal to the pedicle, and persistent enhancement at 6 weeks all suggest the presence of underlying metastases. When metastatic disease is suggested, a whole-body MR imaging technique is employed to localize a site suitable for biopsy, which is usually performed under CT guidance (48–51).

Previously, Yuh et al. (52) divided marrow patterns following fracture into category 1, 2, and 3 types based on the review of parasagittal T1-weighted images. Category 1 pattern is characterized by complete replacement of normal marrow by low-signal material, which, when identified without adjacent disk abnormality or vertebral fragmentation, is secondary to maligancy in up to 80% of cases (Figs. 16 and 17). Category 3 is characterized by increased marrow signal throughout the collapsed vertebral body, reflecting the presence of normal yellow marrow; it is invariably a marker of benignity (Fig. 18). The category 2 marrow pattern is characterized by incomplete replacement of normal marrow, an inhomogeneous pattern. In this group, random distribution of poorly marginated signal hypointensity suggests metastatic or neoplastic infiltration. In contrast, a sharply marginated signal abnormality with preservation of a band of normal marrow posteriorly suggests benign osteoporotic vertebral body collapse.

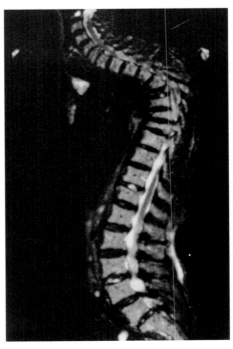

FIG. 16. Sagittal T2-weighted image of the entire spine shows complete replacement of spinal marrow in multiple myeloma, with associated compression wedging in the middorsal spine. (Courtesy of S. Valentine, M.D., Calgary, AB.)

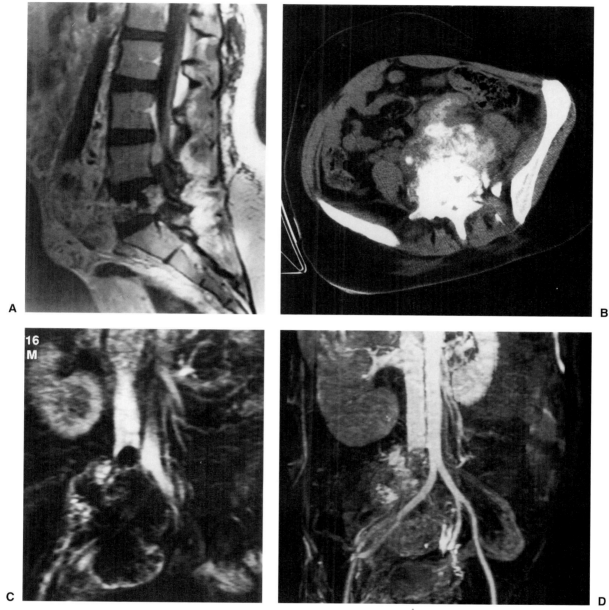

FIG. 17. (A) Category 1 complete replacement of normal marrow with destruction of the L5 vertebral body. There is extension of tumor anteriorly with invasion of the inferior vena cava. **(B)** Axial CT scan shows organized matrix within the tumor, subsequently confirmed as a primary osteosarcoma of the vertebral body. **(C)** This MIP reconstruction from two-dimensional time-of-flight images shows invasion of the vena cava. Loss of signal within the mass corresponds to mineralization in **B**. **(D)** Gadolinium-enhanced image confirms patency of displaced distal aorta and common iliac vessels.

Benign	Malignant
Solitary	Multiple
Some Normal Marrow Signal (Posterior Band)	Complete Loss of Normal Marrow Signal
Superior end plate fracture	Inferior end plate fracture
Enhancement decreases at 6 weeks	Enhancement persists or increases at 6 weeks

Stable Versus Unstable Thoracic Fractures

Unlike the lumbar spine, where the presence of a single intact column may confer stability, such a concept is not applicable to the thoracic spine. Instability in the thoracic spine should be suspected, in the presence of fracture dislocation, posttraumatic kyphosis of more than 40°, posterior rib fractures, costovertebral dislocation, and sternal fractures (32).

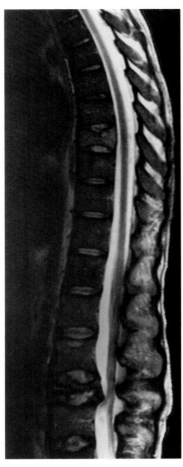

FIG. 18. Sagittal T2-weighted image shows complete collapse at L3 with heterogeneous marrow. Some preservation of normal marrow suggests benign collapse; however, lack of disease at other adjacent levels makes this less likely. There is wedging of the T8 vertebral body with diffuse vertebral body edema and relative preservation of the anatomic configuration. Biopsy at L3 showed metastatic lung carcinoma.

Cord Injury Following Dorsolumbar Fracture

Cord hematoma may be differentiated from edema in the first few hours on T2-weighted sequences.

Hematomas are generally hypointense on T2-weighted sequences, most likely because of the presence of deoxyhemoglobin and intracellular methemoglobin. In contrast, edema and contusion typically present as areas of signal hyperintensity on T2-weighted sequences. There may be no discernible signal abnormaltity on T1-weighted scans (7).

Cord Hematoma Versus Cord Edema

Cord Hematoma: T2 Hypointense
Cord Edema: T2 Hyperintense

Complications of Spinal Injury

In addition to direct injury to the cord, with either hemorrhage or edema, fracture of the dorsolumbar spine may be complicated by dural tear in up to 15% of cases. If the dura is torn, it is possible for nerve roots to become tangled within fracture fragments. When this condition is identified, surgical repair is undertaken from a posterior rather than anterior approach. Dural tear should be suspected in the presence of a laminar fracture or if a hematocrit level is identified within the dependent portion of the thecal sac.

Posttraumatic cord atrophy or central spinal cord cysts may produce progressive neurologic signs several years after spinal injury. Spinal cysts are easily identified at MRI and are an indication for surgical decompression (53).

ANKYLOSING SPONDYLITIS

Pseudarthrosis complicating an end-stage bamboo spine in ankylosing spondylitis occurs at a point of relative instability within an otherwise stable spine, most frequently at the thoracolumbar junction.

As disease progresses, the spine becomes progressively fused. At the dorsolumbar junction, greater motion prevents complete fusion. As the remainder of the spine becomes progressively fixed, motion at this site becomes increasingly more important. Progressive motion leads to degeneration of the intervertebral disk with the development of secondary

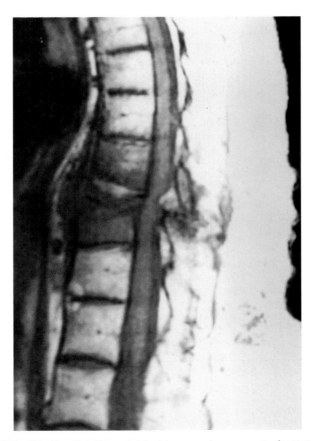

FIG. 19. Sagittal T1-weighted image shows acute fracture through vertebral body and posterior element in a patient with a fused spine of ankylosing spondylitis.

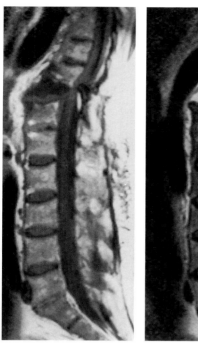
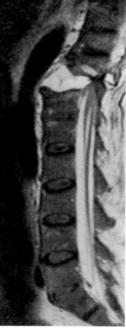

A   B

FIG. 20. Sagittal T1- **(A)** and T2-weighted **(B)** images in a further patient with end-stage ankylosing spondylitis show a catastrophic fracture through a preexisting Anderson lesion.

osteoarthritis at this level, with end plate sclerosis mimicking infection, the Anderson lesion.

Following minor trauma, forced motion is transmitted to the site of the pseudarthrosis, often resulting in catastrophic hyperflexion and fracture through or just above the disk. Extending through the posterior elements, the injury is usually complicated by acute cord impaction, hemorrhage, and edema (Figs. 19 and 20).

It is the role of the radiologist to identify sites of pseudarthrosis before such a catastrophe. Unlike the primary disease, where enthesopathy generates osteophytes oriented to the long axis of the spine, pseudarthrosis is characterized by degenerative osteophytes with an orientation parallel to the end plate.

KUMMEL'S DISEASE

Kummel's disease is an uncommon cause of vertebral body collapse, usually several weeks (6 weeks) following direct spinal trauma. Following insult, serial radiographs or MR scans show progressive vertebral body collapse over 6 weeks, the benign nature of which is suggested by the presence of characteristic intravertebral body gas. Although the etiology is unclear, posttraumatic osteonecrosis appears to be the likeliest cause (54).

REFERENCES

1. Czervionke LF. Lumbar intervetebral disc disease. *Neuroimag Clin North Am* 1993;3:465–485.
2. Hackney DB. Neoplasms and related disorders. *Top Magn Reson Imag* 1992;4:37–61.
3. Watanabe R, Parke WW. Vascular and neural pathology of lumbosacral spinal stenosis. *J Neurosurg* 1986;64:64.
4. Modic MT, Ross JT. Morphology, symptoms, and causality. *Radiology* 1990;175:619.
5. Post MJD, Sze G, Quencer RM, et al. Gadolinium enhanced MR in spinal infection. *J Comput Assist Tomogr* 1990;14:721.
6. Jinkins JR. Magnetic resonance imaging of benign nerve root enhancement in the unoperated and postoperative lumbosacral spine. *Neuroimag Clin North Am* 1993;3:525–541.
7. Hackney DB, Asato R, Joseph PM, et al. Hemorrhage and edema in acute spinal cord compression: demonstration by MR imaging. *Radiology* 1986;161:387–390.
8. Wagner M, Sether LA, Yu S, et al. Age changes in the lumbar intervertebral disc studied with magnetic resonance and cryomicrotomy. *Clin Anat* 1988;1:93–103.
9. Yu S, Haughton VM, Sether LA, Wagner M. Comparison of MR and diskography in detecting radial tears of the annulus. *Am J Neuroradiol* 1989;10:1077–1081.
10. Jinkins JR, Whittemore AR, Bradley WG. The anatomic basis of vertebrogenic pain and the autonomic syndrome associated with lumbar disc extrusion. *Am J Neuroradiol* 1989;10:219.
11. Modic MT, Masaryk TJ, Ross JS, et al. Imaging of degenerative disc disease. *Radiology* 1988;168:177–186.
12. Yu S, Haughton VM, Ho PSP, et al. Progressive and regressive changes in the nucleus pulposus. Part 2. The adult. *Radiology* 1988;169:93–97.
13. Modic MT, Herfkens RJ. Intervertebral disk: normal age related changes in MR signal intensity. *Radiology* 1990;177:332–334.
14. Modic MT, Masaryk T, Boumphrey F, et al. Lumbar herniated disk disease and canal stenosis: prospective evaluation by surface coil MR, CT and myelography. *Am J Roentgenol* 1986;147:757–765.
15. Johnson WJ, Farnum GN, Latchaw RE, et al. MR imaging of the pars interarticularis. *Am J Roentgenol* 1989;152:327.
16. Porter RW, Hibbert CS. Symptoms associated with lysis of the pars interarticularis. *Spine* 1984;9:755.
17. Rauch RA, Jinkins JR. Lumbosacral spondylolisthesis associated with spondylolysis. *Neuroimag Clin North Am* 1993;3:543–555.
18. Alexander E, Kenny DL, Davis CH, et al. Intact arch spondylolisthesis. *J Neuroimag* 1985;63:840.
19. Bailey W. Observations on the etiology and frequency of spondylolisthesis and its precursors. *Radiology* 1947;48:107.
20. Jinkins JR, Matthes JC, Sener RN, et al. Spondylolysis, spondylolisthesis, and associated nerve root entrapment in the lumbosacral spine: MR evaluation. *Am J Roentgenol* 1992;159:799.
21. Pathria M, Sartoris D, Resnick D. Osteoarthritis of facet joints. Accuracy of oblique radiographic assessment. *Radiology* 1987;164:227.
22. Griffiths HJ, Parantainen H, Olson PN. Disease of the lumbosacral facet joints. *Neuroimag Clin North Am* 1993;3:567–575.
23. Wenger DR, Bobechko WP, Gilday DL. The spectrum of intervertebral disc space infection in children. *J Bone Joint Surg [Am]* 1978;60:100.
24. Wiley AM, Trueta J. The vascular anatomy of the spine and its relationship to pyogenic vertebral osteomyelitis. *J Bone Joint Surg* 1959;41B:796.
25. Modic MT, Feiglin DH, Piraino DW, et al. Vertebral osteomyelitis: assessment using MR. *Radiology* 1985;151:157.
26. Post MJD, Bowen BC, Sze G. Magnetic resonance imaging of spinal infection. *Rheum Dis Clin North Am* 1991;17:773.
27. Andriacchi T, Schultz A, Belytschko T, et al. A model for studies of mechanical interactions between the human spine and rib cage. *J Biomech* 1974;7:497–507.
28. El-Khoury GY, Whitten CG. Trauma to the upper thoracic spine. Anatomy, biomechanics and unique imaging features. *Am J Roentgenol* 1993;160:95–102.
29. Denis F. The three column spine and its significance in the classification of acute thoraco lumbar spinal injuries. *Spine* 1983;8:817–831.
30. Fletcher GH. Anterior vertebral wedging—frequency and significance. *Am J Roentgenol* 1947;57:232–238.
31. Hanley EN, Eskay ML. Thoracic spine fractures. *Orthopedics* 1989;12:689–696.
32. Kaye JJ, Nance EP. Thoracic and lumbar spine trauma. *Radiol Clin North Am* 1990;28:361–377.
33. Saifuddin A, Noordeen H, Taylor BA, et al. The role of imaging in the diagnosis and management of thoracolumbar burst fractures: Current

concepts and a review of the literature. *Skeletal Radiol* 1996;25:603–613.

34. Cammisa FP, Eismont FJ, Green BA. Dural laceration occurring with burst fractures and associated laminar fractures. *J Bone Joint Surg [Am]* 1989;71:1044–1052.

35. Daffner RH, Deeb ZL, Rothfus WE. The posterior vertebral body line. Importance in the detection of burst fractures. *Am J Roentgenol* 1987;148:93–96.

36. Chance GQ. Note on type of flexion fracture of the spine. *Br J Radiol* 1948;21:452–453.

37. Manaster BJ, Osborn AG. CT patterns of facet fracture dislocations in the thoracolumbar spine. *Am J Roentgenol* 1987;148:335–340.

38. Fowler AW. Flexion-compression injury of the sternum. *J Bone Joint Surg [Br]* 1957;39:487–496.

39. Gopalakrishnan KC, Masri WS. Fractures of the sternum associated with spinal injury. *J Bone Joint Surg [Br]* 1986;68:178–181.

40. Bolesta MJ, Bohlman HH. Mediastinal widening asssociated with fractures of the upper thoracic spine. *J Bone Joint Surg [Am]* 1991;73:447–450.

41. Rhea JT, Novelline RA, Lawrason J, et al. The frequency and significance of thoracic injuries detected on abdominal CT scans of multiple trauma patients. *J Trauma* 1989;29:502–505.

42. Lauridsen KN, De Carvalho A, Anderson AH. Degree of vertebral wedging of the dorso-lumbar spine. *Acta Radiol* 1984;25:29–32.

43. Benzian SR, Mainzer F, Gooding CA. Pediculate thinnning: a normal variant at the thoracolumbar junction. *Br J Radiol* 1971;44:936–939.

44. Cuenod CA, Laredo JD, Chevret S, et al. Acute vertebral collapse due to osteoporosis or malignancy. Appearance on unenhanced and gadolinium enhanced MR images. *Radiology* 1996;199:541–549.

45. Warnock NG, Yuh WTC. Magnetic resonance imaging in the discrimination of benign from malignant disease of the lumbosacral vertebral column. *Neuroimag Clin North Am* 1993;3:609–623.

46. An HS, Andreshak TG, Nguyen C, et al. Can we distinguish between benign and malignant compression fractures of the spine by magnetic resonance imaging. *Spine* 1995;20:1776–1782.

47. Eustace S, Tello R, DeCarvalho V, Carey J, Wroblicka JT, Melhem ER, Yucel EK. A comparison of whole body turbo short tau inversion recovery MR imaging and planar technetium 99m methylene diphosphonate scintigraphy in the evaluation of patients with suspected skeletal metastases. *Am J Roentgenol* 1997;169:1655–1661.

48. Baker LL, Goodman SB, Perkash I, et al. Benign vertebral pathologic compression fractures of the vertebral bodies: Assessment with conventional spin echo, chemical shift and STIR MR imaging. *Radiology* 1990;174:495–502.

49. Baker LL, Goodman SB. Benign versus malignant vertebral body infiltration. Marrow signal pattern differentiation by means of chemical shift MR images. *Radiology* 1988;169:65.

50. Li KC, Poon PY. Sensitivity and specificity of MRI in detecting malignant spinal cord compression and in distinguishing malignant from benign compression fractures of vertebrae. *Magn Reson Imag* 1988;6:546–556.

51. Fruehwald FX, Tscholakoff D, Schwaighofer B, et al. Magnetic resonance imaging of the lower vertebral column in patients with multiple myeloma. *Invest Radiol* 1988;23:193–199.

52. Yu WTC, Zacher CK, Barloon TJ, et al. Vertebral compression fractures. Distinction between benign and malignant causes with MR imaging. *Radiology* 1989;172:215–218.

53. Keenan TL, Antony J, Benson DR. Dural tears associated with lumbar burst fractures. *J Orthop Trauma* 1990;4:243–245.

54. Steel HH. Kummel's disease. *Am J Surg* 1951;81:161–167.

CHAPTER 10

The Shoulder

Stephen J. Eustace

Optimizing imaging of the shoulder is technically difficult because of the peripheral position, its rounded anatomic configuration, its proximity to pulsating cardiothoracic structures, and the need for high-resolution imaging to adequately visualize complex soft tissue structures. This chapter outlines a practical approach to rapid imaging and then reviews both acute soft tissue and bony injuries complicating trauma.

PATIENT POSITIONING AND IMAGING PROTOCOLS

Positioning

Shoulder imaging is performed in the supine position with the patient introduced to the scanner head first. The arm is positioned at the patient's side in the neutral position with the thumb straight up. Elbow stabilization reduces motion and improves image quality. The flexed arm position with the hand laid over the torso should be avoided in order to

minimize cardiothoracic pulsation and secondary image distortion (Fig. 1).

Receiver Coil

In order to optimize reception of generated signal, imaging requires a molded or tightly apposed surface coil. Commonly, single-loop coils are used, placed along the anterolateral shoulder margin to improve signal from the distal rotator cuff. Quadrature (increasing received signal 1.4 times) and phased-array molded coils are now available allowing both improved tissue coverage and improved image signal.

Imaging Plane

Images are prescribed off an axial localizer such that the coronal oblique plane parallels the supraspinatus muscle and tendon, and sagittal oblique images are prescribed perpendicular to the supraspinatus tendon.

Field of View

Improved spatial resolution is achieved with smaller field of view; however, less than 14 cm is likely to result in incomplete joint coverage.

S. J. Eustace: Department of Radiology, Section of Musculoskeletal Radiology, Boston University School of Medicine and Boston Medical Center, Boston, Massachusetts 02118.

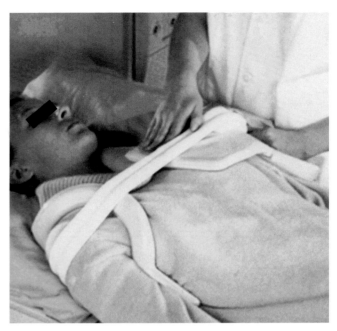

FIG. 1. Positioning of open flexible surface coil around the shoulder. Patient supine and introduced into the magnet head first. (Courtesy of Philips Medical Systems, Shelton, CT.)

Slice Thickness

Improved image signal to noise is yielded by thicker slices greater than 5 mm; nevertheless, improved spatial resolution and detection of subtle abnormalities is yielded by images with thinner slices, generally 3 mm or less in thickness.

Motion Suppression

An obliquely oriented saturation band is routinely placed over the upper thorax for acquisition of coronal and sagittal oblique images, minimizing pulsation artifact.

Imaging Protocol

With an increasing range of excitatory pulse sequences and variations in hardware, it is not possible to dictate what sequence should and should not be used to image the shoulder. Following orthopedic trauma, when evaluation of osseous injury is particularly important, a turbo inversion recovery sequence is often employed to localize the site of injury. A turbo spin-echo T1-weighted sequence is then employed to facilitate evaluation of complex anatomy, in coronal, sagittal, and axial planes. Turbo spin-echo T1- and T2-weighted coronal obliques and a turbo spin-echo T2-weighted sagittal oblique are generally acquired to facilitate detailed evaluation of the rotator cuff. An axial T2-weighted fast field-echo image with off-resonance magnetization transfer is then acquired to evaluate the labrum.

Turbo spin-echo T1 imaging is achieved using a repetition time of 500 msec, an echo time of 15 msec, a short echo train of four, and a low-high echo to view mapping profile. Turbo spin-echo T2-weighted imaging is achieved using a repetition time of 3,000 msec, echo times of 20 and 80 msec, an echo train of six, and linear echo-to-view mapping. Despite potential loss of signal in tendons using turbo spin-echo sequences as a result of magnetization transfer effects, it has not proven to be a source of diagnostic error. Turbo spin-echo T2-weighted images are enhanced by the use of spectral presaturation fat suppression. The efficacy of fat-suppressed turbo spin-echo T2-weighted imaging is now accepted, with fat-suppressed images yielding reported accuracies of up to 95% (1), fat-suppressed images improving both sensitivity and specificity in detection of partial tears relative to conventional sequences, in one series increasing sensitivity from 67% to 92% without a change in specificity (2). Fast field (gradient)-echo images are generally acquired to evaluate the labrum, employing a flip angle of 30°, a repetition time of 700 msec, and an echo time of 15 msec. Contrast between free fluid, cartilage, and labrum is enhanced by an off-resonance magnetization transfer pulse. Turbo inversion recovery sequences are acquired using an inversion time of 160 msec, a repetition time of 2,000 msec, an echo time of 20 msec, an echo train of six, and a linear echo-to-view mapping profile. Partial flip angle (gradient-echo) sequences are rarely employed to evaluate the rotator cuff because the foci of tendinitis and tear both retain signal, making differentiation between the two entities inaccurate (3,4).

In most patients, because of the impact on acquisition time, images are acquired with 256 phase-encode steps, because the perceived difference in image signal to noise between two and three excitations is negligible ($\sqrt{2}$ versus $\sqrt{3}$), and because of the need for rapid imaging, most authors do not employ more than two excitations.

Although faster imaging may be yielded with both GRASE and EPI sequences, their utility in evaluating either the rotator cuff or glenoid labrum are at this time unproven. Gradient-echo components in both sequences are likely to limit the ability to differentiate between cuff tendinopathy and tear. When rapid evaluation of fracture fragments is required, GRASE and EPI sequences must be employed in conjunction with frequency-selective fat saturation to minimize chemical shift artifact (Table 1).

MAGNETIC RESONANCE IMAGING OF SOFT TISSUE INJURIES FOLLOWING ACUTE TRAUMA

The Rotator Cuff

The supraspinatus, infraspinatus, and teres minor tendons insert on the greater tuberosity; the subscapularis tendon inserts on the lesser tuberosity; together they constitute the rotator cuff (Figs. 2 and 3).

The Supraspinatus

Injury to the supraspinatus may be secondary to direct trauma exacerbated by intrinsic factors such as diminished

TABLE 1. *Suggested protocol*

Sequence	Image plane	FOV	TR	TE	ETL	Mapping scheme
TSE T-1	Cor oblique	14	500	15	4	Low-high
TSE T-2 (fat)	Cor oblique	14	2,000	20, 80	6	Linear
TSE T-2 (fat)	Sagittal obl	14	2,000	20, 80	6	Linear
FFE T-2	Axial	14	500	15	30°	Flip angle

vascularity (the "critical zone," 5 mm proximal to the tendon insertion, is thought to be a zone of relative ischemia), overuse, or failure of the tendon's normal healing mechanism or it may occur secondary to chronic impingement. Irrespective of the cause, tendon injury may manifest as tendinosis, partial (incomplete thickness) or full (complete) thickness tears (5).

The term tendinopathy (rather than tendinitis) is used to describe minor tendon injury, as biopsy in these cases often fails to reveal inflammatory cells. Tendinopathy is traditionally graded 1, 2A, or 2B (6). Grade 1 tendinopathy, reflecting mild tendon disruption, is manifest as subtle signal abnormality on short-TE T1 and proton-density-weighted images. Grade 2A tendinopathy, reflecting more marked tendinosis, is manifest by both signal change and smooth tendon swelling (Fig. 4). Grade 2B tendinopathy, the most severe form, is manifest as signal change and tendon swelling with slightly irregular surfaces.

Differentiation of stage 2B tendinopathy from partial tear may be difficult in the absence of intra-articular contrast. Nevertheless, partial tears, in contrast to tendinopathy, retain signal abnormality or hyperintensity on T2-weighted scans, and their visibility is improved by the addition of fat suppression (7,8).

Differentiation of tendinopathy from magic angle phenomenon may be difficult. Magic angle phenomenon reflects an artifact observed in tightly bound tendons throughout the body. Reflecting complex macromolecular structure, tendons are hypointense on T1- and T2-weighted scans. At 55° to the main field or z axis, dipole–dipole interactions between tendon molecules lead to changes in recovery of longitudinal magnetization and loss of transverse magnetization within the tendon, producing slight signal hyperintensity on images acquired at short echo times less than 30 msec, with signal characteristics similar to those of tendinopathy.

In the presence of clinical symptoms, signal changes are frequently assumed to be secondary to tendinopathy. In cases where discrepancy occurs, reimaging the patient in a slightly different position, altering tendon obliquity, may be used to confirm or exclude tendon abnormality (Figs. 5–7) (9–11).

Partial tears of the rotator cuff most frequently arise from the articular surface, particularly along the anterior margin of the tendon. Bursal surface partial tears are less common, and identification in the absence of bursal contrast (bursography) is difficult (Fig. 8) (12). Visibility of these lesions is enhanced by the presence of effusion in the subacromial subdeltoid bursa, although fluid in this site is frequently misinterpreted as the product of a full-thickness tear.

Intrasubstance tear and incomplete tear of tendon from the superior facet represent alternative, less common forms of partial tear (5). At arthrography, partial tears are considered to be grade 1, extending through less than one-fourth of the tendon; grade 2, extending through less than half of the tendon; or grade 3, extending through more than half of the tendon. Visualization may be enhanced at arthrography in the abducted internal rotation position (ABER position) (13).

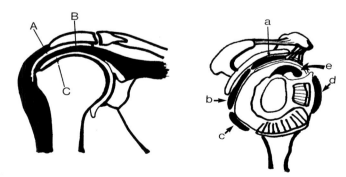

FIG. 2. Coronal oblique image **(left)** of the shoulder shows (A) subacromial bursa, (B) the supraspinatus tendon, and (C) the shoulder joint space. Sagittal oblique image **(right)** shows (a) supraspinatus, (b) infraspinatus, (c) teres minor, (d) subscapularis muscles of the rotator cuff, and (e) the long head of the biceps tendon.

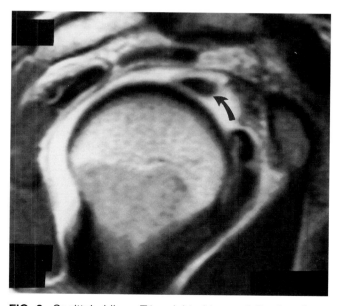

FIG. 3. Sagittal oblique T1-weighted image following direct intra-articular injection of gadolinium shows the muscles of the rotator cuff and the long head of the biceps *(arrow)*.

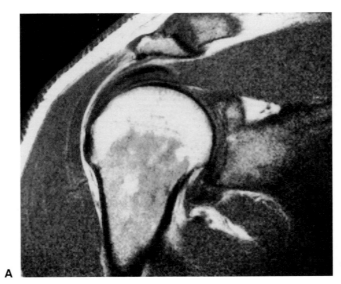
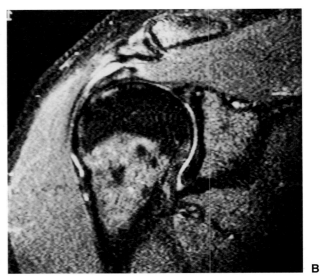

FIG. 4. Coronal oblique TSE T1 **(A)** and IR TSE **(B)** images show smooth swelling of the distal supraspinatus tendon with signal abnormality and trace subacromial fluid secondary to grade 2A tendinitis.

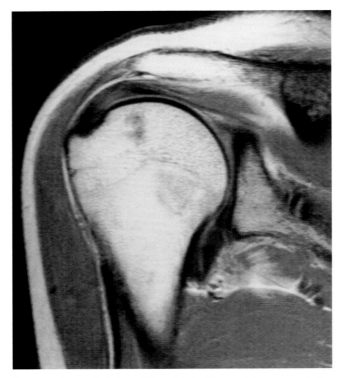

FIG. 5. Coronal oblique T1-weighted image shows focal signal abnormality in the supraspinatus tendon at 55° to B_0, typical of magic angle phenomena.

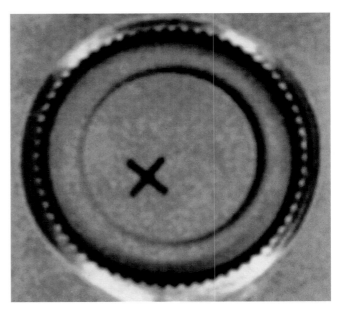

FIG. 6. Image of a cadaveric tendon wrapped around a Petri dish shows signal hyperintensity at four points 55° to B_0 secondary to magic angle phenomenon. (Courtesy of D. Williamson, M.D., Brigham & Women's Hospital, Boston, MA.)

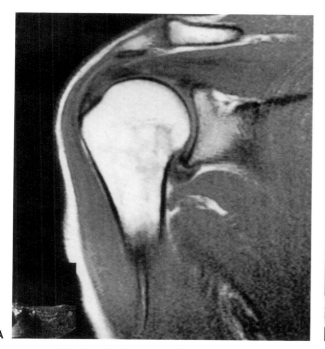
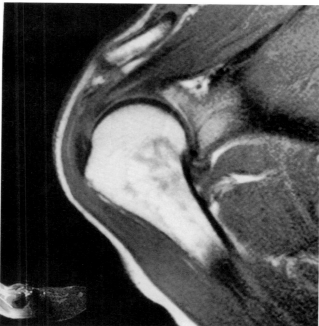

A   B

FIG. 7. (A) Coronal oblique short-TE image shows persistent signal abnormality in the distal supraspinatus tendon despite reimaging in an altered position **(B)**, excluding magic angle phenomena. A diagnosis of grade 2B tendinitis was made.

Partial Supraspinatus Tendon Tears
Articular surface
Bursal Surface
Intrasubstance
Superior facet avulsion

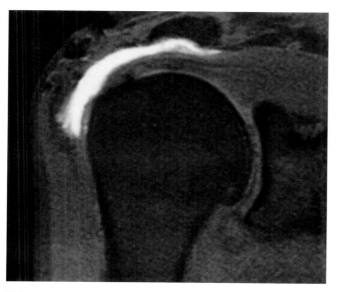

FIG. 8. Coronal T1-weighted conventional spin-echo image with fat suppression shows gadolinium in the subacromial bursa following bursography in a patient referred with a suspected superior surface tear.

Occasionally articular surface partial tears occur at the posterior rotator interval at the junction of the supraspinatus and infraspinatus, secondary to impaction against the posterosuperior glenoid in internal rotation, in throwing athletes such as baseball pitchers (14). In this setting, cuff tears are often associated with the development of cysts in the humeral head, posterosuperior labral tears, and posterior capsular ossification (the Bennet lesion) (15–18) (Fig. 9).

Full-thickness cuff tears allow free communication between the shoulder joint space and the subacromial subdeltoid bursa and are therefore manifest by signal abnormality on T1-, proton-density-, and T2-weighted scans (Fig. 10) (19). Uninterrupted signal abnormality traversing the tendon on T2-weighted scans allows differentiation of partial and complete injuries (20).

Similar to partial tears, complete tears tend to extend posteriorly from the anterior margin of the tendon. Detachment of the distal anterior aspect of the supraspinatus tendon from the greater tuberosity is often the earliest sign of a full-thickness tear (Fig. 11) (20). Uninterrupted tendon fibers are retracted in time, leaving an obvious gap in the tendon. Tears are considered to be small when the retraction is less than 1 cm, medium when the retraction is between 1 and 3 cm, and massive when the retraction is greater than 5 cm (Fig. 12) (21). Both the anteroposterior extent of the tear and the amount of retraction are usually recorded and are useful predictors of outcome following surgical intervention (19–21).

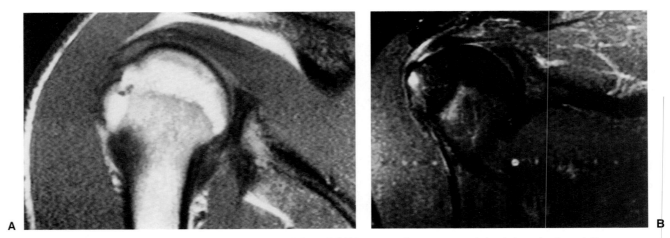

FIG. 9. (A) Coronal oblique TSE T1 and **(B)** IR TSE images show a tear of the infraspinatus at the posterior rotator interval with cystic change most likely secondary to posterior cuff impingement secondary to pitching.

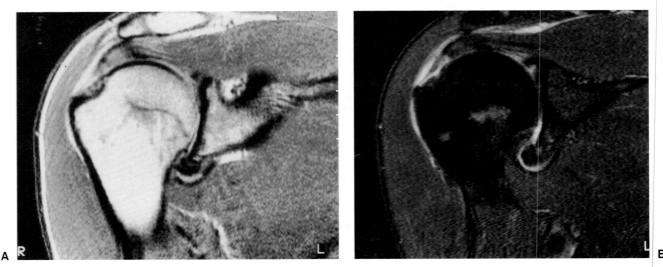

FIG. 10. (A) Coronal oblique TSE T1 and **(B)** IR TSE images show a full-thickness tear of the supraspinatus with minimal retraction, the position maintained by residual intact tendon fibers.

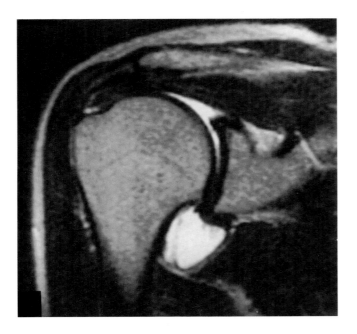

FIG. 11. Coronal oblique TSE T2 image following injection of saline shows an undisplaced tear at insertion of supraspinatus on the humeral head.

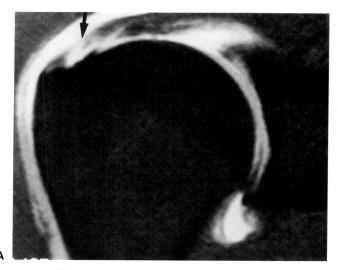
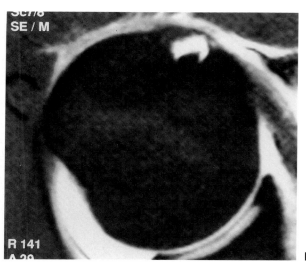

FIG. 12. (A) Coronal oblique and (B) axial TSE T1-weighted images with frequency-selective fat saturation following gaddinium orthrography show free communication of fluid to the subacromial bursa, without tendon retraction.

In chronicity, atrophy of the muscle belly commonly accompanies tendon injury. Secondary elevation of the humeral head with coracohumeral arch impingement results in biceps tendon impaction, shear, and secondary tendinosis (Fig. 13).

Tendinosis versus Tear

Grade 1: Short-TE Hyperintensity
Grade 2A: Short-TE Hyperintensity and Swelling
Grade 2B: Short-TE Hyperintensity and Swelling with Surface Irregularity
Grade 3A: Short- and Long-TE Hyperintensity with Definite Partial Defect
Grade 3B: Short- and Long-TE Hyperintensity with Full-Thickness Defect (Adapted from ref. 6)

Partial Tear

Persistent Hyperintensity on Long-TE Sequences: Bursal Versus Articular Surface
Grade 1: Less Than One-Fourth Tendon Thickness
Grade 2: Less Than One-Half Tendon Thickness
Grade 3: More Than One-Half Tendon Thickness

Full Thickness

Persistent Hyperintensity on Long-TE Sequences, Anterior to Posterior Margins
Small, 1 cm; Medium, 1–3 cm; Massive, 5 cm
Rarely Low Signal Intensity on T1 and T2 in Chronic Atrophic Tears with Tendon Retraction and Atrophy

Magic Angle Phenomenon

Dipole–Dipole Interactions at 55° Resulting in Focal Signal Hyperintensity on T1 and Proton-Density Scans

---

Subscapularis Injury

Subscapularis tendon injury is uncommon, but when it occurs, it is usually as a sequel to anterior dislocation, injury to the shoulder in abduction with external rotation, or chronic subcoracoid impingement. Because it is inserted in the biceps tendon sheath groove, rupture is often accompanied by biceps tendon subluxation, tear, or dislocation (22–24) (Fig. 14).

Infraspinatus

Isolated infraspinatus tendon injury is extremely uncommon, rarely complicating posterior shoulder dislocation (see Fig. 9) (20).

Biceps Brachii

The biceps brachii muscle is composed of a long head and a short head. The two muscle bellies share a single tendon insertion on the bicipital tuberosity of the radius. The short head arises from the apex of the coracoid; the long head arises from the supraglenoid tubercle of the scapula. Injury involving the biceps muscle more frequently involves the tendons than the muscle bellies, and of the tendons, more frequently affects the tendon of the long head (25–27).

Stabilization of the long head biceps tendon within the joint space is by the coracohumeral ligament (the coracohumeral ligament fuses with the supraspinatus tendon); extra-articular stabilization outside the joint within the biceps tendon sheath groove is by the transverse humeral ligament and subscapularis proximally and by the pectoralis major distally (25).

Biceps injury may be secondary to overuse, inflammation, impingement, degeneration, or dislocation. In most cases, injury accompanies significant rotator cuff disease. In such a way, chronic supraspinatus tear with coracohumeral arch impingement may result in intra-articular biceps tendinosis, attenuation, and tear (26). In contrast, subscapularis tendon tear, either secondary to anterior dislocation or secondary to

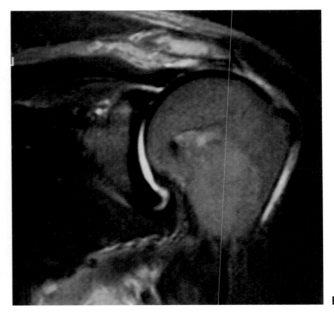

FIG. 13. Chronic rotator cuff tear with retraction (*arrow* indicates the retracted tendon), atrophy, and free communication to the subacromial, subdeltoid bursa. Unlike acute tear, fibrosis and granulation tissue result in signal hypointensity at the site of the tear.

chronic subcoracoid impingement, may be complicated by tendinosis, tear, subluxation, or dislocation of the extra-articular biceps tendon (27) (see Fig. 14).

Impingement

The term *primary impingement* is used to describe extrinsic compression of the rotator cuff by structures of the cora-coacromial arch as a result of either congential or acquired coracoacromial outlet narrowing, leading to cuff tendinopathy, attenuation, and tear. Secondary impingement is the term used to describe dynamic narrowing of the coracoacromial outlet as a result of shoulder instability, as a sequel to labral, capsule, or, most frequently, rotator cuff tear (28–30).

Neer previously proposed that primary impingement accounted for almost 95% of recognized cuff tears (31). It is

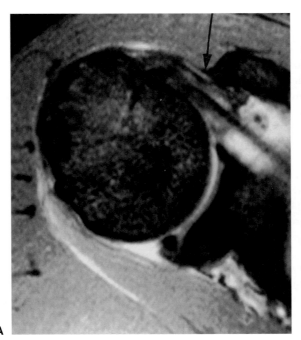

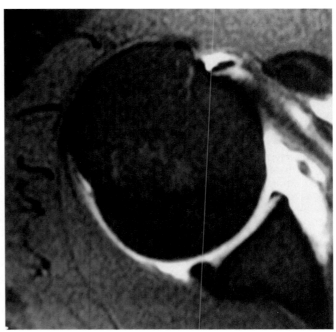

FIG. 14. Axial SE T1-weighted images show subcoracoid impingement *(arrow)*, tear, or split of the subscapularis with medial subluxation of the biceps tendon.

now clear that cuff tears often occur without impingement and that narrowing of the coracoacromial space, producing an appearance of impingement, is a secondary phenomenon, so-called *secondary impingement*.

According to Neer, three distinct stages are observed following cuff injury, each of which is accounted for by primary impingement (31).

Stage 1, occurring between 20 and 30 years, follows acute injury and is characterized by the development of reversible cuff edema. Stage 2, occurring between 30 and 45 years, is the sequel to repetitive trauma and is characterized by the development of irreversible tendon scar and fibrosis. Stage 3 occurs from 45 years onward, following further shoulder trauma, and results in the development of degenerative tear (31).

The coracoacromial arch is formed by the coracoid, the coracoacromial ligament, and the acromion process. Several studies have reviewed anatomic variations in the arch contributing to or promoting impingement. Morrison and Bigliani (32) described three variations in the shape of the acromion: type 1, flat; type 2, curved; and type 3, hooked. Several authors have demonstrated an association between the type 3 shape and rotator cuff impingement and tear (33). The acromion arises from fusion of three ossification centers, which occurs by 25 years of age. Unfused segments, termed os acromiale, occur in up to 3% of the population and, being unstable, are associated with cuff impingement and tear (34–36). Pathologic thickening of the coracoacromial ligament as a degenerative process or the development of traction osteophytes at its insertion (enthesopathy of coracoacromial ligament), both of which are manifest as T1 and T2 signal hypointensity, also lead to cuff impingement and tear (37,38). Similarly, osteoarthritis of the acromioclavicular joint with formation of inferior osteophytes from the distal clavicle may result in cuff impingement (28). Identification of each pathology is crucial, as surgical intervention is tailored to mechanism. Anterior acromioplasty is undertaken in patients with the type 3 hooked acromion; resection of the distal clavicle is undertaken in patients with inferior osteophytes at the acromioclavicular articulation; resection of the coracoacromial ligament is undertaken in patients with thickening or enthesopathy involving the ligament; fusion or resection is undertaken in patients with os acromiale (see Fig. 11).

Subcoracoid Impingement

Subcoracoid impingement may be secondary to altered anatomic configuration following coracoid or lesser tuberosity fracture or reflect dynamic narrowing secondary to anterior instability. In chronicity, impingement leads to attenuation and tear of the subscapularis, often accompanied by biceps tendon subluxation (see Fig. 14) (39,40).

Posterosuperior Glenoid Impingement

Posterosuperior impingement is uncommon and is generally seen only in professional athletes such as pitchers, in whom coracoacromial impingement with tear of the posterior fibers of the supraspinatus and superior fibers of the infraspinatus occurs in the late cocking phase or with internal rotation accompanying tear of the posterosuperior glenoid labrum (see Fig. 9) (41,42).

Contributors to Primary Cuff Impingement
Acromial Downslope
Acromial Shape: Hooked Type 3 Acromion
Unfused Acromion: Os Acromiale
Thickened Coracoacromial Ligament
Coracoacromial Enthesopathy
Abnormal Scapular Motion

Contributors to Secondary Impingement: Coracoacromial Outlet Narrowing
Rotator Cuff Tear
Bicipitolabral Tear

Glenohumeral Instability

The Labral–Ligamentous Complex

The labral–ligamentous complex, which includes the glenoid labrum and the superior, middle, and inferior glenohumeral ligaments, functions to anchor the humeral head to the osseous glenoid. Although visualization of the labral ligamentous complex may be achieved in both coronal oblique and axial planes without intra-articular contrast, visualization and understanding of labral injury is dramatically enhanced using intra-articular contrast (40–48).

The superior and middle glenohumeral ligaments originate together from the superior labrum immediately anterior to the labral–bicipital anchor. The superior ligament courses anteriorly to merge with the coracohumeral ligament; the middle ligament courses inferiorly to merge with the subscapularis. The inferior glenohumeral ligament has three components, including anterior and posterior bands and an intervening axillary pouch. The anterior band is thicker than the other glenohumeral ligaments and has a broader glenolabral origin; therefore, it is the dominant contributor to shoulder stability (between 3 and 9 o'clock) (43–47). Although three types of anterior capsular insertion have been described, they do not predict presence or absence of shoulder stability and may actually reflect the position of rotation in which the examination was performed. Although the middle glenohumeral ligament is usually broad, merging with the subscapularis laterally, it is associated with considerable variation in form, ranging from absence to a cord-like configuration. A cord-like middle glenohumeral ligament is often associated with absence of the anterosuperior glenoid labrum, the Buford complex (48,49). Variations in the structure of the middle glenohumeral ligament are thought to account for six reported variations in the pattern of synovial recesses within the joint space. According to De Palma, a type 1 joint is characterized by one recess above the middle glenohumeral ligament; a type 2 joint is characterized by one recess arising below the middle glenohumeral ligament; a type

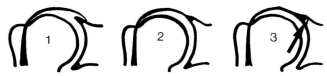

FIG. 15. Diagrammatic representation of the three types of bicipitolabral complex: type 1, insertion of the long head of the biceps to the supraglenoid notch; type 2, insertion to the superior margin of the labrum; type 3, insertion (meniscoid type) to the body of the labrum. Type 3 insertion is commonly associated with a sublabral sulcus *(arrow)*.

3 joint is characterized by two recesses above and below the middle glenohumeral ligament; a type 4 joint is characterized by one large recess and an absent glenohumeral ligament; a type 5 joint is characterized by division of the middle glenohumeral ligament into two synovial folds; and a type 6 joint has no synovial recesses (50).

There are three variations in the pattern of insertion of the tendon of the long head of the biceps into the labrum, the bicipitolabral complex. Most commonly, the biceps inserts at the junction of the superior margin of the labrum and glenoid itself. Less frequently, the biceps inserts into the superior margin of the superior labrum. Less frequently, the biceps inserts into the body of the superior labrum in a meniscoid form (Figs. 15–17) (44).

Articular cartilage normally undercuts the labral fibrocartilage; particularly marked undercutting commonly forms sulci at the labral–bicipital junction (sublabral sulcus and foramen) and between the origins of the middle and inferior glenohumeral ligaments. In old age, sulci become more prominent and frequently mimic labral tears (44) (see Fig. 17).

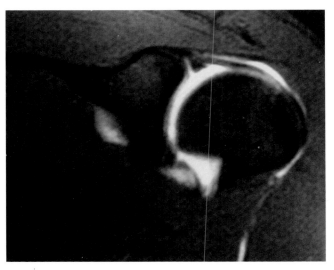

FIG. 17. Coronal oblique fat-suppressed MR arthrogram shows a type 3 meniscoid bicipitolabral complex with a prominent sublabral sulcus.

Variations in Labral Anatomy

Bicipitolabral Complex: Type 1, BLC Adherent to Superior Pole Glenoid; Type 2, BLC Attaches to Superior Labrum; Type 3, Meniscoid Labrum with Large Sulcus
Sublabral Sulcus: Marked in Type 3 BLC Insertion
Absent Middle Glenohumeral Ligament
Cord-Like Middle Glenohumeral Ligament with Absent Anterosuperior Labrum (Buford Complex)
Anterior Capsule Insertion: Type 1, Capsule Arises from Labrum; Type 2, Capsule Arises from Scapular Neck; Type 3, From Neck 1 cm Medial to Labrum

---

Instability reflecting injury to the labral ligamentous complex is primarily classified into two broad categories: traumatic unidirectional anterior inferior or posterior instability with Bankart lesion, usually considered to be correctable by surgical reconstruction (TUBS: traumatic, unidirectional, Bankart, surgical); or multidirectional atraumatic instability, which is rarely correctable by surgical intervention (AMBRI: atraumatic, multidirectional, bilateral instability) (51,53). Multidirectional instability is most frequently characterized by osteoarthritis, osteophytes, and both tear and attenuation of labrum at MR imaging. Unidirectional instability, in contrast, is frequently readily accounted for by either soft tissue or bony Bankart lesions of the anteroinferior labrum at MRI, discussed in detail in the next section.

Isolated Labral Tears

Isolated tears of the anterosuperior, superior, and posterior labrum following shoulder trauma may occasionally present with shoulder pain or impaired shoulder movement.

Snyder et al. (54) described four types of superior labral tear SLAP following trauma: type 1, simple fraying of the articulating surface of the labrum; type 2, fraying and strip-

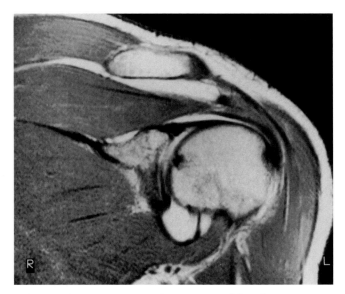

FIG. 16. Coronal oblique T1-weighted SE MR arthrogram shows a type 2 bicipitolabral complex.

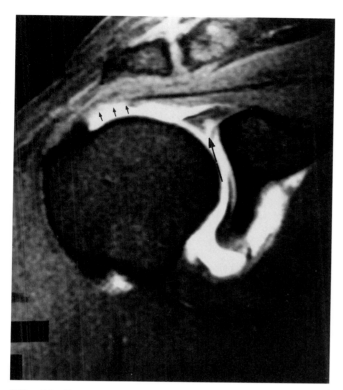

FIG. 18. Coronal oblique fat-suppressed MR arthrogram shows a SLAP tear of the superior labrum *(straight arrow)* associated with a subtle undersurface supraspinatus tendon tear *(small arrows)*. (Courtesy of M. Barish, M.D., Boston Medical Center, Boston, MA.)

insertion of the glenohumeral ligament on the lesser tuberosity (HAGL: humeral avulsion glenohumeral ligament) (Fig. 19) (53,56).

Occasionally soft tissue Bankart lesions reapproximate and resynovialize, making detection before surgery extremely difficult unless imaging in the stressed position (ABER, abducted externally rotated) is employed (sometimes described as a Perthe lesion) (Fig. 20) (57). Similarly, occasionally underlying scapular periosteum remains intact, and the torn labral ligamentous complex rolls up and displaces medially; this is termed an ALPSA (anterior labral periosteal sleeve avulsion) lesion (Fig. 21) (58). As this lesion heals, fibrous tissue heaps up over the displaced labrum and may make detection difficult despite clinical instability.

Rowe and Zarins (59) have classified Bankart lesions into type 1, characterized by a small detachment of the capsulolabral complex without glenoid stripping; type 2, characterized by moderate detachment with glenoid stripping; type 3, characterized by severe detachment; and type 4, in which both labrum and bone are detached.

In practice, although labral injuries may be difficult to detect, identification of impaction marrow edema in the region of the anteroinferior labrum on fat-suppressed images of patients following anterior dislocation should trigger a more rigorous search, or potentially a referral for MR arthrography if identified on noncontrast studies (Fig. 22).

In our experience, osseous Bankart lesions are often identified in young patients with symptoms following anterior dislocation despite normal conventional radiographs (Fig.

ping of the labrum and biceps anchor; type 3, bucket handle tear with displacement of the central portion; and type 4, bucket handle tear with longitudinal extension to the biceps tendon (Fig. 18).

Neviaser (55) described the glenolabral articular disruption (GLAD) lesion, which refers to a partial labral tear associated with an articular cartilage divot that follows acute forced adduction, as seen when one athlete or professional footballer falls on another. The lesion typically involves the anterior margin of the labrum and does not result in instability.

MAGNETIC RESONANCE IMAGING OF OSSEOUS INJURIES FOLLOWING ACUTE TRAUMA

Anterior Dislocation

Because of the anterior obliquity of the glenoid, injury to the shoulder in abduction, external rotation, or by direct impaction yields either anterior subluxation or frank anterior dislocation. The tendency to sublux is prevented predominantly by the anterior labrum and inferior glenohumeral ligament. Under extreme tension, anterior capsular structures tear, typically at the labral ligamentous insertion accompanied by scapular periosteal avulsion with or without a fracture of the underlying glenoid (Bankart injury), rarely at the

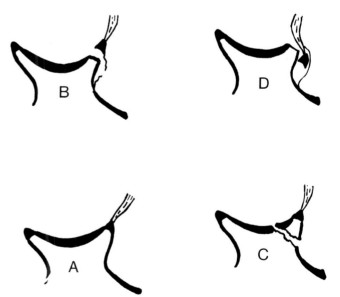

FIG. 19. Diagrammatic representation of the anteroinferior labrum shows **(A)** normal attachment of the inferior glenohumeral ligament to the inferior labrum, **(B)** a soft tissue Bankart lesion or anteroinferior labral avulsion, **(C)** a displaced bony Bankart lesion, and **(D)** medially displaced anteroinferior labrum beneath a periosteal sleeve (ALPSA). Adapted from Tirman et al. (43).

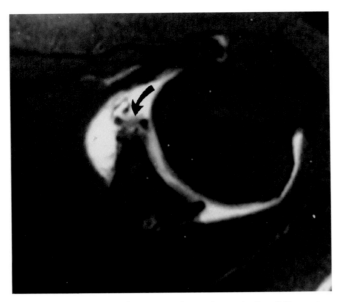

FIG. 20. Axial MR arthrogram shows irregularity of the anteroinferior labrum at a site of undisplaced tear (Perthe lesion) *(curved arrow).*

23). A study comparing MR imaging, radiography, and arthroscopy recently concluded that MR imaging was more accurate than the other two modalities in the diagnosis of Hill Sachs lesions (60).

Sequelae following anterior dislocation in patients over the age of 35 years differ from those in younger patients. Approximately one-third of patients develop tears of the rotator cuff, one-third suffer a fracture of the greater tuberosity (usually treated conservatively) and one third suffer tears

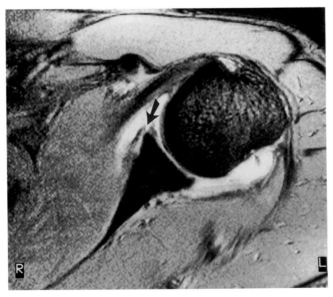

FIG. 21. Axial T2-weighted fast field-echo image shows medial displacement of the labrum beneath a periosteal sleeve (ALPSA).

of the anterior capsule and subscapularis (usually requiring surgical repair) (43) (see Figs. 15 and 23).

Labral Injuries

Anteroinferior Labral Tears (Anterior Band of Inferior Glenohumeral Ligament): Soft Tissue Bankart; Bony Bankart; Perthe Lesion (Undisplaced Labrum, Displaced in ABER Position); ALPSA (Anterior Labral Periosteal Sleeve Avulsion)
Superior Labral Tears (SLAP): Type 1, Fraying; Type 2, Oblique Anteroposterior Tear; Type 3, Oblique Tear Extending to the Biceps Insertion; Type 4, Tear with Bucket Handle
Glenoid Labral Articular Disruption (GLAD Lesion); Forced Adduction Injury

---

Posterior Dislocation

Because of the anteromedial obliquity of the glenoid, posterior dislocation can occur when injury is to the internally rotated adducted shoulder, such as occurs following a fall on an outstretched hand. Altered glenoid angulation or scapula inclination may predispose to such an injury.

In addition to disruption of the posterior labrum (reverse Bankart injury) and occasionally the posterior capsule (Fig. 24), anterior stress on the subscapularis and impaction may lead to avulsion of the lesser tuberosity.

Fractures of the Proximal Humerus

Neer's modified classification of fractures of the head and neck of humerus (dividing the proximal shaft into four segments: greater tuberosity, lesser tuberosity, and anatomic and surgical necks) is widely used to indicate the extent of injury and to plan operative intervention (61). On the basis of this classification, one-part fractures have minimal (less than 1 cm) or no displacement and have minimal (less than 45°) or no angulation (they are common, occurring in approximately 85% of cases); two-part fractures have one fracture segment displaced or angulated; three-part fractures have two fracture segments displaced or angulated; and four-part fractures have three segments displaced including the greater and lesser tuberosities and the surgical neck, with displacement or angulation of all four major fragments (Fig. 25). According to the Neer classification, a fracture dislocation describes a fracture in which the head is displaced outside the joint space, not merely rotated. A head-splitting fracture is an intra-articular fracture involving more than 15% of the articular surface. The AO classification (62) of fractures of the proximal humerus specifically addresses the likelihood of a fracture developing avascular necrosis. In such a way, type A fracture is extracapsular and involves two of the primary four segments, and avascular necrosis is unlikely. A type B fracture is a partially intracapsular fracture involving three of the four primary segments, and avascular necrosis is uncommon. A type C fracture is intra-articular and involves all four segments; avascular necrosis is

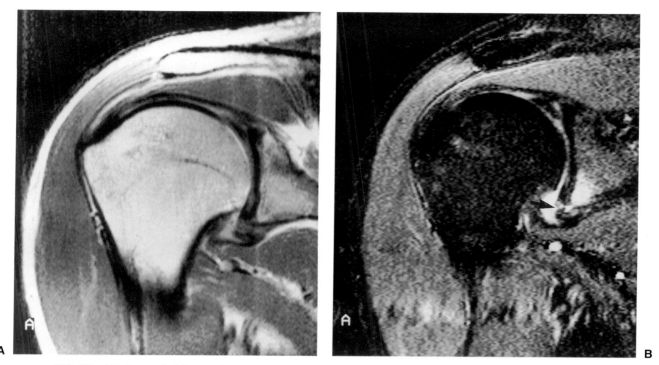

FIG. 22. (A) Coronal oblique TSE T1 and **(B)** IR TSE images of a patient following anterior dislocation show impaction bruise of the anteroinferior labrum with subtle step-off.

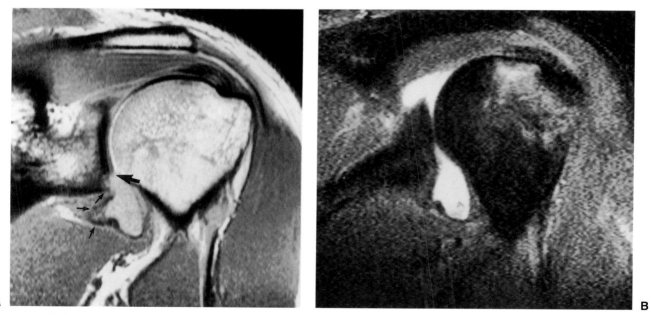

FIG. 23. Coronal oblique TSE T1 **(A)** and IR TSE **(B)** of a patient following anterior dislocation shows a Hill Sachs impaction bruise with edema in the posterolateral humeral head. T1-weighted image shows a *contre-coup* Bankart fracture with an abrupt anteroinferior chondral defect *(straight arrow)* and laxity of the avulsed inferior glenohumeral ligament *(small arrows)*.

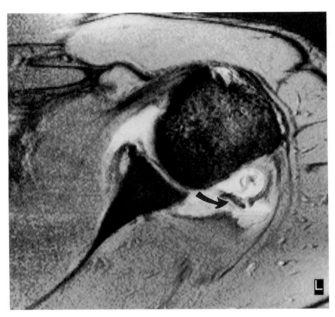

FIG. 24. Axial T2-weighted fast field-echo image shows a posterior capsular avulsion complicating posterior dislocation *(arrow)*.

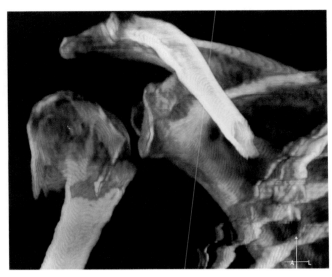

FIG. 26. Inner-view three-dimensional CT scan shows a comminuted fracture of the proximal humerus with gross displacement of bone fragment.

likely. In one study, avascular necrosis occurred in 14% of patients with three-part fractures and in 34% of patients with four-part injuries (63).

Although in routine practice, plain film radiographs allow accurate evaluation of these injuries in most cases, computed tomography is often undertaken before operative intervention to clearly localize the position and number of bone fragments (Fig. 26). When undertaken, multiplanar MR imaging of these fractures not only allows accurate evaluation of bony displacement and angulation, often best perceived in the direct sagittal plane, but also allows evaluation of the rotator

cuff, differentiating cuff tear from cuff avulsion and of vascular integrity of the humeral head (Figs. 27 and 28). Dynamic gadolinium-enhanced keyhole imaging is frequently employed in this setting to evaluate the vascular integrity of the fracture fragments. Unlike scaphoid fractures, where revascularization often occurs within the first 6 weeks of injury, avascular large segments of the proximal humeral head do not revascularize. Early identification of ischemia results in humeral head replacement at the time of injury rather than as a delayed event when severe AVN is manifest or nonunion is evident (64).

Fractures of the Humeral Diaphysis

At the level of the midhumeral diaphysis, the radial nerve crosses the bone posteriorly from medial to lateral within the spiral groove, its proximity accounting for frequently encountered radial nerve palsy in fractures at this site. Up to 18% of humeral shaft fractures have an associated radial nerve injury, most commonly neuropraxia or axonotmesis; 90% resolve in 3 to 4 months. Although it is commonly associated with oblique fracture of the distal third of the humerus (Holstein Lewis fracture), the injury also accompanies fractures of the middiaphysis (65). Although angulation and displacement of a fragment may be corrected by manipulation and cast fixation or delayed internal fixation, operative intervention is undertaken acutely in patients with associated nerve palsy in whom MR images show impaction of the nerve within the fracture margins (Fig. 29) (66). In contrast, delayed operative fixation or conservative management is undertaken if the radial nerve is demonstrated remote from fracture margins, displaced by either hematoma or soft tissue edema, in patients in whom palsy is presumed to be secondary to reversible contusion. Although specific sequences

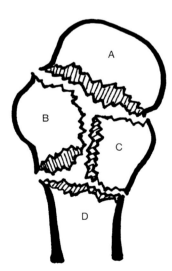

FIG. 25. Diagram shows four parts of humeral head from which the Neer classification is derived: **(A)** humeral head; **(B)** greater tuberosity; **(C)** lesser tuberosity; **(D)** shaft.

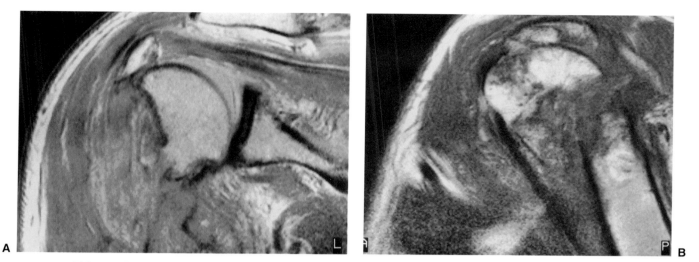

FIG. 27. (A) Three-part fracture of the humeral head with retraction of fragment by the intact supraspinatus. (B) Sagittal image shows minimal anterior displacement of fragment.

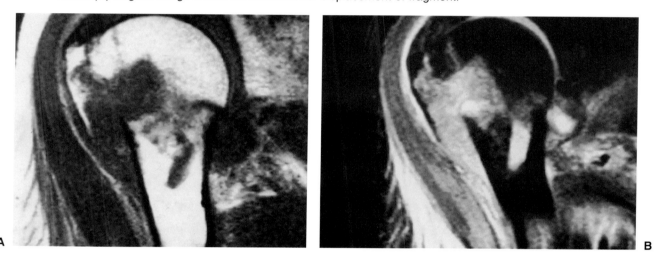

FIG. 28. Coronal TSE T1 (A) and IR TSE (B) images show a three-part fracture of the right proximal humerus without significant soft tissue derangement.

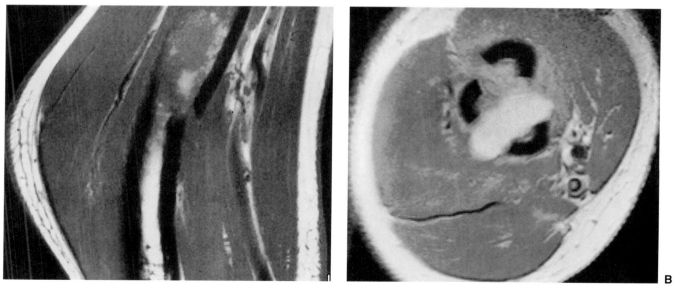

FIG. 29. Coronal (A) and axial (B) proton-density-weighted images show an angulated fracture of the midhumerus in a patient with radial neuropathy. Note matrix hyperintensity secondary to extracellular methemoglobin. Reproduced with permission from Eustace and Denison (79).

clearly defining peripheral nerves are not currently available, conventional spin-echo sequences, particularly in the axial plane, allow identification of isointense nerves based on anatomic location.

Occult Fractures

Similar to other sites, sensitivity of fat-suppressed images to subtle marrow edema reflecting microtrabecular trauma frequently allows identification of occult fractures of the humeral head. Occult undisplaced avulsions are frequently identified at the insertion of the rotator cuff, particularly the supraspinatus, and present with symptoms incorrectly attributed to cuff tendinitis or tear. Direct impaction following a fall, particularly following ski accidents, often results in undisplaced radiographically occult fractures of the greater tuberosity (Fig. 30).

Isolated avulsion fractures of the greater tuberosity, referred to as fissure or eggshell fracture, may occasionally follow acute traction through the supraspinatus tendon (Figs.

31 and 32). The fracture is usually undisplaced, radiographically occult, and presents with impaired shoulder movement; it often results in referral for MR imaging to exclude the presence of rotator cuff tear (67).

Pathologic Fractures

Magnetic resonance imaging is routinely employed in all patients sustaining fractures in the absence of trauma in whom underlying pathologic bone is suspected, in all patients over 35 years presenting with avulsion fractures (in whom the avulsions are considered to reflect an abnormality in underlying bone) and in all patients presenting with recognized pathologic fractures before surgical intervention to determine method of fixation. Occasionally in the presence of an unknown primary tumor, MRI is undertaken to determine the source of metastases using a whole-body turboSTIR technique (68).

Because of the distribution of red marrow around the shoulder, both myelomatous and metastatic deposits are

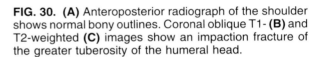

FIG. 30. (A) Anteroposterior radiograph of the shoulder shows normal bony outlines. Coronal oblique T1- (B) and T2-weighted (C) images show an impaction fracture of the greater tuberosity of the humeral head.

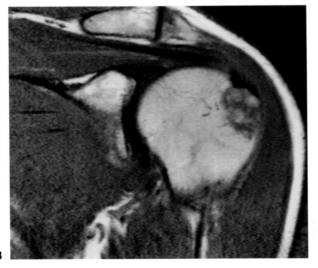

A

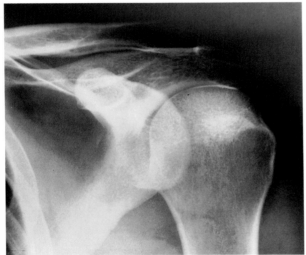

B

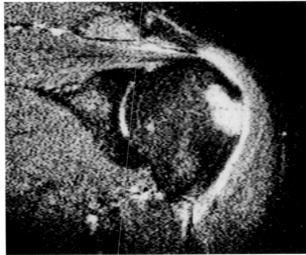

C

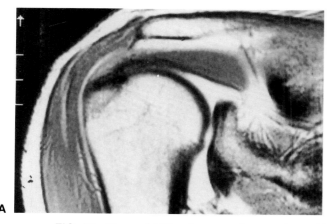
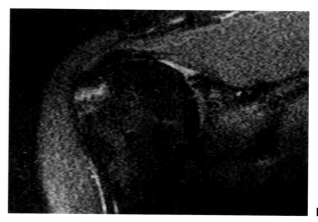

FIG. 31. Coronal MR arthrogram in a patient with a suspected cuff tear, showing a subtle area of osseous irregularity adjacent to the superior facet of the humeral head, secondary to an occult avulsion injury.

most commonly identified in the glenoid and in the metaphysis of the proximal humerus.

Magnetic Resonance Imaging in Pathologic Fractures

Avulsion Fractures in Adults (over 35 Years)
Fracture in the Absence of Trauma
Delayed Union of an Immobilized Fracture
To Localize Source of Primary Tumor in a Recognized Metastatic Deposit

---

Acromioclavicular Subluxation

Acromioclavicular subluxation or dislocation is usually readily identified on conventional radiographs with or with-

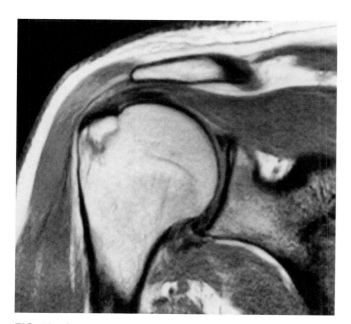

FIG. 32. Coronal TSE T1-weighted image shows an eggshell fracture of the greater tuberosity without displacement.

out the stresses of weight bearing. Occasionally, patients are referred with suspected injury to the rotator cuff in whom pain relates to unrecognized acromioclavicular (AC) joint disease.

Magnetic resonance imaging, although generally unnecessary, may be used to determine integrity of the coracoclavicular ligament in patients in whom surgical intervention is being considered.

Recurrent AC Joint Subluxation: Posttraumatic Osteolysis of the Clavicle

Osteolysis after trauma most commonly occurs at the lateral aspect of the clavicle, distal ulna, and pubis. Osteolysis of the outer clavicle may follow a single episode of blunt trauma (posttraumatic osteolysis) or recurrent minor trauma (stress osteolysis) such as occurs following bench pressing (Fig. 33). In affected patients, repeated subluxation results in the development of para-articular marrow edema readily identified at MRI, usually many weeks before the appearance of radiographic changes. Clinical symptoms include pain, crepitus, and impaired motion. Although poorly understood, similar to algodystrophy, autonomic dysfunction is thought to induce vascular changes in the outer clavicle, resulting in bony resorption. Soft tissue or synovial overgrowth is accompanied by swelling, hyperemia, demineralization, and finally resorption (69–71).

At MRI, osteolysis is noted to be hypointense on T1- and heterogeneous on T2-weighted images. Fat suppression often reveals marrow edema long before osseous change is apparent (72) (see Fig. 33).

The process is self-limiting over 18 months and is followed by bony reconstitution, although surgery and early immobilization may decrease symptoms and amount of bone loss (71).

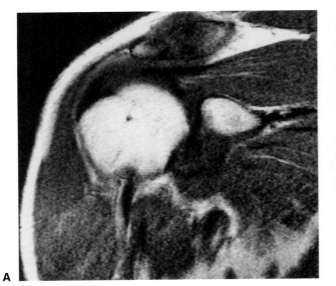
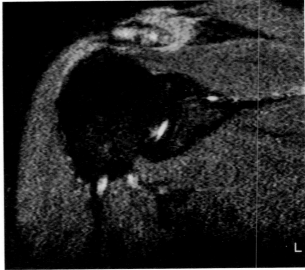

FIG. 33. Coronal TSE T1 **(A)** and IR TSE **(B)** images show hypertrophic inflammatory change in the acromioclavicular articulation, with early posttraumatic osteolysis of the medial clavicle.

Fractures of the Clavicle

Fractures of the clavicle are readily identified on conventional radiographs. Fractures are classified as fractures of the middle third (80% of cases), distal third (15%), and inner third (5%) (73). Commonly accompanying severe trauma to the upper thorax, fractures of the clavicle are often associated with rib fractures, parenchymal lung contusion, and occasionally brachial plexopathy (74). The latter injury is best evaluated with MRI. In this regard, MRI is used to differentiate among compression of the brachial plexus by posttraumatic hematoma requiring evacuation, a displaced fracture fragment requiring decompression, and simple neuropraxia, which may be treated conservatively (Fig. 34). When it occurs, direct injury to the plexus usually involves the lateral cord. Late compression neuropathies usually involve the middle cord and produce ulnar neuropathy, particularly common in fractures of the midclavicle with complicating hypertrophic nonunion (75).

Vascular injury to the subclavian artery and vein is uncommon, primarily because the inner fracture segment is elevated by the action of the sternocleidomastoid away from the vessels. Occasionally, downward traction on the inner segment by the pectoralis muscles impacts on vessels resulting in either spasm or, less frequently, laceration (75) (Fig. 35).

Sternoclavicular Dislocation

Sternoclavicular dislocation is uncommon. When it occurs following a fall on the shoulder, reflecting the anterior obliquity of the joint space, the medial clavicle subluxes anteriorly and is readily apparent clinically. Occasionally, either sec-

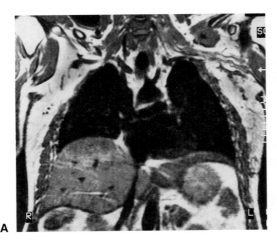
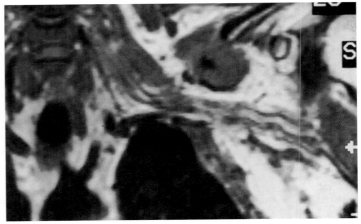

FIG. 34. (A) Coronal T1-weighted image of the thorax with a body coil shows a fracture of the left clavicle with extensive edema and hemorrhage without encroachment of the brachial plexus **(B).**

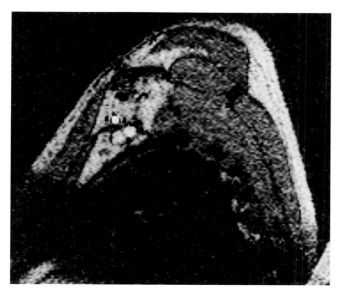

FIG. 35. Sagittal two-dimensional time-of-flight image shows patent axillary vessels.

ondary to direct impaction trauma in a motor vehicle accident or secondary to a sharp blow to the back of the shoulder in which torque is transmitted through to the medial clavicle, the subluxation or dislocation is posterior. In this setting diagnosis is often improved by axial imaging using either CT or MRI. In this setting, dramatic three-dimensional reconstructions using CT are helpful; nevertheless, MR angiography allows noninvasive evaluation of compressed mediastinal vascular structures (76,77) (Fig. 36).

Scapula Fractures

Fractures of the scapula often occur in association with fractures of the clavicle and ribs and contusion to lung parenchyma. Fractures may be confined to the coracoid or the neck of the acromion or extend through the scapular body to the glenoid articular surfaces. Zdravkovic and Damholt (78) (Fig. 37) classify fractures into three types: type 1, fractures of the body; type 2, fractures of the apophysis including the coracoid and acromion; and type 3, fractures of the superior lateral angle including the neck and glenoid. Type 3

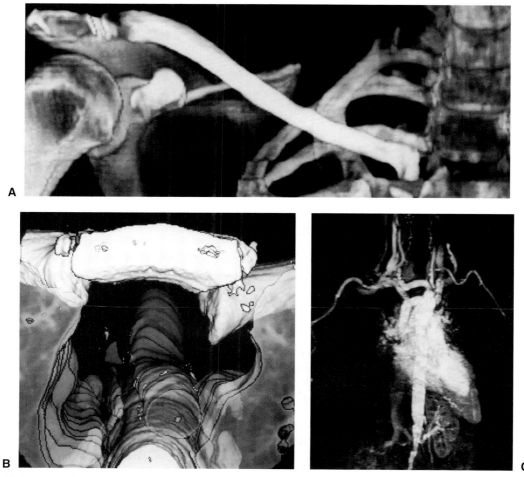

FIG. 36. (A) Three-dimensional CT reconstruction of the right clavicle without focal abnormality. **(B)** Axial inner view reformatted images show encroachment of the underlying bronchial tree secondary to posterior stemoclavicular dislocation. **(C)** Dynamic contrast-enhanced study shows patent arterial structures.

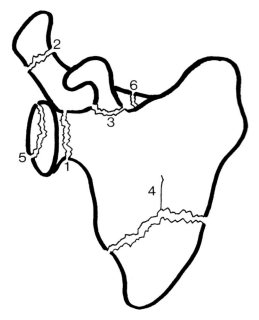

FIG. 37. Diagrammatic representation of the sites of fractures of the scapular: 1, neck of glenoid; 2, acromion; 3, neck coracoid; 4, body; 5, glenoid; 6, the spine.

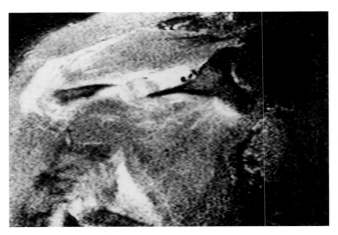

FIG. 39. Coronal oblique IR TSE shows a fracture through the spine of the left scapula without encroachment of the suprascapular notch.

fractures are considerably more difficult to treat and are often associated with other injuries, including pneumothorax in up to 30%, pulmonary contusion, rib fractures, and injuries to both the brachial plexus and vascular structures; both complications are well visualized on MRI (Figs. 38 and 39).

Although CT scanning in the axial plane allows reformatting in both sagittal and coronal oblique planes, direct multiplanar imaging using magnetic resonance overcomes potential reformatting artifacts and allows determination of the relationship between fragment position and adjacent soft tissues (79).

Fractures of the acromion are frequently associated with rotator cuff tears. Intra-articular glenoid fractures are frequently associated with labral tears; coracoid fractures frequently accompany acromioclavicular separations. Because

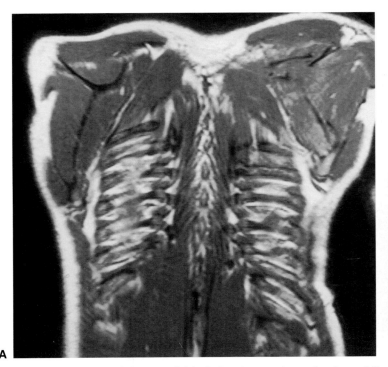

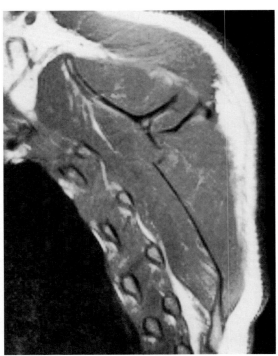

FIG. 38. (A) Large-field-of-view image shows fracture of the left scapula (B) with associated posterior rib fractures.

each structure of the scapula contributes to proximal shoulder girdle motion, body fractures altering scapula inclination are often associated with development of primary rotator cuff impingement, and coracoid fractures predispose patients to subcoracoid impingement and subscapularis tear.

REFERENCES

1. Iannotti JP, Zlatkin MB, Esterhai JL, et al. Magnetic resonance imaging of the shoulder. Sensitivity, specificity and predictive value. *J Bone Joint Surg [Am]* 1991;73:17.
2. Palmer WE, Brown JH, Rosenthal DI. The rotator cuff. Evaluation with fat suppressed MR arthrography. *Radiology* 1993;188:683.
3. Stoller DW. *MR Imaging in Orthopedics and Sports Medicine, 2nd ed.* Philadelphia: Lippincott–Raven, 1997;674.
4. Parsa M, Tuite M, Norris M, et al. MR imaging of rotator cuff tendon tears: comparison of T2* weighted gradient echo and conventional dual echo sequences. *Am J Roentgenol* 1997;168:1519–1524.
5. Uri DS. MR imaging of shoulder impingement and rotator cuff disease. *Radiol Clin North Am* 1997;35:77–96.
6. Zlatkin MB, Iannotti JP, Roberts MC, Esterhai JC, Dalinka MK, Kressel HY, Lenkinski R. Rotator cuff disease. Diagnostic performance of MR imaging: comparison with arthrography and correlation with surgery. *Radiology* 1989;172:223–229.
7. Quinn SF, Sheley RC, Demlow TA, et al. Rotator cuff tendon tears: Evaluation with fat suppressed MR images with arthroscopic correlation in 100 patients. *Radiology* 1995;195:497–501.
8. Reinus WR, Shady KL, Mirowitz SA, et al. MR diagnosis of rotator cuff tears of the shoulder: Value of using T2-weighted fat saturated images. *Am J Roentgenol* 1995;164:1451–1455.
9. Erickson SJ, Cox IH, Hyde JS, et al. Effect of tendon orientation on MR imaging signal intensity. A manifestation of the magic angle phenomenon. *Radiology* 1991;181:389.
10. Erickson SJ, Prost RW, Timins ME. The magic angle effect. Background physics and clinical relevance. *Radiology* 1993;188:23.
11. Timins ME, Erickson SJ, Estowski LD, et al. Increased signal in the normal supraspinatus tendon on MR imaging. Diagnostic pitfall caused by magic angle effect. *Am J Roentgenol* 1995;164:109–114.
12. Fukuda H, Mikasa M, Yamanaka K. Incomplete rotator cuff tears diagnosed by subacromial bursography. *Clin Orthop* 1987;223:51–58.
13. Rafii M, Firooznia H, Sherman O, et al. Rotator cuff lesions: signal patterns at MR imaging. *Radiology* 1990;177:817–823.
14. Gartsman GM, Milne JC. Articular surface partial thickness rotator cuff tears. *J Shoulder Elbow Surg* 1995;4:409–415.
15. Jobe CM. Posterior superior glenoid impingement: expanded spectrum. *Arthroscopy* 1995;11:530–536.
16. Walch G, Boileau P, Noel E, et al. Impingement of the deep surface of the supraspinatus tendon on the posterosuperior glenoid rim: An arthroscopic study. *J Shoulder Elbow Surg* 1992:1:238–245.
17. Tirman PFJ, Bost FW, Steinbach LS, et al. Posterosuperior glenoid impingement of the shoulder: findings at MR imaging and MR arthrography with arthroscopic correlation. *Radiology* 1994;192:851–856.
18. Ferrari JD, Ferrari DA, Coumas J, et al. Posterior ossification of the shoulder. The Bennet lesion. Etiology, diagnosis and treatment. *Am J Sports Med* 1994;22:171–176.
19. Zlatskin MB, Reicher MA, Kellerhouse LE, McDade W, Vetter L, Resnick D. The painful shoulder: MR imaging of the glenohumeral joint. *J Comput Assist Tomogr* 1988;12:995–1001.
20. Fritz RC, Stoller DW. MR imaging of the rotator cuff. *Magn Reson Imag Clin North Am* 1997;5:735–754.
21. Post M, Silver R, Singh M. Rotator cuff tears. Diagnosis and treatment. *Clin Orthop* 1983;173:78–91.
22. Nevasier TJ. The role of the biceps tendon in impingement syndrome. *Orthop Clin North Am* 1987;18:383–386.
23. Patten RM. Tears of the anterior portion of the rotator cuff (the subscapularis tendon): MR imaging findings. *Am J Roentgenol* 1994;162:351–354.
24. Gerber C, Hersche O, Farron A. Isolated rupture of the subscapularis tendon. *J Bone Joint Surg [Am]* 1996;78:1015–1023.
25. Van Leersum M, Schweitzer ME. Magnetic resonance imaging of the biceps complex. *Magn Reson Imag Clin North Am* 1993;1;77–86.
26. Klug JD, Moore SL. MR imaging of the biceps muscle tendon complex. *Magn Reson Imag Clin North Am* 1997;5:755–765.
27. Erickson SJ, Fitzgerald SW, Quinn SF, et al. Long bicipital tendon of the shoulder: Normal anatomy and surgical implications. *Am J Roentgenol* 1992;158:1091.
28. Cone RO III, Resnick D, Denzig L. Shoulder impingement syndrome. Radiographic evaluation. *Radiology* 1984:150:29.
29. Fu FH, Harner CD, Klein AH. Shoulder impingement syndrome. A critical review. *Clin Orthop* 1991;289:162.
30. Brossman J, Preidler KW, Pedowitz RA, et al. Shoulder impingement syndrome: influence of shoulder position on rotator cuff impingement—an anatomic study. *Am J Roentgenol* 1996;167:1511.
31. Neer CS II. Anterior acromioplasty for the chronic impingement syndrome in the shoulder. *J Bone Joint Surg [Am]* 1972;54:41.
32. Bigliani LU, Morrison DS, April EW. The morphology of the acromion and its relationship to rotator cuff tears. *Orthop Trans* 1986;10:228.
33. Peh WCG, Farmer THR, Totty WG. Acromial arch shape: assessment with MR imaging. *Radiology* 1995;195:501.
34. Norris TR, Fischer J, Bigliani LU, et al. The unfused acromial epiphysis and its relationship to impingement syndrome. *Orthop Trans* 1983;7:505.
35. Neer CS. Rotator cuff tears associated with os acromiale. *J Bone Joint Surg [Am]* 1984;66:1320–1321.
36. Park JG, Lee JK, Phelps CT. Os acromiale associated with rotator cuff impingement: MR imaging of the shoulder. *Radiology* 1994;193:255–257.
37. Tuite MJ, Toivonen DA, Orwin JF, et al. Acromial angle on radiographs of the shoulder: correlation with the impingement syndrome and rotator cuff tears. *Am J Roentgenol* 1995;165:609–613.
38. Ogata S, Uhthoff HK. Acromial enthesopathy and rotator cuff tear. A radiologic and histologic portmortem investigation of the coracoacromial arch. *Clin Orthrop* 1990;254:39–48.
39. Patte D. The subcoracoid impingement. *Clin Orthop* 1990;254:55–59.
40. Gerber C, Terrier F, Ganz R. The role of the coracoid process in the chronic impingement syndrome. *J Bone Joint Surg Clin Orthop* 1987;215:132–138.
41. Banas MP, Miller RJ, Totterman S. Relationship between the lateral acromial angle and rotator cuff disease. *J Shoulder Elbow Surg* 1995;4:454–461.
42. Jobe CM, Bradley JP, Pink M. Impingement syndrome in overhand athletes. *Surg Rounds Orthop* 1990;4:19–24.
43. Tirman FJP, Palmer WE, Feller JF. MR arthrography of the shoulder. *Magn Reson Imag Clin North Am* 1997;5:811–839.
44. Palmer WE, Caslowitz PL, Chew FS. MR arthrography of the shoulder: Normal intra-articular structures and common abnormalities. *Am J Roentgenol* 1995;164:141–146.
45. Tirman PFJ, Applegate GR, Flannigan BD, et al. Shoulder MR arthrography. *Magn Reson Clin North Am* 1993;1:125–142.
46. Palmer WE, Brown JH, Rosenthal DI. Labral ligamentous complex of the shoulder: evaluation with MR arthrography. *Radiology* 1994;190:645–651.
47. Neumann CH, Peterson SA, Jahnke AH. MR imaging of the labral-capsular complex: Normal variations. *Am J Roentgenol* 1991;157:1015–1021.
48. Tirman PFJ, Feller J, Palmer WE, et al. The Buford complex—a variation of normal shoulder anatomy. MR arthrographic imaging features. *Am J Roentgenol* 1996;166:869–873.
49. Williams MM, Snyder SJ, Buford D. The Buford complex—the cordlike middle glenohumeral ligament and absent anterosuperior labral complex: A normal anatomic capsulolabral variant. *Arthroscopy* 1994;10:241–247.
50. De Palma AF, Callery G, Bennet GA. Variational anatomy and degenerative lesions of the shoulder joint. *Am Acad Orthop Surg Instruct Course Lect* 1949;6:255–281.
51. Lippit S, Matsen F. Mechanisms of glenohumeral joint stability. *Clin Orthop* 1993;291:20–27.
52. Silliman J, Hawkins R. Classification and physical diagnosis of instability of the shoulder. *Clin Orthop* 1993;291:7–19.
53. Bankart ASB. The pathology and treatment of recurrent dislocation of the shoulder joint. *Br J Surg* 1938;26:23–29.
54. Snyder SJ, Karzel RP, Del Pizzo W, et al. SLAP lesions of the shoulder. *Arthroscopy* 1990;6:274–279.
55. Neviaser TJ. The glad lesion: Another cause of anterior joint pain. *Arthroscopy* 1993;9:22–23.
56. Tirman PFJ, Steinbach LS, Feller JF, et al. Humeral avulsion of the

anterior shoulder stabilizers after anterior shoulder dislocation: Demonstration by MRI and MR arthrography. *Skeletal Radiol* 1996;25:743–748.

57. Cvitanic O, Tirman PFJ, Feller JF, et al. Using abduction and external rotation of the shoulder to increase the sensitivity of MR arthrography in revealing tears of the anterior glenoid labrum. *Am J Roentgenol* 1997;169:837.

58. Neviaser TJ. The anterior labroligamentous periosteal sleeve avulsion lesion: A cause of anterior instability of the shoulder. *Arthroscopy* 1993;9:17.

59. Rowe CR, Zarins B. Recurrent transient subluxation of the shoulder. *J Bone Joint Surg [Am]* 1981;63:863–871.

60. Workman TL, Burkhard TK, Resnick D, et al. Hill Sachs lesion: Comparison of detection with MR imaging, radiography and arthroscopy. *Radiology* 1992;185:847–852.

61. Neer CS. Displaced proximal humeral fractures: 1. Classification and evaluation. *J Bone Joint Surg [Am]* 1970;52:1077–1089.

62. Jakob RP, Kristianson T, Mayo K, Ganz R, Muller ME. Classification and aspects of treatment of fractures of the proximal humerus. In: Bateman JE, Welsh RP, eds. *Surgery of the Shoulder*. Philadelphia: BC Decker, 1984;40–59.

63. Gerber C, Berberat C. The clinical relevance of post traumatic avascular necrosis of the humeral head. An anatomic study. *J Bone Joint Surg [Am]* 1990;72:1486–1494.

64. Hagg O, Lundberg B. Aspects of prognostic factors in comminuted and dislocated proximal humeral fractures. In: Bateman JE, Welsh RP, eds. *Surgery of the Shoulder*. Philadelphia: BC Decker, 1984;51–59.

65. Garcia A Jr, Maeck BH. Radial nerve injuries in fractures of the shaft of the humerus. *Am J Surg* 1960;99:625–627.

66. Kettlekamp DB, Alexander H. Clinical review of radial nerve injury. *J Trauma* 1967;7:424–432.

67. Patten RM, Mack LA, Wang KY, et al. Nondisplaced fractures of the greater tuberosity of the humerus. Sonographic detection. *Radiology* 1992;182:201–204.

68. Eustace S, Tello R, DeCarvalho V, Carey J, Wroblicka JT, Melhem ER, Yucel EK. A comparison of whole body turbo short tau inversion recovery MR imaging and planar technetium 99m methylene diphosphonate scintigraphy in the evaluation of patients with suspected skeletal metastases. *Am J Roentgenol* 1997;169:1655–1661.

69. Jacobs P. Post traumatic osteolysis of the outer end of the clavicle. *J Bone Joint Surg [Br]* 1964;46:705.

70. Levine AH, Pais MJ, Schwartz EE. Posttraumatic osteolysis of the distal clavicle with early emphasis on early radiologic changes. *Am J Roentgenol* 1976;127:781.

71. Madsen B. Osteolysis of the acromial end of the clavicle following trauma. *Br J Radiol* 1963;36:822.

72. Murphy SJ, Kneeland JB, Komorowski RA, et al. Post traumatic osteolysis of the clavicle. MR features. *J Comput Assist Tomogr* 1990;14:835.

73. Allman FL. Fractures and ligamentous injuries of the clavicle and its articulation. *J Bone Joint Surg [Am]* 1967;49:774–784.

74. Rumball KM, DaSilva VF, Preston DN, Carruthers CC. Brachial plexus injury after clavicular fracture. Case report and literature review. *Can J Surg* 1991;34:264–266.

75. Koss SD, Giotz HT, Redler NR, et al. Non union of a midshaft clavicle fracture associated with subclavian vein compression. A case report. *Orthop Rev* 1989;18:431–434.

76. Nettles JL, Linscheid R. Sternoclavicular dislocations. *J Trauma* 1968;8:158–164.

77. Mehta JC, Sachdev A, Collins JJ. Retrosternal dislocation of the clavicle. *Injury* 1973;5:79–83.

78. Zdravkovic D, Damholt VV. Comminuted and severely displaced fractures of the scapula. *Acta Orthop Scand* 1974;45:60–65.

79. Eustace S, Denison B. MR imaging of acute orthopedic trauma to the upper extremity. *Clin Radiol* 1997;52:338–344.

CHAPTER 11

The Elbow

Stephen J. Eustace

Successful MR imaging of the elbow can be obtained on both dedicated extremity magnets and on mid- and high-field superconducting units. This section outlines a practical approach to imaging the elbow, reviews potential diagnostic pitfalls, and finally outlines commonly encountered bone and soft tissue injuries.

PATIENT POSITIONING AND IMAGING PROTOCOLS

Positioning

Effective MR imaging of the elbow is usually acheived with the patient supine, with the arm at the side, elbow extended and supinated. In such a position there is minimal

rotation of the forearm, allowing visualization of the medial and lateral collateral ligaments and the common flexor and the extensor tendon insertions in a single coronal (oblique) acquisition (Fig. 1).

In large adult patients or patients following cast fixation, bore diameter of the magnet may mitigate against comfortable imaging of the elbow by the patient's side in the supine position, even in the swimmer's-type position (the contralateral normal elbow placed above the head). In this setting, the patient is either obliqued or imaged with the elbow above the head (Fig. 2).

In the oblique position, the elbow is dependent, and the extended supinated position is maintained. In the above-head position, the arm is often slightly flexed and pronated. In such a position, collateral ligaments and the extensor and flexor tendons are obliqued, making image interpretation extremely difficult.

Following cast fixation, the elbow is fixed in either flexion or extension, which further dictates patient positioning for

S. J. Eustace: Department of Radiology, Section of Musculoskeletal Radiology, Boston University School of Medicine and Boston Medical Center, Boston, Massachusetts 02118.

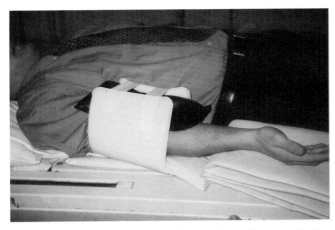

FIG. 1. Flexible wraparound surface coil positioned with the patient supine and the arm by the side.

successful imaging. Flexed fixation necessitates imaging in the above-head position.

Receiver Coil

In order to optimize reception of generated signal, imaging requires either a molded or tightly apposed surface coil or the use of a dedicated quadrature coil. In routine practice, a flexible surface coil molded to the contour of the elbow is employed to receive generated signal. Dedicated phased-array coils improve image signal to noise and have the potential to decrease the number of excitations required to yield diagnostic images, particularly using extremity systems.

Volumetric coils are used to image patients following cast fixation, as loss of apposition secondary to the presence of a cast dramatically decreases received signal with flexible surface coils.

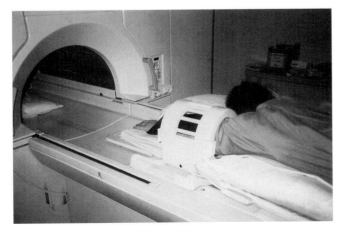

FIG. 2. Swimmer's position with the patient prone and the arm extended above the head.

Imaging Plane

Successful elbow imaging with the arm by the side requires off-central axis imaging capability, which is available on all modern machines.

Coronal images are prescribed off axial and sagittal localizers. An axial image is typically acquired at the level of the medial and lateral epicondyles of the distal humerus. Coronals are prescribed parallel to a line drawn between these two anatomic points; sagittals are prescribed perpendicular to this line.

Field of View

Similar to other sites, a preliminary image, usually a coronal fast inversion recovery image, is often acquired with extended coverage, or a field of view of 15 to 20 cm, before the dedicated images, allowing global perception of the extent of trauma to precede high-resolution imaging of internal joint structures.

To image patients with suspected soft tissue injury to either tendons or ligaments, images are subsequently acquired with a 14-cm field of view.

Slice Thickness

Detailed evaluation of collateral ligaments and common extensor and flexor tendon origins necessitates imaging with a slice thickness not greater than 3 mm. When magnets have gradient strengths up to 26 mT/m, 1-mm slices may be routinely acquired through regions of particular interest, although improved resolution is at the expense of coverage.

Contiguous 3-mm slices generally allow adequate evaluation of osseous injury.

Motion Suppression

In the hand-by-the-side supine and obliqued projections, respiratory and cardiac motion may be problematic. Saturation bands are routinely applied parallel to the long axis of the arm through the lateral margin of the abdomen to minimize this effect.

In infants referred with suspected growth plate injury, imaging is achieved using chloral hydrate sedation (75 mg/kg up to 10 kg weight, 50 mg/kg for each additional 1 kg) with the arm by the side.

Imaging Protocol

Following trauma, a turbo inversion recovery sequence with an extended field of view (20 cm) is often employed (applied in the coronal plane) to localize and determine the extent of injury (1 min 15 sec acquisition time). Subsequent imaging is performed using a combination of turboSTIR and turbo spin-echo T1-weighted sequences in coronal, sagittal,

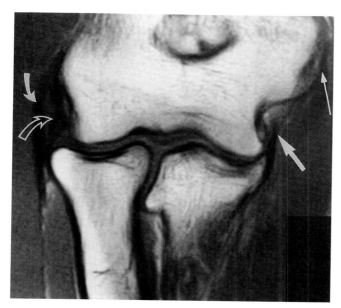

FIG. 3. Coronal T1-weighted image of the elbow shows the insertion of the common extensor tendon *(curved solid arrow),* the radial collateral ligament *(open curved arrow),* the ulnar collateral ligament *(straight solid arrow),* and the insertion of the common flexor tendon *(straight thin arrow).*

and axial planes (1 min 5 sec for each acquisition) with a field of view of 14 cm, although this is dictated by patient size (Fig. 3).

Inversion recovery is usually employed rather than spectrally acquired frequency-selective fat saturation in the elbow, as field homogeneity at the periphery of the main field is often heterogeneous (although this is less marked on high-gradient systems). As has been discussed in Chapter 2, proximity of frequency peaks of fat and water at low field strength (less than 40 Hz) mitigates against the use of frequency-selective fat saturation when images are acquired with dedicated extremity units (Lunar Artoscan).

Turbo spin-echo T1 imaging, similar to that in all other joints, is achieved using a repetition time of 500 msec, an echo time of 15 msec, a short echo train of up to six, and a low-high echo to view *k*-space mapping profile. Use of a short echo train facilitates the use of a short repetition time, enhancing T1 weighting and further decreasing acquisition time. Turbo inversion recovery sequences are acquired using an inversion time of 160 msec, a repetition time of 2,000 msec, an echo time of 20 msec, an echo train of six, and a linear echo to view *k*-space mapping profile. Multiple excitations are generally unnecessary using inversion recovery sequences, as diagnostic decisions are generally made on the basis of contrast afforded by fat-suppressed images rather than on the basis of signal to noise.

When collateral ligament or common extensor or flexor tendon injury is suspected, the site of trauma is localized using a turboSTIR image in the coronal plane; evaluation of complex anatomy is based on review of turbo spin-echo

T1-weighted images, in both axial and direct coronal planes (Fig. 4). When fine resolution is required, a three-dimensional (3D) gradient-echo image is acquired in the coronal plane, allowing thin 1-mm section reconstruction in multiple oblique planes.

To image suspected biceps brachialis or triceps tendon disruption, a dual-echo turbo spin-echo T2-weighted and a turboSTIR sequence are acquired in the sagittal plane. Dual-echo turbo spin-echo T2-weighted imaging is achieved using a repetition time of 2,000 to 3,000 msec (actual TR is a function of the coverage required), echo times of 20 and 80 msec, an echo train of six, and linear echo to view *k*-space mapping.

When a patient is referred with a suspected osteochondral abnormality, such as Panner's disease, turbo inversion recovery and T2-weighted fast field-echo (gradient-echo) with off-resonance magnetization transfer saturation images are acquired in coronal and sagittal planes. Fast field-echo T2 weighting is achieved with a low flip angle of 30°, a long repetition time of 500 msec, and an echo time of 15 msec. With such a sequence, the off-resonance pulse saturates partially bound protons, reducing signal in cartilage.

The same T2-weighted gradient- or fast field-echo sequence with off-resonance magnetization transfer saturation is used to image suspected pediatric growth plate injury, particularly before growth plate mineralization.

In most patients, an image matrix with 256 phase-encodes is employed, and because the perceived difference in image signal to noise between two and three excitations is negligi-

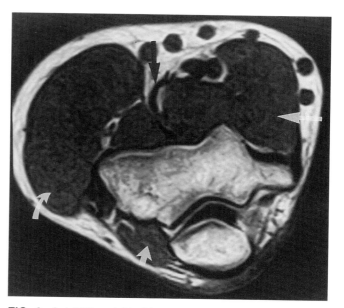

FIG. 4. Axial T1-weighted image of the elbow at the level of the distal humerus (acquired on a dedicated low-field extremity magnet, courtesy of Lunar Artoscan, Madison, WI) shows the extensor compartment *(curved arrow),* the anconeus *(short straight arrow),* the biceps tendon *(black arrow),* and the flexor compartment *(straight white arrow).*

TABLE 1. *Protocol to image the elbow following trauma*

Sequence	Image plane	FOV	TR	TE	ETL	Mapping scheme
Occult or documented fracture evaluation						
IR TSE	Cor direct	14	2,000	20	6	Linear
TSE T1	Cor direct	14	500	15	4	Low-high
+ or − additional planes						
IR TSE	Sag direct	14	2,000	20	6	Linear
TSE T2	Axial	14	2,000	20, 80	6	Linear
Pediatric growth plate injury						
T-2 FFE	Multiple Planes	14	500	15		With off-resonance MT

ble ($\sqrt{2}$ versus $\sqrt{3}$, a relative improvement in signal to noise by 1.4- versus 1.6-fold), more than two excitations are rarely employed in a drive for rapid imaging.

Magnetic resonance arthrography, with a single contrast injection into the elbow (radiocapitellar) joint space, improves the visibility of articular cartilage and may improve the evaluation of both collateral ligament injury and loose intra-articular bodies. Detection of loose bodies is fraught with difficulty as a result of numerous fatty folds around the margin of the joints. When this approach is employed, 4 to 5 cc of a gadolinium, 1% lidocaine, and renografin solution is injected into the radiocapitellar joint space using a 25-gauge needle (0.1 ml of gadolinium DTPA to 5 ml of 1% lidocaine and 15 cc of renografin 60) (Table 1).

Anatomic Variants and Pitfalls in MR Evaluation of the Elbow

Five commonly identified anatomic features of the normal elbow are frequently misinterpreted as being abnormal or incorrectly attributed to disease.

Pseudodefect of Capitellum

In the normal elbow, there is an apparent osteochondral abnormality (often mistaken as being caused by Panner's disease) in the sagittal plane along the posterior half of the perceived articular surface of the capitellum. In cadaveric specimens, this has been shown to represent the junction of capitellum and lateral epicondyle (Fig. 5) (1).

Pseudodefect of Trochlear Groove and Ridge

The junction of the coronoid and olecranon is marked by a ridge 3 to 5 mm thick, devoid of overlying cartilage, routinely identified traversing across the joint space on sagittal images of the elbow. At this junction, bone extends to appose the surfaces created by articular cartilage (ridge), occasionally not quite to the level of the articular cartilage (notch), but never beyond. At the far medial and lateral margins of the ridge, the bone flares to form marginal grooves (see Figs. 5 and 6) (2).

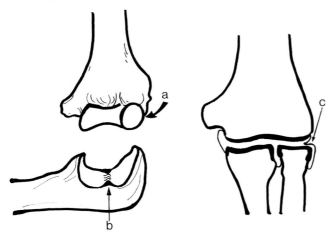

FIG. 5. Diagrammatic representation of anatomic variants in the elbow including the pseudodefect of the capitellum at the junction with the lateral epicondyle **(a)**, the trochlear ridge or notch **(b)**, and the lateral synovial fringe **(c)**. Adapted from Rosenberg et al. (4).

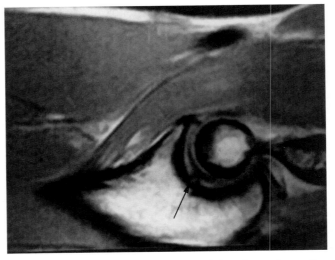

FIG. 6. Sagittal T1-weighted image of the elbow shows the trochlear ridge *(arrow)* between articular cartilage of the coronoid and the olecranon.

The Lateral Synovial Fringe or Meniscus

A triangular-shaped circumferential marginal fold of capsule and synovium is interposed between the radial head and the capitellum in the normal elbow. It may become more prominent in patients with Panner's disease secondary to friction imposed by irregular articular surfaces or in patients with inflammatory arthritis (see Fig. 5) (3).

Skin Thickening over the Extensor Surface of the Elbow

Skin overlying the olecranon appears thickened at MR imaging as a result of a paucity of underlying subcutaneous fat, particularly on images acquired in the sagittal plane (4).

Distal Triceps Tendon Signal Heterogeneity

In the axial plane, the fibers of the distal triceps are loosely packed, resulting in signal heterogeneity, even in health. In the hyperextended position, sagittal images show triceps tendon laxity and folds, and these should not be mistaken for partial tears (5).

Additional infrequently encountered variants, which include asymptomatic subluxation of the ulnar nerve (secondary to an absent arcuate ligament); an accessory muscle in the region of the cubital tunnel fixing the ulnar nerve, termed the *anconeus epitrochlearis;* an accessory osseous process extending from the anteromedial border of the distal humerus oriented toward the joint, the *supracondylar process;* or an accessory ossicle in the posterior joint space, termed the *os supratrochlare,* are rarely identified. Each variant is reported to occur in fewer than 1% of patients (6–9).

ACUTE SOFT TISSUE INJURIES

Collateral Ligament Injury

Similar to the knee, injury to the medial or ulnar collateral ligament occurs considerably more frequently than injury to the lateral or radial collateral ligament (10).

The Ulnar Collateral Ligament

The ulnar collateral ligament is responsible for medial elbow joint stability and resistance to valgus strain. It is composed of three discrete tendon bundles: the anterior bundle, the posterior bundle, and the transverse bundle (Fig. 7). Despite anatomic complexity, the anterior bundle is the most important contributor to stability and is therefore most frequently injured. Fortuitously, the anterior bundle (the A-UCL) is taut in the extended-elbow position and is therefore readily visualized on direct coronal images running from the undersurface of the medial epicondyle, just deep to the common flexor tendon origin, distally to its attachment to the medial aspect of the ulnar coronoid process. The anterior bundle blends with the fibers of the overlying flexor digitorum superficialis muscle. The posterior and transverse

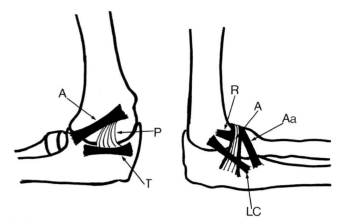

FIG. 7. Diagrams of the medial **(left)** and lateral collateral **(right)** ligaments of the elbow. The medial or ulnar collateral ligament **(left)** is composed of the anterior bundle (A), the posterior bundle (P), and the transverse bundle (T). The lateral or radial collateral ligament is composed of the radial collateral ligament (R), the annular ligament (A), the accessory annular ligament (Aa), and the lateral ulnar collateral ligament (LC).

bundles may be identified in the axial plane forming the floor of the cubital tunnel (11,12).

At MR imaging, similar to other tendons with organized structure, the ulnar collateral ligament is hypointense on all sequences. Following injury, intrasubstance hemorrhage and edema result in localized signal changes or loss of hypointensity. Tendon strain following valgus injury results in associated edema both within and around the collateral ligament, often extending to the overlying flexor digitorum superficialis muscle belly. In severe injury, complete rupture occurs, which is most frequently midsubstance (87%) (13). Avulsion is extremely uncommon (Fig. 8).

The sensitivity of MR imaging to complete collateral ligament injury is reported to be as high as 100%. The sensitivity of MR imaging to partial tears, particularly undersurface tears, is considerably less, with surgically proven undersurface partial tears identified in as few as 14% of cases. When partial tears are suspected, MR arthrography dramatically improves the sensitivity to almost 86%; partial tears manifest by extension of fluid along the medial margin of the coronoid process (Fig. 9) (13,14).

When repair is undertaken in proven cases, graft is usually harvested from either the palmaris longus or achilles tendons.

The Lateral Collateral Ligament

Injury to the lateral radial collateral occurs less frequently than injury to the medial ulnar collateral ligment, complicating either acute varus strain or elbow dislocation.

The lateral collateral ligament has four components: the radial collateral ligament, which is primarily responsible for lateral joint line stability; the lateral ulnar collateral liga-

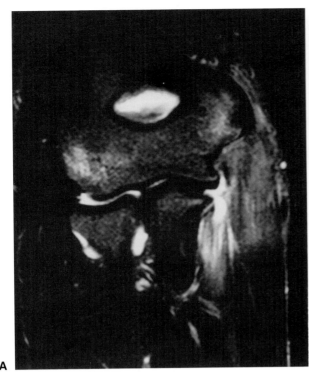
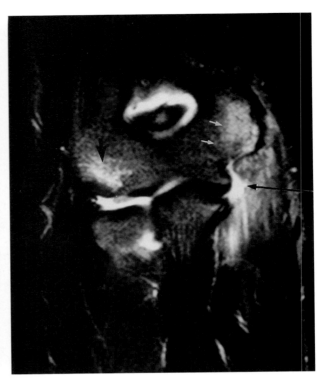

FIG. 8. Coronal T2-weighted images with fat suppression show **(A)** a tear of the ulnar collateral ligament with associated avulsion and incomplete tear of the common flexor tendon *(arrow)*. **B:** Following valgus injury, there is marrow edema within the medial epicondyle at the site of common flexor avulsion and within the capitellum at the site of radial head impaction.

ment, which is primarily responsible for posterolateral stability; and the annular and accessory annular ligaments, which are responsible for stability of the proximal radioulnar joint (see Fig. 7) (15,16).

At MR imaging the radial collateral ligament, being taut throughout elbow flexion, is readily identified on coronal images approximately at the same level as the A-UCL. The lateral ulnar collateral ligament is identified on posterior coronal images. It runs obliquely from the lateral epicondyle to the posterolateral aspect of the ulnar and is identified on serial images. It is taut when varus strain is applied. The annular ligaments are best visualized in the axial plane, and injury to them should be suspected in patients with either acute or repeated radial head subluxation or dislocation.

Similar to the ulnar collateral ligament, injury ranges from subtle signal abnormality through periligonentous edema to complete ligament disruption. Radial collateral ligament injury, because it often reflects long-term overuse, is commonly accompanied by extensor tendon injury, epicondylitis, or tennis elbow (most frequently with partial tear of the extensor carpi radialis brevis) (Fig. 10) (17).

The sensitivity of MR imaging in the detection of LCL complex injury is currently unclear, as injury is less common than injury to the ulnar collateral ligament and, therefore, surgery, which would allow a correlation to be made, is infrequently undertaken.

Tendon Injuries

Tendon injuries at the elbow most frequently follow forced eccentric contraction but are more common in patients with connective tissue diseases on long-term steroids, in patients debilitated by chronic renal impairment or hyperparathyroidism, or in individuals on anabolic steroids. In the latter group, with excessive muscle strength, additional stress is transmitted to the tendon unit (18,19).

Biceps Muscle Injury

The biceps brachii muscle is composed of a long head and a short head. The two muscle bellies share a single tendon insertion on the bicipital tuberosity of the radius. The short head arises from the apex of the coracoid; the long head arises from the supraglenoid tubercle of the scapula. Injury involving the biceps muscle more frequently involves the tendons than the muscle bellies, and of the tendons, most frequently affects the tendon of the long head.

Injury to the distal biceps tendon is less common and, when it occurs, is usually secondary to acute macrotrauma or eccentric overload as occurs attempting to catch or carry a heavy object. In such a way, attempted elbow flexion through the biceps tendon is counterposed by forced extension induced by the object. The resulting tear occurs most frequently at or just proximal to the tendon insertion on the

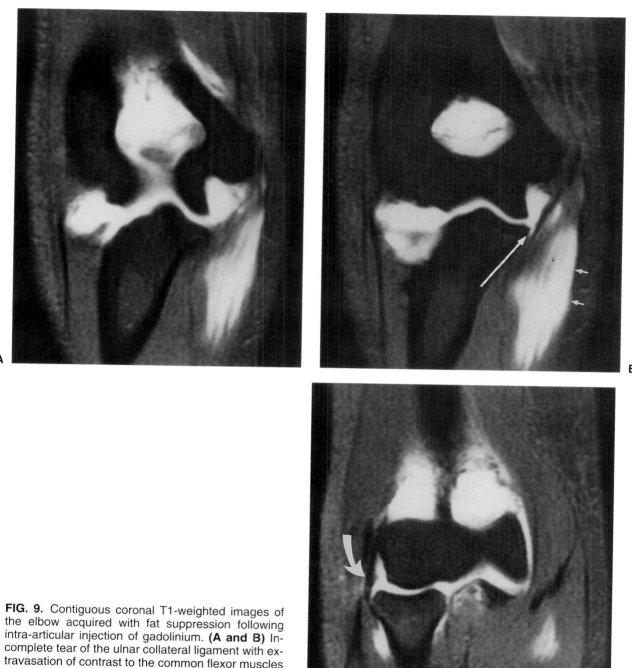

FIG. 9. Contiguous coronal T1-weighted images of the elbow acquired with fat suppression following intra-articular injection of gadolinium. **(A and B)** Incomplete tear of the ulnar collateral ligament with extravasation of contrast to the common flexor muscles *(small arrows)* and extension of contrast along the medial margin of the coronoid process *(straight arrow).* **(C)** *Curved arrow* indicates an intact radial collateral ligament. (Courtesy of M. Barish, M.D., Boston Medical Center, Boston, MA.)

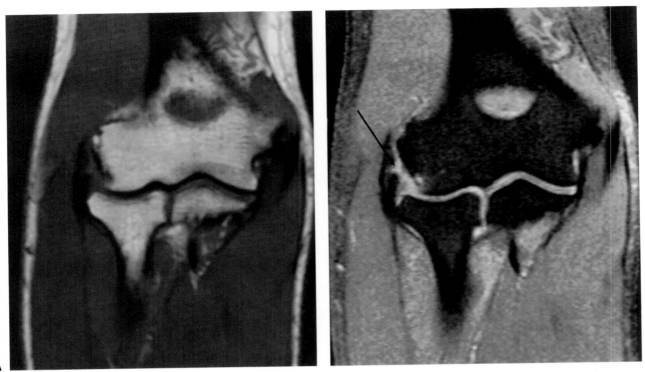

FIG. 10. Coronal T1 **(A)** and inversion recovery **(B)** images show a tear of the radial collateral ligament with interposition of fluid *(arrow)*. (Courtesy of Arthur Newberg, M.D., New England Baptist Hospital, Boston, MA.)

radial tuberosity (20,21). Following rupture, the main muscle belly retracts proximally to the midarm with extensive residual hemorrhage and edema at the site of tear (Figs. 11 and 12). Although such an injury is usually clinically apparent,

manifest as an obvious mass, compensatory flexion incurred by the brachialis may obscure the diagnosis. When the injury is apparent, MR imaging is used before surgical repair to determine the extent and site of the retracted tendon.

The distal biceps tendon is best visualized in the axial and sagittal planes, the axial images clearly depicting the normal insertion site on the radial tuberosity, the sagittal images

FIG. 11. Sagittal IR TSE image shows an incomplete tear of the biceps muscle with retraction of the muscle belly *(arrow)* and extensive soft tissue edema.

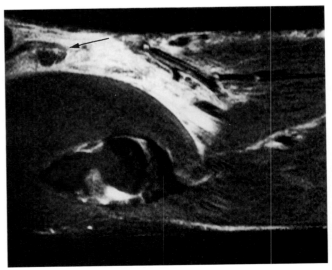

FIG. 12. Sagittal IR TSE image shows a complete tear of the biceps muscle *(arrow)*. There is extensive hemorrhage and edema within the adjacent soft tissues.

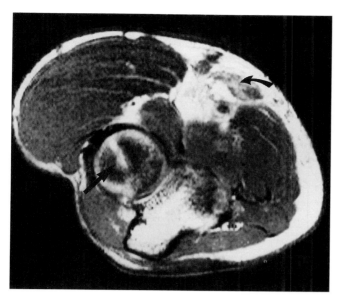

FIG. 13. Axial proton-density SE image shows a partial tear of the distal biceps at the musculotendinous junction with characteristic signal heterogeneity secondary to hemorrhage *(curved arrow)*. Acute eccentric contraction has been complicated by an oblique crack fracture of the radial head *(straight arrow)*.

allowing an appreciation of the extent of retraction (see Figs. 11 and 12).

Partial tears of the distal biceps or tendinosis are less common and are usually a sequel to overuse (Figs. 13 and 14), often induced by weight lifting. Magnetic resonance imaging is helpful, as it allows differentiation of primary tendon abnormality, manifest as tendon thickening or partial tear, from either brachialis tendon injury or bicipitoradial bursitis, which may accompany or occur in isolation in overuse syndromes. In practice, each entity is treated conservatively, although steroid injection to the bicipitoradial bursa may be undertaken if it is identified (21,22).

Triceps Tendon Injury

The triceps muscle lies in the posterior compartment of the arm and is composed of three heads, the long head arising from the infraglenoid tubercle, the lateral head arising from the lateral and posterior aspect of the humerus, and the medial head arising distally from the medial and posterior aspect of the humerus. The three heads unite to form the triceps tendon in the midarm; the tendon is composed of a dominant deep component that merges with a superficial component before inserting on the posterosuperior surface of the olecranon (24).

Triceps tendon injury is extremely uncommon and most frequently occurs secondary to forced flexion against a contracting muscle (attempting to extend the elbow) as occurs following a fall on an outstretched hand (forced eccentric contraction). Rarely, injury may follow a direct blow or com-

plicate olecranon bursitis where steroid injections, synovitis, and superimposed infection conspire to weaken the tendon (Fig. 15) (25).

In most cases, tear is complete and associated with avulsion of a small fragment of bone from the posterior aspect of the olecranon, readily visualized on conventional radiographs. Rupture of the muscle belly or at the myotendinous junction in the absence of an avulsion is extremely uncommon (Fig. 16) (26).

Acute rupture of the triceps tendon is readily visualized in both the sagittal and axial planes at MR imaging, manifest by both morphologic and signal changes of hemorrhage and edema. Tendinosis secondary to overuse is manifest by tendon thickening with loss of normal signal hypointensity. Partial tear, which is extremely uncommon, is manifest by disruption of fibers, usually within the middle third of the tendon.

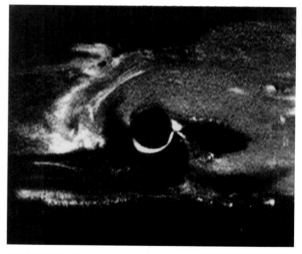

A

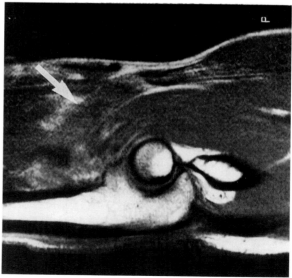

B

FIG. 14. Sagittal IR TSE **(A)** and TSE T1 **(B)** images show hemorrhage and swelling of the distal biceps tendon secondary to a surgically proven partial tear of the distal biceps tendon.

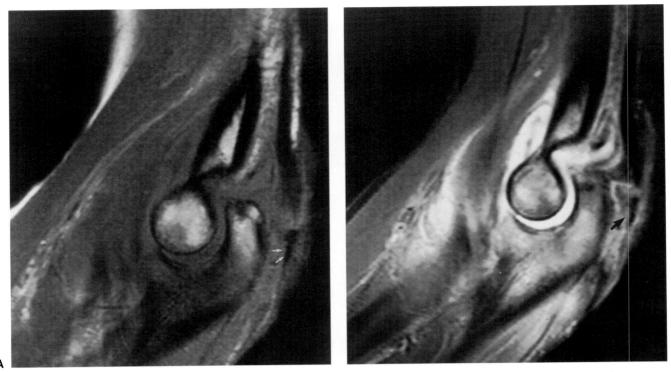

FIG. 15. (A) Sagittal TSE T1 and **(B)** IR TSE image of the elbow shows heterogeneous signal abnormality in the olecranon with superficial hemorrhage and edema secondary to osteomyelitis complicating chronic bursal steroid injection. Note is made of an associated avulsion at the insertion of the distal triceps tendon *(arrows)*.

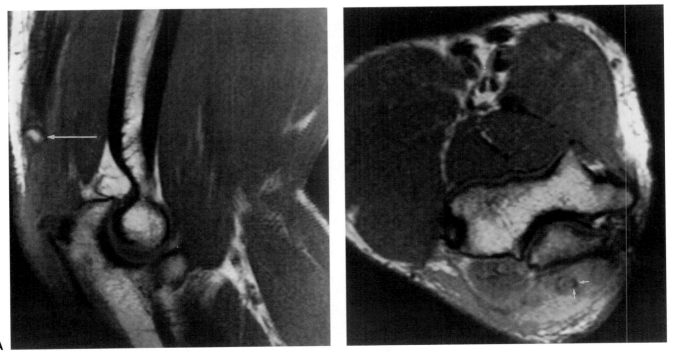

FIG. 16. (A) Sagittal and **(B)** axial TSE T1-weighted images show a distal triceps avulsion fracture in an adult complicating a fall on the outstretched hand with proximal retraction of fragment *(arrows)* and extensive hemorrhage and edema at the site of rupture between the avulsed fragment and the olecranon.

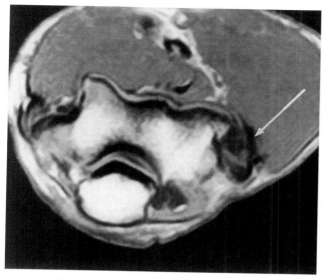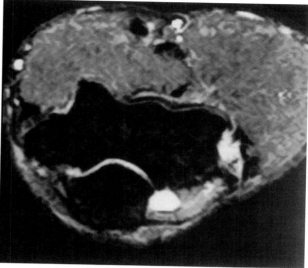

FIG. 17. **(A)** Axial T1- and **(B)** T2-weighted gradient-echo images at the level of the distal humerus show avulsive and inflammatory changes at common extensor origin on the lateral epicondyle complicating chronic epicondylitis. (Images acquired on a dedicated extremity 0.3-T magnet courtesy of Lunar Artoscan, Madison, WI.)

Pitfall

Laxity of Triceps Tendon when Imaged in Full Extension

SOFT TISSUE INJURY ACCOMPANYING CHRONIC REPETITIVE TRAUMA

Lateral Epicondylitis

Lateral epicondylitis or "tennis elbow" is the most common cause of elbow pain in the adult population. The term epicondylitis is misleading, as the disorder is characterized by soft tissue changes in the absence of epicondylar bony edema or inflammation. It is thought to reflect degeneration and tearing of the common extensor tendon as a result of chronic microtrauma secondary to traction forces, as it is most frequently identified in athletes (26). Resected specimens show fibrillary, hyaline, and myxoid degeneration with angiofibroblastic proliferation within the tendon origin with minimal associated inflammatory change (27).

Reflecting tendon degeneration, MR images show local tendon thickening with low to intermediate signal change. Acute injuries are less common but manifest as local edema and hemorrhage, which appear as poorly defined increased signal on T2-weighted images. More often, acute partial tears are superimposed on chronic tendon thickening, particularly of the extensor carpi radialis brevis muscle tendon unit (Fig. 17). Occasionally, edema is identified in the adjacent anconeus (posterolateral) muscle belly unit (28).

Medial Epicondylitis

Medial epicondylitis or "golfer's elbow" is considerably less common than lateral epicondylitis. Its descriptive term is also misleading, as the injury is primarily to the common flexor tendon rather than to the underlying bone (29).

Repetitive valgus stress at the elbow in overhead racquet games, in golfers, and in adolescent baseball pitchers results in chronic microtrauma to the common flexor tendon with secondary degenerative rather than inflammatory changes. Swelling of the flexor carpi ulnaris within the cubital tunnel may lead to secondary ulnar nerve compression (Fig. 18) (30).

At MR imaging, medial epicondylitis is manifest as tendon swelling with associated intermediate signal abnormality within the common extensor tendon, superficial to the ulnar collateral ligament, on all sequences. Superimposed partial tears, which frequently accompany medial epicondylitis, generate foci of signal hyperintensity on T2-weighted sequences.

Pitfall

Recent Intramuscular Steroid Injection Producing Muscle Edema

---

Nerve Injury Following Elbow Trauma

Elbow trauma may lead to injury to the median nerve within the anteromedial soft tissues (most frequently following anterior dislocation), the radial nerve anterior to the lateral epicondyle (most frequently following lateral epicondylar fracture), or injury to the ulnar nerve within the cubital tunnel immediately posterior to the medial epicondyle.

Intimately related to the medial epicondyle, the ulnar nerve is the most frequently injured nerve about the elbow. Direct impaction leading to nerve contusion, fracture result-

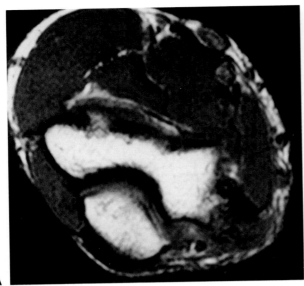
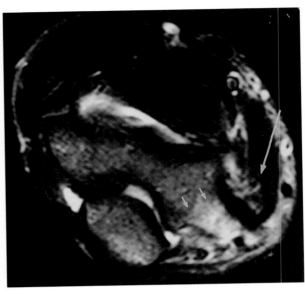

A

B

FIG. 18. (A) Axial T1- and (B) T2-weighted images show acute inflammatory change at the common flexor insertion on the medial epicondyle. Note edema within and immediately behind the medial epicondyle *(short arrows)* and at the insertion site of the common flexor tendon *(long arrow).*

ing in nerve compression or traction, and muscle or ligament tear allowing nerve subluxation may all lead to reversible nerve deficit.

Magnetic resonance imaging allows clear visualization of the course of the nerve and potential sites of nerve compression. Injury to the nerve is manifest as nerve displacement, nerve swelling, and intraneural signal hyperintensity on T2-weighted scans. Muscle denervation is manifest by signal hyperintensity within the affected muscle group on both frequency-selective and inversion recovery fat-saturated images (31).

OSSEOUS INJURY FOLLOWING ACUTE ORTHOPEDIC TRAUMA

Pediatric Growth Plate Injury

The Development of the Elbow

An understanding of the stages in the development of the elbow allows accurate interpretation of images acquired following trauma. At birth, the distal humerus is composed of a single cartilaginous epiphysis separated from the metaphysis by an arched physis. Injury at this time results in complete epiphyseal separation. The primitive epiphysis differentiates into four ossification centers: two epiphyses, the capitellum and the trochlea; and two apophyses, the medial and lateral epicondyles. Following such a division, subsequent injury is usually confined to individual ossification centers in contrast to the gross injury or displacement that occurs in infancy (32).

The cartilage of the proximal ulna develops a single ossification center, the olecranon, which eventually leads to min-

eralization of the coronoid. The cartilage of the radial head develops into a further single ossification center.

The appearance of ossification centers occurs 1 to 2 years earlier in girls than boys and follows an orderly progression with appearance of the capitellar ossification center first at 1 to 2 years, the radial head at 3 to 6 years, the inner or medial epicondyle at 4 years, the trochlea at 8 years, the olecranon at 9 years, and the external epicondyle at 10 years (33).

Appearance of Ossification Centers	
Capitellum	1–2 years
Radial Head	3–6 years
Inner (Medial) Epicondyle	4 years
Trochlea	8 years
Olecranon	9 years
External (Lateral) Epicondyle	10 years

In adolescence, usually between 10 and 12 years, the three lateral ossification centers fuse, followed by closure of their associated physis at 13 to 16 years. The medial epicondyle physis is the last to close between 16 and 18 years.

Inappropriately treated injury to any of the ossification centers around the elbow may lead to deformity; however, because the elbow physes contribute to only 20% of final length, shortening is often subtle (34).

Pediatric Elbow Fractures

Salter and Harris originally classified growth plate injuries in 1963 (35). Although the understanding of growth plate

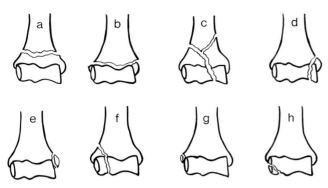

FIG. 19. Diagrammatic representation of fractures of the distal humerus: **a,** supracondylar; **b,** transcondylar; **c,** intercondylar; **d,** medial condylar; **e,** medial epicondylar; **f,** lateral condylar; **g,** lateral epicondylar; **h,** capitellar.

injury has improved since that time, these injuries have continued to present special problems in both diagnosis and management.

The growth plate is considerably weaker than both adjacent ligaments and bone, making it susceptible to injury, particularly during growth spurts at puberty (36). In most cases, callus formation and subsequent healing of fractures are uneventful. Rarely persistent motion at the fracture margins or the development of bone bridges impairs healing and leads to long-term complications such as growth arrest or deformity (37–39). It is only by complete and accurate imaging, allowing appropriate orthopedic intervention, that these complications may be avoided (Fig. 19).

Although plain radiographs allow adequate evaluation of growth plate injuries in most cases, additional imaging is occasionally undertaken in patients in whom radiographic appearances fail to explain symptoms or when surgical intervention is planned and an improved preoperative road map is required (Fig. 20). In this regard, previously, authors have reviewed use of both planar and computed tomography, ultrasound, and scintigraphy in evaluation of the growth plate. Planar and computed tomography allow better visualization of cartilaginous growth plates than conventional radiographs. However, despite the ability to improve contrast resolution by windowing at computed tomography, visibility of low-density cartilage at both conventional and computed tomography is still relatively poor (40). Similarly, although recent studies have emphasized the ability of ultrasound to detect and evaluate growth plate injury, it is an operator-dependent modality, and the images are in a form not readily interpreted by referring orthopedic colleagues. Scintigraphy, although widely used in adults with suspected fractures, is not widely favored for this purpose in children, as intense physiological osteoblastic response concentrating radiopharmaceutical at the margin of the growth plate can mask an underlying fracture (35). Although many radiologists prefer to employ spiral CT to evaluate growth plate injuries, on the premise that displacement of fracture fragments is the

principal issue in treatment planning, MR imaging, when employed, allows evaluation of injury to both bone and unossified cartilage (see Fig. 20). Visualization of unossified cartilage is of importance as identification of fracture extension through unossified cartilage changes the fracture description from Salter 2 to Salter 4. Type 2 supracondylar fractures are treated conservatively, whereas type 4 fractures generally require open reduction and internal fixation (Fig. 21) (37).

Although conventional T2-weighted spin-echo images afford excellent contrast between growth plate cartilage and joint fluid, our experience suggests that application of an off-resonance pulse to a T2-weighted gradient-echo sequence (fast field-echo, Philips Medical Systems) (T2* contrast) affords the best visualization of unossified growth plate cartilage (Fig. 22). The precession frequency of partially bound water within growth plate cartilage differs from that in free synovial fluid, facilitating selective saturation by a finely tuned radiofrequency pulse (1,500 Hz off resonance) (see Fig. 19). In such a way, partially bound fluid becomes hypointense or saturated relative to free fluid, enhancing contrast between growth plate cartilage and free joint fluid.

When occult osseous injury rather than injury to unossified growth plate cartilage is dominant, it is best evaluated by a spin-echo-based sequence in which a refocusing 180° pulse minimizes the effects of susceptibility differences between trabeculae and marrow components. Susceptibility differences between these components may lead to obscuring of subtle osseous injury on gradient- or fast field-echo sequences, particularly when long-echo-time T2* weighting is employed. Dramatic contrast afforded by short-tau inversion recovery sequences (STIR), enhancing visibility of marrow edema, facilitates rapid fracture localization, although differentiation of the identified bone bruise from a true fracture is best made by review of spin-echo sequences (fracture manifest as linear hypointensity).

Fractures of the elbow most frequently involve the distal humerus, classified as supracondylar or epiphyseal; the olecranon; and rarely the radial head.

Supracondylar Fractures

Supracondylar fractures account for up to 60% of pediatric fractures of the distal humerus, most frequently complicating a fall on the outstretched hand with the elbow in extension (although a significant number of fractures complicate a fall in flexion). They occur most frequently between 3 and 10 years of age.

Supracondylar fractures are easily diagnosed on conventional radiographs as they extend through the ossified metaphysis and are usually associated with dorsal angulation of the distal fragment. Inadequate reduction and malunion predispose to subsequent deformity, posterior elbow dislocation, and occasionally nerve injury (38–40).

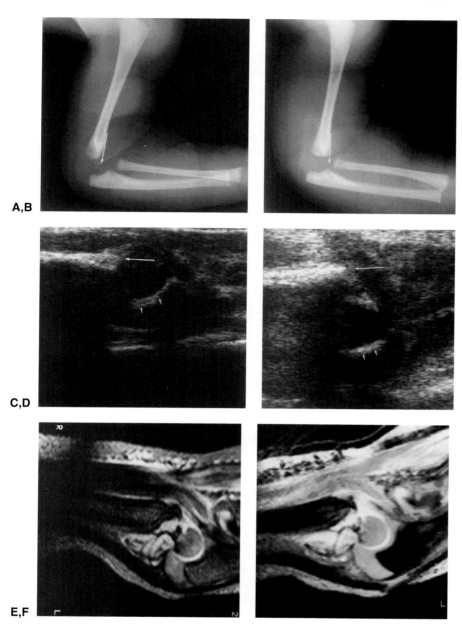

A,B

C,D

E,F

FIG. 20. A 4-day-old child delivered hand first, with a suspected complicating growth plate injury. **(A)** Lateral radiograph of the normal elbow shows the anterior humeral line intersecting the unossified capitellar cartilage *(arrow)*. **(B)** Lateral radiograph in abnormal elbow shows the anterior humeral line intersecting the unossified radial head *(arrow)*, worrisome for fracture. **(C)** Ultrasound of normal elbow, performed with a linear array 10-MHz high-resolution probe, shows anterior humeral line *(long arrow)* derived from the echogenic anterior cortex of the distal humerus intersecting the hypoechoic unossified growth plate cartilage. *Small arrows* indicate the anterior cortex of the coronoid process. **(D)** Ultrasound of the abnormal elbow shows marked anterior displacement of the anterior humeral *(arrows)* line, which passes well anterior to the unossified growth plate cartilage, indicating fracture. **(E)** Sagittal T2-weighted fast field-echo image shows a supracondylar fracture with dorsal displacement of distal fragments. **(F)** Sagittal T2-weighted fast field-echo image of the same patient with improved contrast obtained by the application of an off-resonance magnetization transfer saturation pulse. Reproduced with permission from ref. 56.

Occasionally, potential extension of the fracture through unossified cartilage cannot be excluded on a conventional radiograph alone. Beltran et al. have reported four such cases, in whom extension was radiographically suspected but excluded in three by MR imaging (see Fig. 21).

Epiphyseal Fractures

Lateral Condylar Fractures

Lateral condylar fractures are the most common of the epiphyseal fractures of the elbow, occurring between 5 and 10 years of age. Similar to supracondylar fractures, they most frequently complicate a fall on the outstretched hand in both extension and varus. Fractures extending through unossified cartilage are inadequately evaluated by conventional radiographs, and in this setting, ultrasound, arthrography, or direct visualization of cartilage with MRI are of particular value.

With MR imaging, fractures may be classified according to the Rutherford system into type 1 fractures, in which the distal articular cartilage is intact and the fragment is hinged; type 2 fractures, where the fracture extends to involve the distal articular surface, although the fragment remains undisplaced; and type 3 fractures, in which the fragment is both displaced and rotated. The latter group, type 3 fractures, in which there is more than 2 mm of displacement, require surgical fixation (Fig. 23) (41).

Medial Epicondylar Fractures

Medial epicondylar avulsions represent 10% of pediatric elbow fractures, third in frequency after supracondylar and

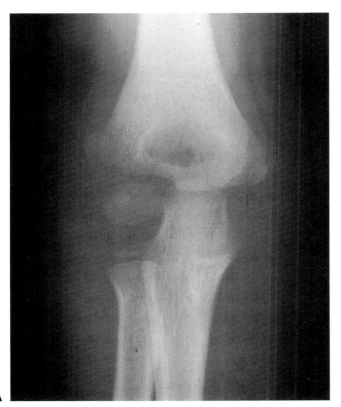
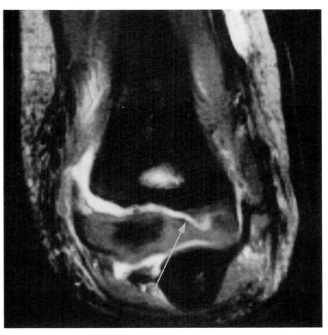

A   B

FIG. 21. (A) Anteroposterior radiograph shows a Salter 2 fracture of the lateral epicondyle of the distal humerus, with early callus formation. **(B)** Coronal T2-weighted fast field-echo image with off-resonance magnetization transfer saturation pulse shows an oblique fracture *(arrow)* extending from the metaphysis across the lateral physis and into the unossified cartilage of the trochlea (Rutherford type 1 fracture). Reproduced with permission from ref. 56.

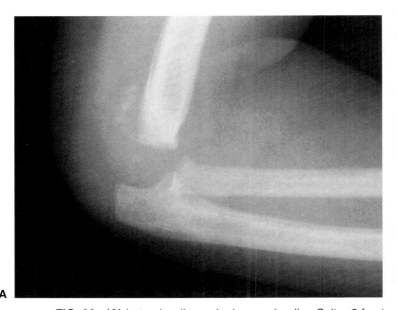
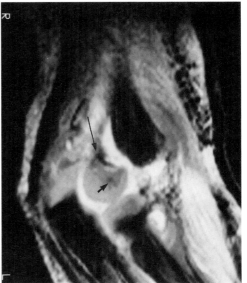

A   B

FIG. 22. (A) Lateral radiograph shows a healing Salter 2 fracture of the distal humerus with persistent deformity; anterior humeral line intersects the unossified radial head. **(B)** Sagittal fast field-echo image with off-resonance magnetization transfer confirms persistent deformity with metaphyseal extension *(long arrow)*. Note early mineralization within the capitellum *(small arrow)*. Reproduced with permission from ref. 56.

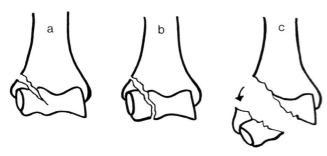

FIG. 23. Diagrammatic representation of the Rutherford classification of lateral condylar fractures: **a,** undisplaced with extension to unossified capitellar cartilage; **b,** undisplaced with extension through unossified capitellar cartilage; **c,** displaced fracture.

lateral condylar fractures. The injury is a complication of acute valgus stress either in isolation or accompanying elbow dislocation.

The avulsion usually involves the growth plate of the medial epicondyle and may extend through the physis of the distal humerus, the latter defining whether it is a Salter 3 or 4 injury. Most cases are minimally displaced and can be treated conservatively. Displaced fractures require surgical fixation (42).

Medial Condylar Fracture (Trochlea Fractures)

Medial condylar fractures are uncommon and often unrecognized as the fracture extends through the unmineralized trochlea cartilage and is not perceived on conventional radiographs. Management of these fractures is usually surgical (Fig. 24).

Capitellar Fractures

Capitellar fractures are uncommon and classified as types 1 to 3 (Fig. 25). Types 1 and 2, described by Kocher and Lorenz (43,44), are readily visualized as they involve the mineralized capitellar ossification center, displacement of which is readily identified on radiographs. Type 3 fractures, described by Wilson (45), are chondral and are characterized by subtle fractures of the cartilage of the articular surface identified only at MR imaging or arthrography. These fractures generally complicate impaction and shear transmitted through the radial head.

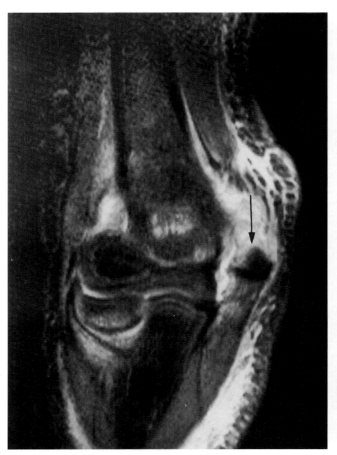

A

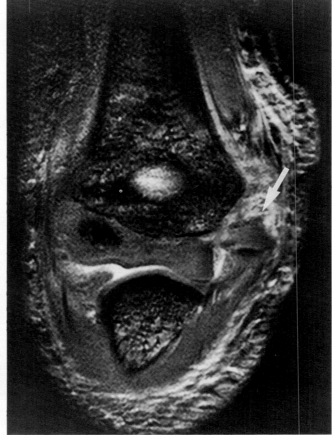

B

FIG. 24. (A) Coronal IR TSE and **(B)** coronal T2-weighted FFE image with off-resonance magnetization transfer saturation shows a displaced medial condylar fracture through unossified trochlear cartilage *(arrows).*

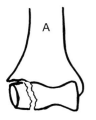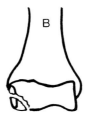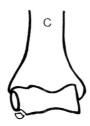

FIG. 25. Diagrammatic representations of capitellar fractures: **A** and **B** involve the mineralized portion of the capitellar cartilage and are radiographically apparent; **C** involves unmineralized cartilage.

Distal Humeral Epiphyseal Separation: Transcondylar Fractures

The physis between the distal humerus and the unossified epiphysis represents a plane of potential weakness. Up to 2 years of age, fracture may extend through this plane alone (Salter 1); after 2 years of age, the fracture may also involve the metaphysis (Salter 2).

Although the diagnosis is readily made on conventional radiographs both by analyzing the anterior humeral line and by comparison with the asymptomatic elbow, difficulty obtaining a true lateral film may create diagnostic difficulty. Although ultrasound is often employed when diagnosis is uncertain, MR provides a roadmap readily employed by referring surgeons (see Fig. 20).

Radial Head Fractures

Radial head fractures are uncommon in childhood and, when they occur, most commonly complicate posterior dislocation, where they are often associated with fracture of the coronoid. Displaced fractures may be complicated by avascular necrosis.

Elbow Fractures In Adulthood

In general, fractures of the elbow in adulthood, involving bone without soft tissue derangement, are readily identified on conventional radiographs. Magnetic resonance imaging in adulthood is undertaken to evaluate suspected occult or pathologic fractures or to evaluate complex condylar fractures or dislocations.

Occult Fractures

The most common occult fracture of adulthood is a posttraumatic undisplaced fracture of the radial head, complicating a fall on the outstretched hand. In most cases, the injury is heralded by the presence of a joint effusion, usually attributed to the presence of an undisplaced fracture, and no further imaging is undertaken. In athletes or patients with confusing symptoms, MR images reveal extensive marrow edema throughout the proximal radius, with or without an identifiable fracture line (Figs. 26 and 27). Occasionally imaging demonstrates associated injury of the coronoid pro-

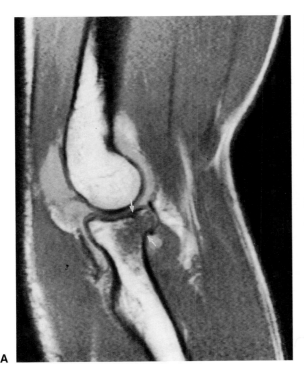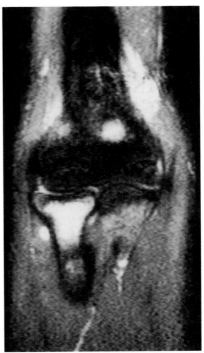

FIG. 26. (A) Sagittal TSE T1 and **(B)** coronal IR TSE image shows a type 1 radiographically occult fracture of the radial head *(arrows)* with extensive marrow edema secondary to impaction or compression forces.

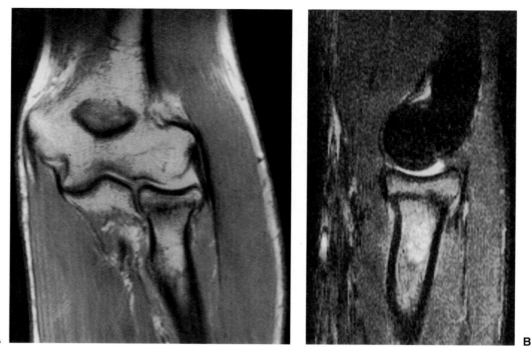

FIG. 27. (A) Coronal TSE T2 and **(B)** sagittal IR TSE show an undisplaced radiographically occult impaction fracture of the radial head. Note suppressed signal within the distal humerus with extensive marrow edema in the proximal radius.

cess, although this does not result in any change in patient management.

As a result of chronic triceps traction, stress fractures are occasionally identified through the olecranon process in professional athletes, pitchers, and occasionally weight lifters. Rarely, stress fractures or edema is identified at the insertion of the medial collateral ligament on the medial epicondyle in pitchers.

Chronic olecranon bursitis may be complicated by osteomyelitis or olecranon insufficiency fracture (hyperemic induced demineralization of bone), readily identified at MRI.

Fractures of the Coronoid

The coronoid process is responsible for anterior joint stability. Fracture, although uncommon, usually complicates elbow dislocation or subluxation.

Type 1 fractures are small shear fractures and do not lead to joint instability (Figs. 28 and 29). Type 2 fractures involve less than 50% of the coronoid but generally require fixation. Type 3 fractures involve more than 50% of the coronoid and, despite fixation, are often associated with long-term instability (46).

Condylar Fractures

Fractures of the condyles in adulthood usually complicate trauma in hyperextension with superimposed abduction or adduction forces.

Milch classifies medial condylar fractures according to whether or not the fracture involves the lateral trochlear ridge (Fig. 30) (47). Type 1 fractures spare the ridge, thereby maintaining ulnohumeral stability; type 2 fractures involve the ridge, resulting in ulnohumeral instability and subluxation, often associated with disruption of the lateral collateral ligament and capsular disruption.

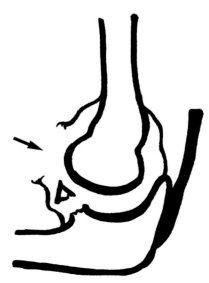

FIG. 28. Diagram showing type 1 fracture of the tip of the coronoid process *(arrow)* complicating an anterior dislocation with an associated disruption of the anterior capsule.

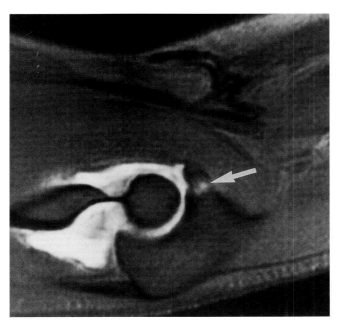

FIG. 29. Sagittal T1-weighted image with fat suppression, following direct intra-articular gadolinium arthrography, shows a type 1 undisplaced fracture of the tip of the coronoid *(arrow)*.

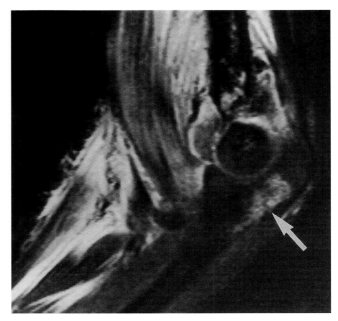

FIG. 31. Sagittal IR TSE image shows an undisplaced intra-articular fracture of the olecranon *(arrow)* accompanying a minimally displaced supracondylar fracture and joint effusion. Signal hypointensity within the joint effusion is secondary to hemorrhage with a short T1 value similar to that of fat.

In a similar way, fractures of the lateral condyle are divided into types 1 and 2 on the basis of preservation or disruption of the lateral trochlear ridge. Type 2 fractures, extending from the lateral condyle through the trochlear ridge, are usually associated with medial collateral ligament tear.

Olecranon Fractures

Fracture of the olecranon complicating direct trauma and impaction are divided into two types according to Colton:

type 1 fractures are nondisplaced; type 2 fractures are displaced. Nondisplaced fractures show no change in position on gentle flexion-extension and less than 2 mm articular step-off (Fig. 31) (48).

DISLOCATIONS

Posterior Elbow Dislocation

Elbow dislocation is the second most common major joint dislocation in adults and the most common dislocation in children less than 10 years, most frequently accompanying a fall on an outstretched hand in hyperextension.

Posterior forces imposed by a fall are opposed in adulthood by ossified coronoid, which is invariably fractured in such an injury. In childhood, constraining forces of the mineralized coronoid are absent up to the age of 10 years, allowing dislocation and often accompanying spontaneous reduction in childhood. Magnetic resonance imaging, following reduction, usually reveals hemorrhage and edema within the brachialis muscle, joint effusion, and often contusion or bone bruise in the capitellum. Imaging in adulthood invariably indicates hemorrhage and edema within the brachialis muscle, disruption of the anterior capsule, and fracture of the coronoid in the sagittal plane with disruption of the radial and lateral ulnar collateral ligament in the coronal plane (49).

Elbow instability is reported to occur as a spectrum. Stage 1 is characterized by posterolateral subluxation of the radius and ulna relative to the humerus secondary to disruption of

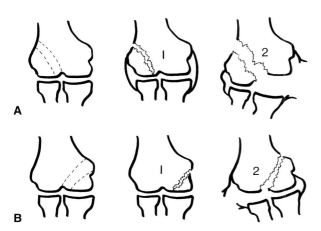

FIG. 30. Diagrammatic representation of the Milch classification of condylar fractures shows **(A)** lateral condylar fractures sparing **(1)** and involving the notch **(2)** (unstable) and shows **(B)** medial condylar fractures sparing **(1)** and involving the notch **(2)** (unstable).

the lateral ulnar collateral ligament. Stage 2 is characterized by further subluxation such that the trochlea is perched on the coronoid with disruption of the anterior and posterior joint capsules. Stage 3 is characterized by complete dislocation with disruption of joint capsule and both the radial and ulnar collateral ligaments (50).

Elbow Instability

Stage 1: Posterolateral Instability; Lateral Ulnar Collateral Ligament Rupture

Stage 2: Subluxation with Rupture of Capsule and Lateral Collateral Ligament

Stage 3: Dislocation with Additional Injury to Ulnar Collateral Ligament; Posterior UCL, Stage A; Anterior UCL, Stage B

Anterior Dislocation

Anterior dislocation rarely occurs complicating a blow to the dorsal aspect of the olecranon or forearm in the flexed position. Medial and lateral dislocations complicate condylar fractures secondary to applied abduction or adduction forces in extension.

Radioulnar Dislocation

Isolated dislocation of either ulna or radius may occur in patients with combined injury to collateral ligaments, specifically the annular ligaments of the radioulnar articulation. If the radial head is dislocated anteriorly, a Monteggia fracture should be suspected (associated fracture of the proximal ulna); if the radial head is dislocated posteriorly, disruption of the lateral ulnar collateral ligament should be suspected.

MAGNETIC RESONANCE IMAGING OF OSSEOUS INJURY FOLLOWING REPETITIVE TRAUMA

Panner's Disease Versus Little Leaguer's Elbow

Osteochondral injury to the radial head and capitellum commonly accompanies repetitive valgus strain with impaction in adolescent baseball pitchers or direct impaction in young female gymnasts (51).

Trauma-induced osteochondral injury may be isolated and self-limiting but, when recurrent, is often accompanied by disruption of a tenuous blood supply to the capitellum, resulting in osteochondritis. Persistent ischemia results in infarction and fragmentation of the capitellum with the development of articular cysts and loose bodies (Fig. 32). Up to 50% of affected individuals ultimately develop osteoarthritis.

Magnetic resonance imaging, best performed in the coronal plane, reveals local edema, manifest as loss of T1 signal and as signal hyperintensity on inversion recovery sequences, adjacent to the articular surface of the capitellum, often before the appearance of any radiographic abnormality (Fig. 33). Rest and splinting may result in resolution of the changes over 6 weeks. Following breakdown of the articular surface, which is often radiographically apparent, MR imaging is undertaken to determine relative stability of associated osteochondral fragments. In the absence of loose fragments, abrasion chondroplasty is occasionally undertaken to promote vascular reperfusion and a healing response at the site of injury. When fluid is identified encircling fragments on T2-weighted scans, surgery is undertaken to either fix or remove fragments and occasionally to reconstruct with bone graft (52).

A pseudodefect at the junction of the capitellum and the lateral epicondyle should not be mistaken for osteochondral defects, which are usually identified along the anterior margin of the capitellum.

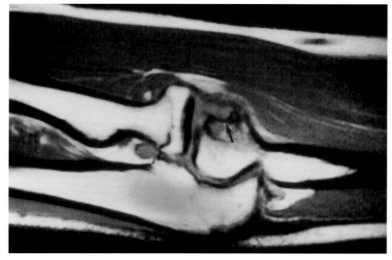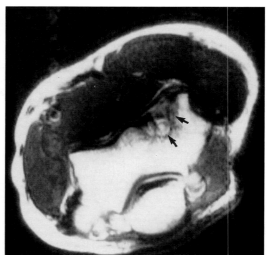

FIG. 32. (A) Sagittal and **(B)** axial TSE T1 show osteochondral lesion of the capitellum in a professional pitcher *(arrows)*.

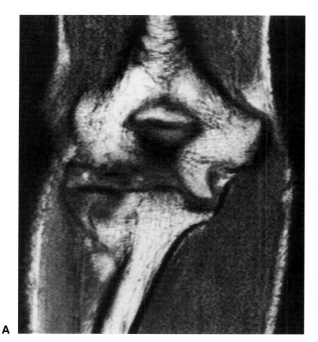
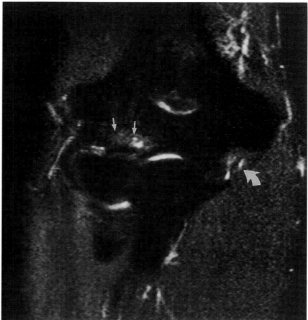

A   B

FIG. 33. (A) Coronal TSE T1 and **(B)** IR TSE images show osteochondral abnormality in the capitellum *(small arrows)* accompanied by subtle edema in the medial collateral ligament *(large arrow)* in a patient with little leaguer's elbow.

Panner's disease is an osteochondrosis that occurs before ossification of the capitellum, between 5 and 11 years. Unlike posttraumatic osteochondritis or little leaguer's elbow, cartilaginous fragmentation occurring in Panner's disease resolves during mineralization of the capitellum without sequelae (53,54).

REFERENCES

1. Rosenberg ZS, Beltran J, Cheung Y. Pseudodefect of the capitellum: Potential MR imaging pitfall. *Radiology* 1994;191:821–823.
2. Rosenberg ZS, Beltran J, Cheung Y, et al. MR imaging of the elbow: Normal variant and potential diagnostic pitfalls of the trochlear groove and cubital tunnel. *Am J Roentgenol* 1995;164:415–418.
3. Clarke RP. Symptomatic lateral synovial fringe (plica) of the elbow joint. *Arthroscopy* 1988;4:112–116.
4. Rosenberg ZS, Bencardino J, Beltran J. MR imaging of normal variants and interpretation pitfalls of the elbow. *Magn Reson Clin North Am* 1997;5:481–499.
5. Apfelberg DB, Larson SJ. Dynamic anatomy of the ulnar nerve at the elbow. *Plast Reconstr Surg* 1973;51:79–81.
6. Childress HM. Recurrent ulnar nerve dislocation at the elbow. *J Bone Joint Surg [Am]* 1956;38:978–984.
7. Hodgkinson PD, McLean NR. Ulnar nerve entrapment due to epitrochleo-anconeus muscle. *J Hand Surg [Br]* 1994;19:706–708.
8. Kessel L, Rang M. Supracondylar spur of the humerus. *J Bone Joint Surg [Br]* 1966;48:765–769.
9. Gudmundsen TE, Ostensen H. Accessory ossicles in the elbow. *Acta Orthop Scand* 1987;58:130–132.
10. Desharnais L, Kaplan PA, Dussault RG. MR imaging of ligamentous abnormalities of the elbow. *Magn Reson Clin North Am* 1997;5:515–528.
11. Fritz RC. MR imaging of the elbow. *Semin Roentgenol* 1995;30:241.
12. Herzog RJ. Magnetic resonance imaging of the elbow. *Magn Reson Q* 1993;9:188.
13. Schwartz ML, Al-Zahrani S, Morwessel RM, et al. Ulnar collateral

ligament injury in the throwing athlete. Evaluation with saline enhanced MR arthrography. *Radiology* 1995;197:297–299.
14. Timmerman LA, Andrews JR. Undersurface tears of the collateral ligament in baseball players: A newly recognized lesion. *Am J Sports Med* 1994;22:33–36.
15. Morrey BF, An KN. Functional anatomy of the ligaments of the elbow. *Clin Orthop* 1985;201:84–90.
16. Morrey BF, An KN. Articular and ligamentous contributions to the stability of the elbow joint. *Am J Sports Med* 1983;11:315–319.
17. Ho CP. Sports and occupational injuries of the elbow. MR imaging findings. *Am J Roentgenol* 1995;164:1465–1471.
18. Seiler JG, Parker LM, Chamberland PDC, Sherbourne GM, Carpenter WA. The distal biceps tendon: two potential mechanisms involved in its rupture. Arterial supply and mechanical impingement. *J Shoulder Elbow Surg* 1995;4:149.
19. Bourne MH, Morrey BF. Partial rupture of the distal biceps tendon. *Clin Orthop* 1991;271:143.
20. Falchook FS, Zlatskin MB, Erbacher GE, Moulton JS, Bisset GS, Murphy BJ. Rupture of the distal biceps tendon: evaluation with MR imaging. *Radiology* 1994;190:659.
21. Fitzgerald SW, Curry DR, Erickson SJ, Quinn SF, Friedman H. Distal biceps tendon injury: MR imaging diagnosis. *Radiology* 1994;191:203.
22. Bourne MH, Morrey BF. Partial rupture of the distal biceps tendon. *Clin Orthop* 1991;271:143.
23. Tarsney FF. Rupture and avulsion of the triceps. *Clin Orthop* 1972;83:177.
24. Sonin AH, Fitzgerald SW. MR imaging of sports injuries in the adult elbow. A tailored approach. *Am J Roentgenol* 1996;167:325.
25. Ho CP. MR imaging of tendon injuries in the elbow. *Magn Reson Clin North Am* 1997;5:529–543.
26. Tiger E, Mayer DP, Glazer R. Complete avulsion of the triceps tendon: MRI diagnosis. *Comput Med Imag Graph* 1993;17:51.
27. Patten HG. Overuse syndromes and injuries involving the elbow: MR imaging findings. *Am J Roentgenol* 1995;164:1205.
28. Potter HG, Hannafin JA, Morwessel RM, et al. Lateral epicondylitis: correlation of MR imaging surgical and histopathologic findings. *Radiology* 1995;196:43.
29. Kaplan PA, Dussault RG. MR imaging of the elbow. In: Weissman BN, ed. *Advanced Imaging of Joints: Theory and Practice.* Chicago: Radiologic Society of North America, 1993;97–105.

30. Kuroda S, Sakamaki K. Ulnar collateral ligament tears of the elbow joint. *Clin Orthop* 1986;208:266–271.
31. Rosenberg ZS, Beltran J, Cheung YY, et al. The elbow: MR features of nerve disorders. *Radiology* 1993;188:235.
32. Jaramillo D, Waters PM. MR imaging of the normal developmental anatomy of the elbow. *Magn Reson Clin North Am* 1997;5:501–513.
33. McCarthy S, Ogden J. Radiology of postnatal skeletal development: Distal humerus. *Skeletal Radiol* 1982;7:239–249.
34. McCarthy S, Ogden J. Radiology of postnatal skeletal development. Elbow joint, proximal radius and ulna. *Skeletal Radiol* 1982;9:17–26.
35. Ogden J. The uniqueness of growing bones. In: Rockwood CA Jr, Wilkins K, King R, eds. *Fracture in Children, ed. 3.* Philadelphia: JB Lippincott, 1991;50–51.
36. Salter RB, Harris WR. Injuries involving the epiphyseal plate. *J Bone Joint Surg [Am]* 1963;45:587–622.
37. Rogers LF, Poznanski AK. Imaging of epiphyseal injuries. *Radiology* 1994;191:297–308.
38. Beltran J, Rosenberg ZS, Kawelblum M, et al. Pediatric elbow fractures: MRI evaluation. *Skeletal Radiol* 1994;23:277–281.
39. O'Brien T, Millis MB, Griffin PP. The early identification and classification of growth plate disturbances of the proximal end of the femur. *J Bone Joint Surg [Am]* 1986;68:237–253.
40. Ogden JA. The evaluation and treatment of partial physeal arrest. *J Bone Joint Surg [Am]* 1987;69:1297–1302.
41. Murray K, Nixon GW. Epiphyseal growth plate: evaluation with modified coronal CT. *Radiology* 1988;166:263–265.
42. Foster DE, Sullivan JA, Gross RH. Lateral humeral condyle fractures in children. *J Pediatr Orthop* 1985;62:1159–1163.
43. Resnick CS. Diagnostic imaging of pediatric skeletal trauma. *Radiol Clin North Am* 1989;27:1013–1022.
44. Kocher T. *Beitrage zur Kenntniss einiger Tisch wichtiger Frachturformen.* Basel: Sallman, 1896;585–591.
45. Lorenz H. Zur kenntniss der fractura humeri (eminentiae capitatae). *Dtsch Z Chir* 1905;78:531–545.
46. Wilson PD. Fractures and dislocations in the region of the elbow. *Gynecol Obstet* 1933;56:335–359.
47. Regan W, Morrey BF. Fractures of the coronoid process of the ulna. *J Bone Joint Surg [Am]* 1989;71:1348–1354.
48. Knight RA. Fractures of the humeral condyles in adults. *South Med J* 1955;70:1165–1173.
49. Colton CL. Fractures of the olecranon in adults: classification and management. *Injury* 1973;5:121–129.
50. O'Driscoll SW, Bell DF, Morrey BF. Posterolateral rotatory instability of the elbow. *J Bone Joint Surg [Am]* 1991;73:440–446.
51. O'Driscoll SW, Morrey BF, Korinek S, et al. Elbow subluxation and dislocation: a spectrum of instability. *Clin Orthop* 1992;280:186–197.
52. Singer KM, Roy SP. Osteochondrosis of the humeral capitellum. *Am J Sports Med* 1984;12:351–360.
53. Kramer J, Stiglbauer R, Engel A, et al. MR contrast arthrography (MRA) in osteochondrosis dessicans. *J Comput Assist Tomogr* 1992;16:254–260.
54. Mitsunaga MM, Adashian DA, Bianco AJJ. Osteochondritis dessicans of the capitellum. *J Trauma* 1982;22:53–55.
55. Brogden BG, Crow NE. Little leaguer's elbow. *Am J Roentgenol* 1960;83:671–675.
56. Carey J, Spence L, Blickman H, Eustace S. MR imaging of pediatric growth plate injury: correlation with plain film radiographs and clinical outcome. *Skeletal Radiol* 1998;27:250–255.

CHAPTER 12

The Wrist and Hand

Stephen J. Eustace

Although traditional imaging, integrating radiographs, tomography, and arthrography, allows detailed evaluation of traumatic wrist injuries, the ability to directly visualize both bones and soft tissues afforded by MRI as a single investigation makes it an attractive alternative in patient evaluation. Magnetic resonance imaging of the wrist may be successfully performed on both whole-body and dedicated low-field extremity systems.

PATIENT POSITIONING AND IMAGING PROTOCOLS

Positioning

Magnetic resonance imaging of the wrist and hand is usually performed with the hand placed flat at the patient's side.

S. J. Eustace: Department of Radiology, Section of Musculoskeletal Radiology, Boston University School of Medicine and Boston Medical Center, Boston, Massachusetts 02118.

Following trauma and bracing, positioning may be more complex, particularly when fixation casts extend across both the wrist and elbow joint. When possible, if MR imaging is anticipated, referring orthopedists are encouraged either to delay casting or to use a half cast to the midforearm until after successful imaging has been undertaken. Because of the negative impact of wet plaster on image signal, fixation with dry materials is encouraged when possible.

Following cast fixation, patient positioning is variable, and although the hand-by-the-side position is favored, the hand above the head in both prone and supine positions is often employed (Fig. 1). In patients with fixed flexion at the elbow because of a plaster cast, imaging may be successfully performed only with the hand across the abdomen. In such a position, respiratory gating or triggering must be employed to limit motion, although even when this is employed, acquired images are still often degraded.

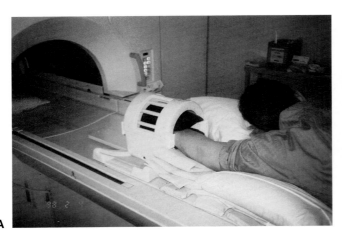
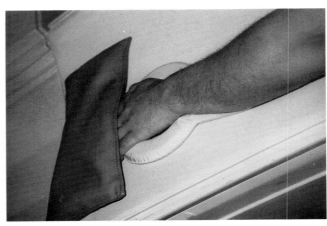

FIG. 1. (A) Magnetic resonance imaging of the wrist in the prone position using a quadrature coil, often favored following cast fixation. **(B)** Magnetic resonance imaging of the wrist using an oval surface coil with the palm flat and motion suppressed by sandbagging.

Receiver Coil

In order to optimize reception of generated signal, imaging requires either a molded or tightly apposed surface coil or the use of a dedicated quadrature coil. Quadrature coils increase image signal to noise by 1.4 times by acquiring signal simultaneously in two perpendicular planes. To improve signal acquisition, dedicated phased-array wrist coils are used, which have the potential to dramatically improve quality of acquired images; they are now widely used, particularly for imaging with low-field permanent extremity magnets.

Volumetric coils are used to image patients following cast fixation, as loss of apposition secondary to the presence of cast dramatically decreases received signal using flexible surface coils (see Fig. 1).

Imaging Plane

Coronal images are prescribed off both axial and sagittal localizers. In the axial plane, images are parallel to a line drawn between both styloid processes; in the sagittal plane, images are parallel to the long axis of the radius.

Axial images are prescribed off coronal and sagittal localizers extending through the distal radius to the bases of the metacarpals; in the sagittal plane, images are prescribed perpendicular to the radiolunatocapitate line.

Sagittal images are prescribed off coronal and axial localizers parallel to the lunatocapitate line.

Field of View

Similar to imaging the knee, a preliminary image is often acquired with extended coverage, a field of view of 15 to 20 cm, before dedicated images with an 8- to 10-cm field of view. In such a way, an overview of the extent of trauma is obtained before high-resolution imaging of internal joint structures is done.

Slice Thickness

Detailed evaluation of intrinsic and extrinsic wrist ligaments necessitates imaging with a slice thickness not greater than 3 mm. With magnets having gradient strengths up to 26 mT/m, 1-mm slices may be routinely acquired. Acquisition of 1-mm slices using conventional systems, employing 10- to 13-mT/m gradients, is usually successfully achieved only by three-dimensional gradient-echo imaging.

Motion Suppression

High-resolution images can be acquired only by completely immobilizing the wrist using sandbags. Images acquired without sandbagging techniques are often degraded despite patient compliance and every attempt to maintain a fixed position.

Pulsation artifact from the radial and ulnar arteries may distort acquired images. Orientation of the phase-encode gradients parallel to the long axis of the digits orients artifact away from the joint space on coronal images (1).

Imaging Protocol

Following acute orthopedic trauma, a turbo inversion recovery sequence is usually initially employed to determine the extent of the trauma, followed by turbo spin-echo T1-weighted sequences in coronal, sagittal, and axial planes. If a turboSTIR image shows no edema or bruising, no further additional imaging (such as occurs in patients referred with suspected scaphoid fractures) is undertaken.

Turbo inversion recovery sequences are acquired using an inversion time of 160 msec, a repetition time of 2,000 msec, an echo time of 20 msec, an echo train of six, and a linear echo to view mapping profile. Such images are acquired in 2 min with two excitations. Multiple excitations are unnecessary with inversion recovery sequences because diagnosis is made in most cases on the basis of contrast

TABLE 1. *Protocol to image the wrist following trauma*

Sequence	Image plane	FOV	TR	TE	ETL	Mapping scheme
Occult fracture detection						
TSE T1	Cor Direct	14	500	15	4	Low-high
IR TSE	Cor Direct	14	2,000	20	6	Linear
Intrinsic or extrinsic ligament or TFCC disruption						
TSE T1 in coronal and sagittal planes						
FFE T2	Cor direct	14	500	15	30°	Flip angle
TSE T2	Axial	14	2,000	20, 80	6	Linear

afforded by fat-suppressed images. Turbo spin-echo T1 imaging is achieved using a repetition time of 500 msec, an echo time of 15 msec, a short echo train of four, and a low-high echo to view mapping profile. Use of a short echo train facilitates the use of a short repetition time, enhancing T1 weighting and further decreasing acquisition time. With such parameters, images are acquired in 1 min 5 sec.

When intrinsic or extrinsic ligament disruptions are specifically sought, a T2-weighted fast field-echo sequence with off-resonance magnetization transfer in both coronal and sagittal planes is usually employed. T2 weighting is achieved with a low flip angle of 30°, a long repetition time of 500 msec, and an echo time of 15 msec. With such a sequence, fluid is bright, articular cartilage is isointense to fluid as a result of the off-resonance pulse, and intercarpal ligaments and triangular fibrocartilage are predominantly hypointense. Other authors routinely favor the use of fat-saturated dual-echo turbo T2-weighted images to evaluate internal joint structures. Turbo spin-echo T2-weighted imaging is achieved using a repetition time of 3,000 msec, echo times of 20 and 80 msec, an echo train of six, and linear echo to view mapping. Evaluation of intrinsic ligament disruption may be enhanced by imaging in radial deviation or with a clenched fist (scapholunate ligament) or in ulnar deviation (lunatotriquetral ligament).

When either fracture of the hook of hamate or median nerve compression is suspected, a dual-echo turbo T2-weighted sequence is employed in the axial plane in addition to sequences previously described.

In most patients, because of the impact on acquisition time, a matrix with 256 phase-encode steps is employed, and because the perceived difference in image signal to noise between two and three excitations is negligible ($\sqrt{2}$ versus $\sqrt{3}$), to obtain rapid imaging, only two excitations are employed.

Similar to the knee and shoulder, both GraSE and multishot EPI images with fat saturation may be used to image internal joint structures. In the absence of fat suppression, chemical shift artifact results in dramatic image distortion, limiting utility. It is likely that single-shot EPI with fat suppression allowing image acquisition in less than 15 sec will form the basis for successful trauma imaging of the wrist in the years ahead.

Magnetic resonance arthrography with single contrast injection to the radiocarpal joint space improves visibility of soft tissue structures including the scapholunate and lunatotriquetral ligaments and the triangular fibrocartilage. In addition to allowing improved visualization of soft tissues, distribution of contrast improves detection of subtle tears. When employed, 4 to 5 cc of a gadolinium, 1% lidocaine, and renografin solution is injected to the radiocarpal joint space alone (0.1 ml of gadolinium DTPA to 5 ml of 1% lidocaine and 15 cc of renografin 60) (Table 1) (2).

WRIST BIOMECHANICS: STABLE VERSUS UNSTABLE EQUILIBRIUM

The biomechanics of the wrist are complex and involve the integrated motion of two intercalated segments (carpal bones linked by intercarpal ligaments), the proximal and distal rows of carpal bones, which articulate with the bases of the metacarpals and the distal radius at the radiocarpal articulation, facilitating wrist flexion and extension, ulnar and radial deviation, and minimal pronation and supination (although this is most marked at the distal radiocarpal articulation).

Within the proximal carpal row, there is a delicate balance between the opposing forces of the volarly angulated scaphoid and the mildly dorsally angulated lunate, transmitted through the scapholunate ligament. Such a balance allows smooth integrated movement of the proximal intercalated segment. In such a way, in the sagittal plane, the scapholunate angle, or angle between the volarly angulated scaphoid and mildly dorsally angulated lunate, is 30° to 60°, whereas the angle between the lunate and capitate is 0° to 30°. The angle of the distal radial articular surface is 10° volar angulation. Although it slightly decreases the range of dorsiflexion at the radiocarpal articulation, it is an evolutionary attempt to stabilize the radiocarpal articulation and limit the tendency to dislocate dorsally at the radiocarpal articulation following a fall and dorsally oriented impaction forces (3–8) (Fig. 2).

Following a fall on an outstretched hand, combined dorsal shear and axial loading forces are applied to the wrist, the induced deformity depending on whether the forces are applied in radial or ulnar deviation. Depending on the balance between axial load and dorsal shear, applied forces may result in a range of both displaced and undisplaced carpal bone fractures including perilunate dislocation (in which all bones distal to the midcarpal articulation sublux dorsally), lunate dislocation (in which axial loading, against the volarly angu-

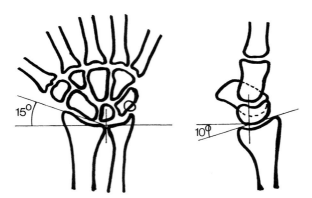

FIG. 2. Diagrammatic representation of normal radial inclination to 15° **(A)** and of normal volar tilt to 10° **(B)**, evolutionary variations conferring stability and resistance to displacement following a fall on the outstretched hand.

lated distal radial articular surface, forces the lunate to sublux volarly), rupture of intrinsic ligaments and stabilizing fibrocartilage within the wrist, and both displaced and undisplaced fractures in the distal radius (9,10).

Fracture, dislocation, or disruption of stabilizing ligaments at any site may neutralize applied forces. In such a way, impaction fracture of the distal radius may neutralize axial loading forces and result in an isolated injury. More often, such applied forces are dissipated by both soft tissue and osseous structures, resulting in extremely complex injury.

When forces are applied to the wrist, induced deformity may be constrained by both osseous and soft tissue ligamentous plasticity so that, following removal of forces, original alignment is restored; this is termed stable equilibrium. If either osseous or soft tissue structures fracture or rupture, original alignment is not restored following removal of applied forces, but forces induced by the deformity displace osseous structures even further from equilibrium, producing an unstable equilibrium (11).

Although evaluation with conventional radiographs has emphasized the impact of osseous injury on wrist function, it is now clear, using MRI, that injury to the wrist is usually more complex and frequently relates to the combined impact of deformity and derangement of both bones and soft tissues accurately evaluated at MRI.

Extrinsic Ligaments of the Wrist

The extrinsic ligaments of the wrist bind the distal radius to the carpal bones and the carpal bones to the bases of the metacarpals (Fig. 3).

Three extrinsic volar ligaments are crucial to wrist stability. Being extrasynovial, they most likely represent thickenings of the capsule itself. The radioscaphocapitate ligament courses obliquely from the radial styloid through the scaphoid to the capitate. The long radiolunate is the largest ligament of the wrist and courses obliquely from the radial sty-

loid through the lunate to the triquetral bone. Both ligaments are routinely identified on coronal images through the volar aspect of the wrist. The short radiolunate ligament runs from the lunate facet of the radius to the volar aspect of the lunate.

The most important extrinsic dorsal ligament is the dorsal radiocarpal ligament, which has three parts—radioscaphoid, radiolunate, and radiotriquetral—connecting the dorsal aspect of the distal radius to the dorsal aspect of the proximal row of carpal bones. Although visualized on coronal images, the dorsal radiocarpal ligament is routinely identified in the sagittal plane (12–14).

Classification of Wrist Injuries

Injury to intrinsic ligaments (scapholunate and lunatotriquetral ligaments) disrupts coordinated movement of carpal bones within intercalated segments and is considered to be dissociative (carpal instability dissociative, CID). In contrast, injury leading to disruption of extrinsic ligaments or bones also results in instability, although movement of intercalated segments remains coordinated (carpal instability nondissociative, CIND) (15–18).

Wrist injuries can be classified as perilunar (perilunate and lunate dislocations), midcarpal, or proximal carpal instabilities (11).

Perilunate injuries can be subdivided into greater and lesser arc injuries. Lesser arc injuries involve disruptions of the scapholunate and lunatotriquetral ligaments and complete perilunate instabilities. Greater arc injuries are divided into scaphoid fractures, scaphoid fracture with perilunate dislocation, and transscaphoid transtriquetral perilunate dislocation.

Midcarpal instability is classified as intrinsic or extrinsic in origin. Intrinsic instabilities include palmar midcarpal instability secondary to laxity of the volar arcuate ligament and dorsal midcarpal instability secondary to malunion of a distal radial fracture with persistent dorsal angulation. Volar arcuate ligament laxity leads to an audible clunk in the clenched-fist position as the capitate subluxes over the volarly angulated lunate to the space of Poirier.

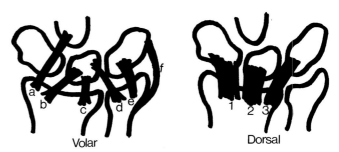

FIG. 3. Diagram showing volar and dorsal extrinsic radiocarpal ligaments. Volar ligaments: a, radioscaphocapitate; b, radioscapholunate; c, radiolunate; d, ulnolunate; e, ulnotriquetral; f, ulnar collateral ligament. Dorsal ligaments: 1, radioscaphoid; 2, radiolunate; 3, radiotriquetral.

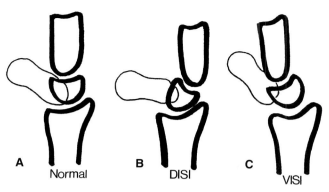

FIG. 4. (A) Diagram showing normal balance between volar tendancy of the scaphoid and dorsal tendency of the lunate balanced by the scapholunate ligament. **(B)** Diagram showing dorsal tilt of the lunate and volar tilt of the scaphoid following scapholunate ligament disruption. **(C)** Diagram showing volar tilt of lunate with the scaphoid following disruption of the lunatotriquetral ligament.

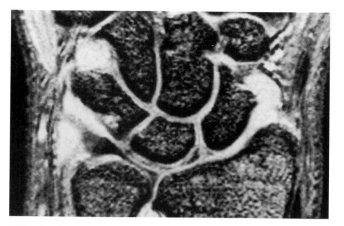

FIG. 5. Coronal fast field-echo image with off-resonance magnetization transfer saturation shows a tear through the scapholunate ligament, which is noted to have a delta configuration.

Proximal carpal instabilities include ulnar translocation of the carpus in which more than 50% of the lunate is medial to the lunate, dorsal instability (secondary to a dorsal rim fracture of the radius, nondissociative, CIND) or secondary to scapholunate ligament disruption (dissociative, CID), and volar instability secondary to a volar rim fracture (volar Barton, nondissociative) or lunatotriquetral ligament disruption (dissociative) (Fig. 4).

PRIMARY SOFT TISSUE INJURY FOLLOWING WRIST TRAUMA

Scapholunate Ligament Disruption

In health, the scapholunate ligament balances opposing forces of the volarly angulated scaphoid and the dorsally angulated lunate. At MRI, the ligament is delta shaped in 75% of cases and linear in approximately 25% and is hypointense in approximately 75% versus heterogeneous with areas of isointensity in 25% of cases. The ligament is usually less than 3 mm in maximal transverse diameter in the coronal plane and is interposed between the scaphoid and lunate in the axial plane as thick dorsal (responsible for stability) and volar fibers plus an interposed membranous portion (19).

Following a fall on the outstretched hand, impaction forces through the long axis of the capitate are transmitted to the scapholunate interspace and the scapholunate ligament. Under the action of such forces, the scapholunate ligament may acutely rupture, most commonly from the proximal pole of the scaphoid, or may stretch before rupture, in either case resulting in widening of the scapholunate interspace (Figs. 5–7) (20). In the absence of restraint, the scaphoid tilts volarly, the lunate tilts dorsally. Induced changes in biomechanics following ligament rupture result in previously described radiographic signs: widening of the scapholunate interspace greater than 4 mm, the Terry Thomas sign, volar angulation, and flattening of the scaphoid, producing the ring

sign (the distal pole of scaphoid projected over the waist and proximal pole) and dorsal tilt of the lunate relative to both the capitate (lunatocapitate angle greater than 30°) and scaphoid (scapholunate angle greater than 60°), producing a dorsal intercalated segmental instability pattern (DISI) (Fig. 8) (21–24).

At MR imaging following injury, the delta configuration (see Fig. 8) of an intact ligament is lost as the ligament elongates before rupture, and frequently intrasubstance edema results in apparent swelling or thickening of the ligament. The lunate attachment has more Sharpey fibers, and hence, when it occurs, tear is usually from the base of the scaphoid. Following rupture, hyperintense fluid is noted to

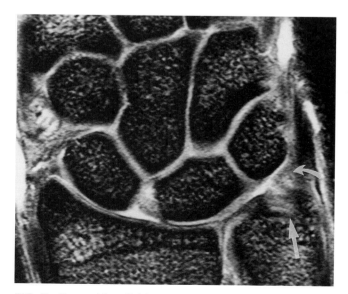

FIG. 6. Coronal fast field-echo image shows intrasubstance rupture of the scapholunate ligament. Note normal loss of signal in the triangular fibrocartilage as fibers become more loosely bound adjacent to the ulnar insertion *(straight arrow). Curved arrow* indicates the meniscal homolog.

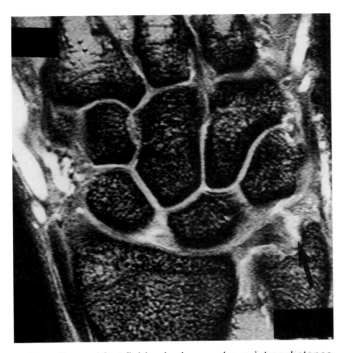

FIG. 7. Coronal fast field-echo image shows intrasubstance rupture of the scapholunate ligament *(arrow)*. Note intact lunatotriquetral ligament, which has a linear configuration. There is a degenerative tear of the triangular fibrocartilage *(arrow)* at the ulnar insertion.

pass freely between radiocarpal and midcarpal joint spaces. Induced instability promotes further deformity before establishing the DISI pattern, which is considered to be unstable equilibrium (23,24).

Although MR imaging may accurately detect scapholunate ligament disruption, the clinical significance of observed abnormalities must always be established before intervention, as central perforations through the membranous portion of the ligament may not result in biomechanical changes, and fenestration establishing contact between radiocarpal and midcarpal joint spaces may occur in health. Because, in many circumstances, fenestrations are symmetric, some advocate imaging both symptomatic and asymptomatic wrists simultaneously using an extended surface coil (25).

Acute scapholunate ligament disruption identified within 4 weeks of initial injury is treated operatively with considerable success. In addition to primary repair, dorsal capsulodesis (Blatt's procedure) (26,27) is often employed to reestablish stability. Chronic scapholunate ligament disruption, in contrast, is usually treated conservatively with customized wrist support braces (Fig. 9). When surgery is undertaken in the minority with persistent symptoms, delayed ligament repair, scaphotrapeziotrapezoid fusion (28), or implant arthroplasty, the results are inconsistent, and although pain is often reduced, it is at the expense of wrist mobility.

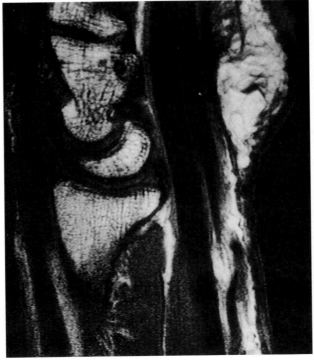

A

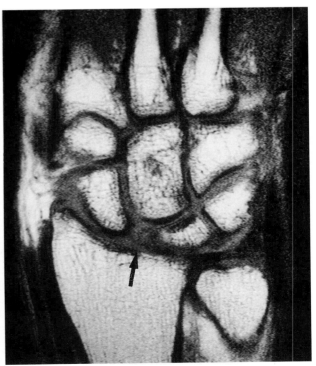

B

FIG. 8. Sagittal **(A)** and coronal TSE T1-weighted **(B)** images show marked dorsal tilt of the lunate (normal lunatocapitate angle is between 0° and 30° of dorsal tilt) secondary to chronic scapholunate ligament disruption *(arrow)*.

Lunatotriquetral Ligament Disruption

The lunatotriquetral ligament, similar to the scapholunate, is comprised of both volar and dorsal components that attach directly to bone rather than to hyaline cartilage overlying carpal bones. The ligament establishes continuity between radial and ulnar structures of the proximal carpal row of bones or intercalated segment (29,30).

Following a fall in ulnar deviation, impaction forces are transmitted through the ulnar side of the wrist with acute shear manifest as rupture of the lunatotriquetral ligament, disruption of components of the triangular fibrocartilage complex, subluxation of the distal radioulnar joint, or fracture (Fig. 10).

Shearing forces lead to acute tear of the lunatotriquetral ligament, which, in contrast to the scapholunate ligament, does not stretch and widen the interspace before actual rup-

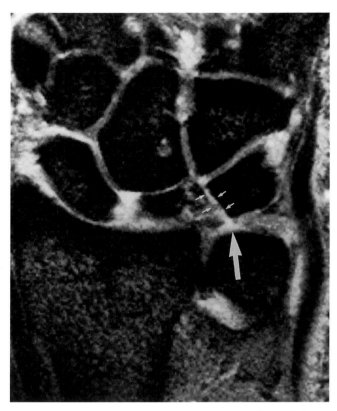

FIG. 10. Coronal IR TSE image shows the effect of shear forces through the ulnar side of the joint with tear of the lunatotriquetral ligament *(small arrows)* and of the triangular fibrocartilage from the radial insertion *(large arrow)*.

ture. Identification of acute rupture requires high-resolution imaging, and even with meticulous attention to detail, the sensitivity of MR imaging in this setting is as low as 50% (29,30).

In chronicity, in an attempt to establish stable equilibrium, the lunate tilts volarly under the influence of the unopposed volar tendency of the scaphoid, establishing a volar intercalated segmental instability pattern. The scapholunate angle decreases to an angle often less than 30° while the lunatocapitate angle increases to as much as 30° (31–33).

Although the results of surgical repair are inconsistent, when undertaken, direct suture repair of the ligament and lunatotriquetral fusion are undertaken (lunatotriquetral coalition is the most common congenital fusion anomaly in the wrist and is uniformly asymptomatic).

Triangular Fibrocartilage Complex

The triangular fibrocartilage complex (TFCC) is a complex anatomic structure composed predominantly of a triangular wedge-shaped fibrocartilaginous disk bridging the distal radioulnar joint supported anteriorly and posteriorly by radioulnar ligaments, distally by attachments to the lunate through the volar ulnocarpal ligaments (the ulnolunate and ulnotriquetral ligaments), and laterally by the ulnar collateral

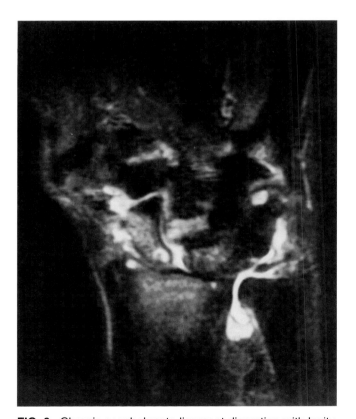

FIG. 9. Chronic scapholunate ligament disruption with laxity and impaction of scaphoid against the radial facet of the distal radius and secondary bone bruising. There is a tear of the triangular turbocartilage with communication to the distal radio-ulna joint.

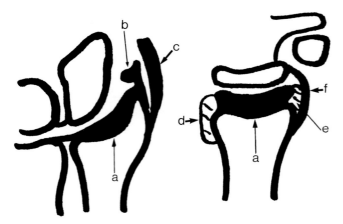

FIG. 11. Diagrammatic representation of the triangular fibrocartilage complex: a, the body of the fibrocartilage; b, the meniscal homolog; c, the ulnar collateral ligament; d, the dorsal radioulnar ligament; e, the volar radioulnar ligament; f, the ulnotriquetral ligament.

ligament and the extensor carpi ulnaris (Figs. 11 and 12). The complex is completed by an additional fold in the medial capsule interposed between the ulnar styloid and the triquetrum termed the meniscal homolog. The meniscal homolog is interposed between the prestyloid recess and the triquetropisiform recess.

The triangular fibrocartilage is a biconcave disk separating the radiocarpal from the distal radioulnar joint spaces. It has attachments to both the ulnar styloid and the lunate fossa of the radius (34).

En bloc, the triangular fibrocartilage complex functions to buttress forces transmitted to the distal ulnar and distal radioulnar articulations secondary to impaction during ulnar deviation. Thus, injury is manifest as atypical pain and tenderness localized to the region of the ulnar styloid, often worse in ulnar deviation. Such discomfort often limits pronation and supination at the distal radioulnar articulations. In old age, as a result of cartilage degeneration, asymptomatic tears of the triangular fibrocartilage are common.

At MR imaging, the triangular fibrocartilage is the only structure of the TFC complex consistently identified, although three-dimensional gradient-echo sequences now allow visualization of both the volar and dorsal radioulnar ligaments (35–39).

Magnetic resonance imaging has a reported sensitivity of 72% to 100% in the detection of tears, with associated specificities of 89% to 100% (35–39).

The TFC tears may be either traumatic (Palmer class I), subdivided according to site of tear, or degenerative (Palmer class II), subdivided according to extent of degeneration (40).

Traumatic tears most commonly occur within 1 to 2 mm of the radial origin of the fibrocartilage where vascular supply is poor. In contrast, reflecting microvascular supply, tears at the ulnar attachment, where vascular supply is rich, have a greater propensity to heal. Fortuitously, MR imaging

is accurate in detection of radial tears, which heal poorly, but is relatively inaccurate in the detection of ulnar-sided tears, which frequently heal without intervention.

At MR imaging, TFC tears are manifest by linear signal abnormality on T1-, proton-density-, and T2-weighted sequences. Identification of hyperintense fluid communicating between radiocarpal and distal radioulnar joint spaces is considered to be definitive evidence of tear (see Figs. 10, 13, and 14).

Degenerative tears of the triangular fibrocartilage occur most commonly at the ulnar attachment and most likely reflect a combination of both chronic impaction and age-related ischemia. Consequently, degenerative tears are most frequently identified in patients with positive ulnar variance or positive ulnar impaction syndrome and are often accompanied by disruption of the lunatotriquetral ligament. Reflecting alteration in vascular supply to the periphery of the triangular cartilage, age-related mucoid degeneration occurs most frequently in the central horizontal portion of the disk and adjacent to the ulnar attachment. In contrast to tear, mucoid degeneration is manifest as signal hyperintensity on T1- and proton-density-weighted images and becomes iso-

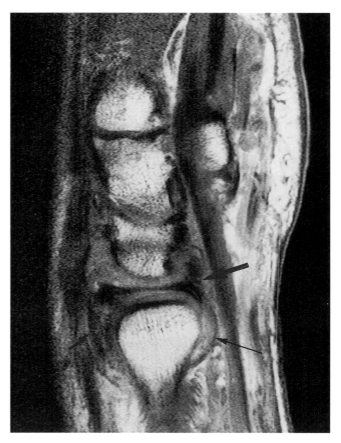

FIG. 12. Sagittal TSE T1-weighted image shows the normal alignment of the ulna, lunate, and capitate bones. *Large arrow* indicates the triangular fibrocartilage; the *short arrow* indicates the dorsal radioulnar ligament; the *thin arrow* indicates the volar radioulnar ligament.

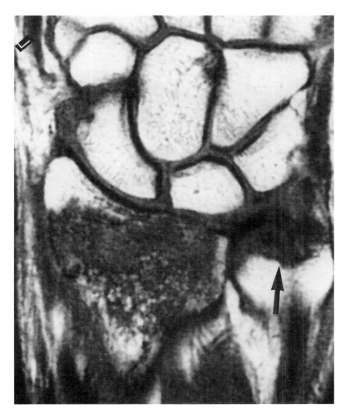

FIG. 13. Coronal TSE T1-weighted image shows an undisplaced impaction fracture of the distal radius with a complex stellate tear of the triangular fibrocartilage *(arrow)*.

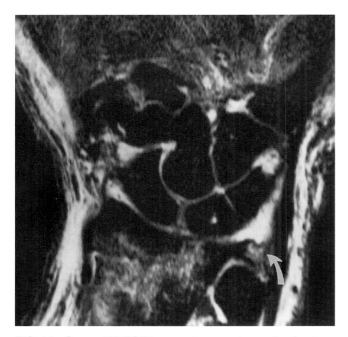

FIG. 14. Coronal IR TSE image shows an impaction fracture of the distal radius with acute tear of triangular fibrocartilage from the ulnar insertion *(curved arrow)*.

intense on T2-weighted images in contrast to true tears. Triangular fibrocartilage perforations were documented in 50% of patients over 60 years in one study (41,42).

Palmer Class I: Traumatic TFC Tears

Type A: Tear of the Disk
Type B: Tear at Ulnar Insertion
Type C: Tears at lunate attachments (ulnolunate or ulnotriquetral ligaments)
Type D: Tear at the Radius Insertion

Palmer Class II: Degenerative TFC Tears

Type A: TFC Wear
Type B: TFC Wear with Ulnar or Lunate Chondromalacia
Type C: TFC Wear with Perforations and Ulnar or Lunate Chondromalacia
Type D: Type C and Disruption of Lunatotriquetral Ligament
Type E: Additional Ulnocarpal Arthritis

In acute symptomatic tears in young patients, surgical repair is often undertaken with success. In this setting, surfaces are either debrided or reconstructed. In patients with positive ulnar variance, ulnar shortening or osteotomy is often undertaken (43,44).

TENDON INJURY AT THE WRIST

Tendon injury of either the flexor or extensor tendons of the wrist may be secondary to an underlying inflammatory process (arthritis, infection), occupational or recreational overuse, or secondary to acute trauma accompanying fracture of the distal radius (Figs. 15 and 16).

Chronic overuse may lead to mucoid degeneration, occasionally cartilage metaplasia, and ultimately tear and rupture.

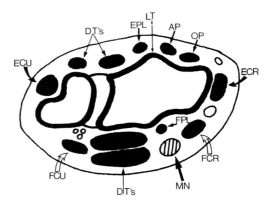

FIG. 15. Diagrammatic representation of tendons of the wrist in the axial plane. Extensors: ECU, extensor carpi ulnaris; DTs, extensor digitorum and digiti minimi tendons; EPL, extensor pollicis longus; LT, Lister's tubercle; AP, abductor pollicis; OP, opponens pollicis; ECR, extensor carpi radialis. Flexors: FCR, flexor carpi radialis; FPL, flexor pollicis longus; MN, median nerve; DTs, digitorum tendons; FCU, flexor carpi ulnaris.

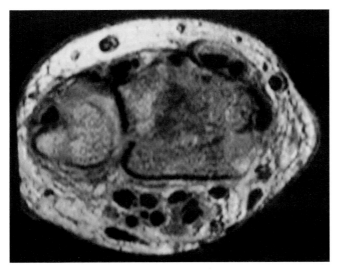

FIG. 16. Axial proton-density-weighted image shows an intra-articular fracture to the distal radioulnar articulation with extensor tendon posttraumatic tenosynovitis, particularly involving the abductor and opponens pollicis tendons.

Trauma most frequently results in a traumatic synovitis with peritendinous fluid; less often results in an acute tear and rupture (44).

Extensor Carpi Ulnaris Syndrome

Extensor carpi ulnaris tenosynovitis usually complicates chronic occupational overuse, presenting as ulnar-sided wrist pain mimicking TFC tear in chronicity commonly accompanying TFC tear. At MR imaging, the tendon sheath is noted to be thickened, associated with peritendinous hyperintense fluid on T2-weighted sequences. In chronicity, foci of mineralization within the tendon are often noted to be hyperintense. Extension of chronic synovitis at the level of the radiocarpal articulation often leads to TFC degeneration in chronicity (Fig. 17) (45).

First Extensor Compartment Syndrome: De Quervain's Tenosynovitis

Repetitive wrist flexion and extension, particularly repetitive extension of the thumb, may promote chronic tenosynovitis within the first dorsal compartment or fibro-osseous tunnel at the level of the radial styloid surrounding the extensor pollicis brevis and abductor pollicis longus tendons. At MR imaging, there is focal peritendinous fluid and apparent soft tissue thickening. Changes are noted to resolve following immobilization and treatment with anti-inflammatories (46).

Flexor Carpi Radialis Syndrome

Within the carpal tunnel, the flexor carpi radialis is separated from other tendons by a thick septum. Being closely

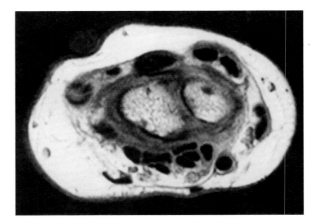

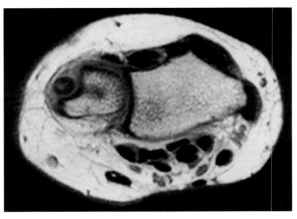

FIG. 17. Axial TSE T1-weighted images show swelling and signal abnormality within the extensor carpi ulnaris tendon secondary to chronic tenosynovitis.

apposed to the scaphoid and its articulations, the flexor carpi radialis tendon is occasionally injured following fracture of the scaphoid in addition to fracture of the distal radius (47).

OSSEOUS INJURY FOLLOWING ACUTE TRAUMA TO THE HAND AND WRIST

Fractures of the Distal Radius

Fractures of the distal radius account for one-sixth of all fractures seen in the emergency room. They are a significant cause of patient morbidity and result in a significant loss of industrial manpower hours. In most cases, fractures heal following simple cast fixation. Surgical fixation is undertaken when external manipulation fails to restore alignment or when extension of fracture to an articular surface is associated with a significant step-off, greater than 2 mm (48).

Posteroanterior, lateral, and oblique conventional radiographs allow accurate evaluation of bony alignment and angulation in most cases. However, as a composite representation, conventional radiographs often fail to detect subtle articular margin step-off and hence limit detailed surgical planning. When diagnostic uncertainty persists or operative fixation is planned, computed tomography in direct sagittal and coronal 2-mm planes is currently most frequently employed to evaluate articular margins and fracture fragment position and number (49,50). Although favored by orthopedic colleagues, neither modality facilitates evaluation of concomitant soft tissue injury, and hence, when undertaken following such imaging, surgical intervention aims to restore osseous integrity alone.

Reviewing impact of soft tissues, Cooney et al. (51) reported complications including median nerve dysfunction, tendon and ligament rupture, carpal instability, avascular necrosis, and radiocarpal and distal radioulnar joint arthritis in 31% in a large retrospective series of 565 patients with fractures of the distal radius (52). Trumble et al. (53) analyzed functional outcome in patients following displaced intra-articular distal radial fractures and found that, despite restoration of anatomic alignment and articular congruity, grip strength averaged only 69%, and range of movement 75%, of that of the opposite side following fracture of the distal radius. While recognizing that restoration of skeletal integrity is crucial, several authors believe that associated soft tissue injuries may explain why such patients continue to have reduced grip strength, reduced range of movement, and pain despite anatomically healed fractures (54,55).

Geissler et al. (56), in a prospective arthroscopic study, examined 60 patients with displaced intra-articular distal radial fractures and found that 41 patients (68%) had associated injuries to soft tissues.

Classification

Traditional classifications of fractures of the distal radius are based on early clinical descriptions by Colles in 1814, Barton in 1838, and Smith in 1854 (57–59).

Colles described the most common fractures of the distal radius characterized by fracture through the distal radial metaphysis within 2 cm of the distal articular surface associated with dorsal angulation and displacement and radial angulation and shortening, often associated with fracture of the ulnar styloid, thought to be secondary to TFC avulsion or traction effect.

Smith described fracture of the distal radius with volar angulation with or without intra-articular extension.

Barton described a fracture of the dorsal rim of the distal radius with radiocarpal subluxation and fracture of the volar rim of the distal radius (reverse Barton) with radiocarpal subluxation.

Two further types of fracture are commonly specifically described.

Chauffeur's fracture (Hutchinson's fracture) describes an intra-articular fracture through the base of the radial styloid, often associated with disruption of the scapholunate ligament or scaphoid fractures.

Die punch fracture describes an isolated intra-articular fracture through the lunate facet with variable degrees of displacement, depression, and comminution.

Although these observations are of value, attempts to de-

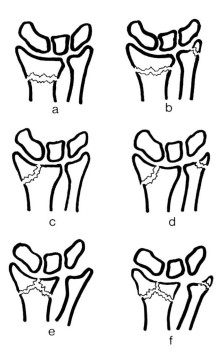

FIG. 18. Modified Frykman classification of distal radial fractures: **a,** extra-articular fracture of the distal radius; **b,** extra-articular fracture of the distal radius with a fracture of the ulnar styloid; **c,** intra-articular fracture to the radiocarpal joint; **d,** intra-articular fracture to radiocarpal joint with a fracture of the ulnar styloid; **e,** comminuted intra-articular fracture to the radiocarpal and radioulnar joints; **f,** intra-articular fracture to the radiocarpal and radioulnar joints with fracture of the ulnar styloid.

fine an approach to management led to the evolution of several complex classifications, including those described by Frykman (most frequently employed) (Fig. 18) (60) and by Mayo and Melone (61). A universal classification has been proposed by Rockwood and Green (62). According to this classification, type 1 fractures are nondisplaced and stable; type 2 fractures are displaced and unstable. In contrast, intra-articular fractures are classified as type 3, undisplaced, and type 4, displaced. Type 4 displaced fractures are further classified as (a) reducible stable, (b) reducible unstable, and (c) complex irreducible. Under this classification, instability is defined as more than 20° of dorsal angulation, marked dorsal comminution, and radial shortening of 10 mm or more. Primary external fixation is recommended for all universal type 3 and 4 fractures (except 4c). Percutaneous pinning is recommended to restore articular integrity in type 2, 3, and 4a fractures. Open reduction is recommended in intra-articular fractures with more than 2 mm distraction; bone graft reconstruction is recommended when there is more than 5 mm residual impaction following attempted restoration of alignment.

Magnetic Resonance Imaging in Distal Radial Fractures

Traditionally radiologists have advocated the use of computed tomography to supplement conventional radiographic evaluation of fractures on the premise that 2-mm slices afford improved spatial resolution and hence evaluation of both fragment position and articular margin integrity. Multiplanar thin-slice imaging afforded by MRI represents an alternative to CT, providing equivalent evaluation of bone (Fig. 19). When undertaken for this purpose, fast field- or gradient-echo sequences should be interpreted with caution, as associated susceptibility effects may lead to obscuring of fractures, particularly in patients with osteoporosis (see Fig. 19).

Previous studies have emphasized the limitations of conventional radiographs in evaluating osseous injury, empha-

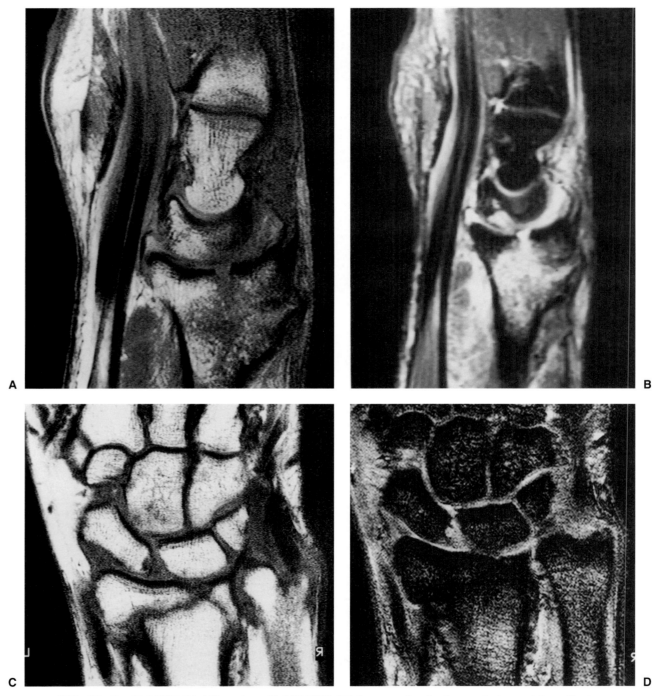

FIG. 19. Sagittal TSE T1 **(A)** and sagittal IR TSE **(B)** images clearly demonstrate an intra-articular fracture of the distal radius with minimal distraction of fragment and with billowing of volar and dorsal radiocarpal ligaments within joint fluid. Coronal TSE T1-weighted image **(C)** shows a healing fracture of the distal radius, which is not identified on the fast field-echo (gradient-echo) image as a result of susceptibility artifact **(D)**. With permission from ref. 64.

sizing the need for additional imaging. Doczi et al. (63) found that conventional radiographs failed to detect 39 out of 626 fractures of the distal radius at the first examination. In our own study (64), comparing radiographs and MR imaging in 21 patients, MR imaging afforded either equivalent or improved osseous evaluation in each of the 21 patients. Imaging in contiguous 3-mm thin slices allowed detection of radiocarpal extension in three patients on MRI alone, in each case leading to surgical intervention and fixation. Distal radioulnar joint extension was identified in a further three patients not recognized despite retrospective review of conventional radiographs. Surgical intervention was undertaken in five of the 21 patients following MR imaging in whom conservative management had initially been planned following review of conventional radiographs (three intra-articular fractures, one scapholunate ligament disruption, one tear of triangular fibrocartilage). Although it would be inappropriate to define indications for MR imaging of distal radial fractures on the basis of this experience in a small group of patients, it is clear that, when employed, MR imaging frequently improves interpretation of the extent of the underlying injury.

As found by Geissler et al. using MRI, it is clear that soft tissue injury frequently accompanies distal radial fractures. It is recognized that conventional radiographs allow the detection of scapholunate ligament disruption in most cases on the basis of well-described radiographic signs (widening of the scapholunate interspace more than 4 mm, volar tilt of the scaphoid, dorsal tilt of the lunate); nevertheless, it is only using MRI that direct visualization of the soft tissue injury may be achieved. Scapholunate ligament rupture has been identified in almost a third of patients referred for MR imaging with distal radial fractures in our institution (Figs. 20–22). According to the mechanism of injury postulated by Mudgal and Jones (65) (as the lunate is driven proximally, a shearing stress is imposed on the scapholunate ligament), scapholunate ligament disruption is commonly identified in patients with intra-articular fractures extending to the junction of the radial and lunate facets (Fig. 23). When identified, the scapholunate ligament is frequently avulsed from its scaphoid rather than its lunate insertion.

Injuries to the triangular fibrocartilage complex (TFCC) are relatively common in patients with distal radial fractures with reported rates of 45% to 66% (53–55). Unlike ligamentous disruption, conventional radiographic evaluation of the TFCC is unhelpful unless there is either wide diastasis or dislocation at the distal radioulnar joint, and its evaluation can therefore be achieved only by arthrography, arthroscopy, or MRI (66,67).

In contrast to published data, we have not observed disruption of the TFC in patients with fracture of the ulnar styloid, even when it is displaced (Figs. 24 and 25). More often, TFC tear appears to accompany complex intra-articular impaction fractures.

Although it is a source of controversy at the time of this writing, many believe that combined primary repair of both osseous and soft tissue components of distal radial fractures is likely to reduce the prevalence of morbidity following this injury.

Soft Tissue Complications of Fractures of the Distal Radius

Scapholunate Ligament Disruption
Lunatotriquetral Ligament Disruption
Triangular Fibrocartilage and Associated Ligaments Tear
Median Nerve Compression
Extrinsic Volar and Dorsal Radiocarpal Ligament Tear
Flexor and Extensor Tendon Injury
(68—70)

Median Nerve Injury

Median nerve injury commonly accompanies distal radial fractures secondary either to the tension of forceful hyperextension or to direct impaction by fracture fragment in forced flexion injury, Smith's fracture.

Chronic median neuropathy was identified in 23% in 536 patients with fractures of the distal radius in one study (51). Median neuropathy is also identified in patients with acute and chronic DISI, with compression of carpal tunnel structures by the body of the lunate, which displaces volarly as it angulates dorsally (such an injury is often occupationally acquired or the sequel to recreational overuse as occurs in oarsmen) (Fig. 26).

Compression of the median nerve, carpal tunnel syndrome, has been extensively studied using MRI. Neuropathy is accompanied by swelling of the median nerve, best evaluated at the level of the pisiform, by flattening of the median nerve, best evaluated at the level of the hamate, and by increased signal within the nerve on T2-weighted images and volar bulging of the retinaculum (71).

Posttraumatic Epiphysiolysis

Although fracture of the distal radius is frequently identified in childhood, long-term impact differs and necessitates the use of the Salter Harris classification. In addition to direct trauma, injury to the developing growth plate may follow repetitive minor trauma such as occurs to the radial and ulnar epiphyses in adolescent gymnasts. Repeated minor trauma may lead to physeal widening, metaphyseal irregularity, and sclerosis without epiphyseal displacement, which is usually reversible by removing the stressor.

Magnetic resonance imaging has been used in these patients and allows earlier and more detailed evaluation of the growth plate. Similar to radiographs, MR images show irregularity of the growth plate with periarticular marrow edema reflecting chronic stress and microtrabecular trauma (Fig. 27) (72).

Distal Radioulnar Joint Injury

Distal radioulnar joint (DRUJ) injury may follow either pronation or supination injury, accompanying fracture of the

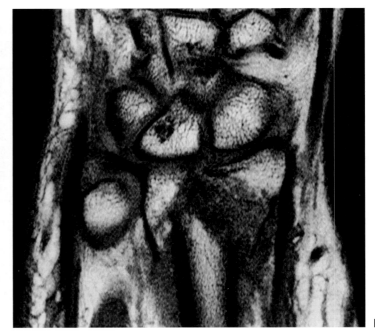

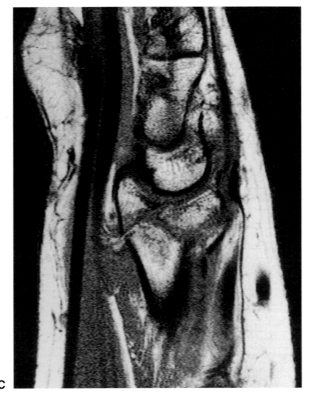

FIG. 20. (A) Radiograph shows an intra-articular fracture to the radiocarpal and the radioulnar articulations. **(B)** Tomographic-type image at MRI shows more marked displacement of bone fragment at the radioulnar articulation **(C)** with 5° of dorsal tilt in the sagittal plane.

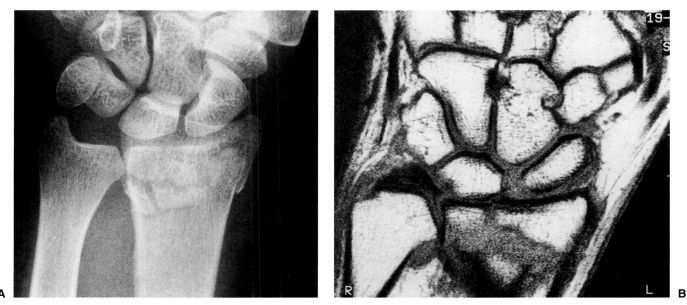

FIG. 21. (A) Radiograph shows a comminuted intra-articular impaction fracture. **(B)** Magnetic resonance image shows intra-articular fracture with scapholunate ligament disruption.

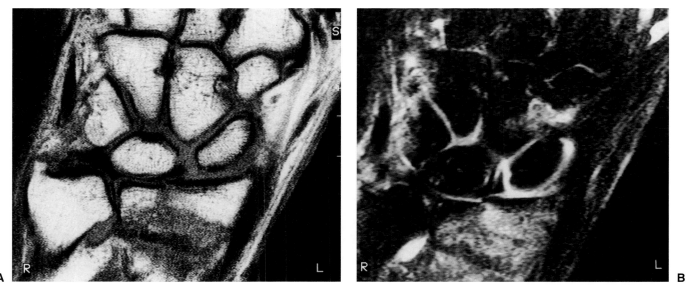

FIG. 22. (A) Coronal TSE T1- and **(B)** IR TSE-weighted images show distal radial fracture with intra-articular extension to the radiocarpal articulation and avulsion of the scapholunate ligament from the proximal pole of the scaphoid. With permission from ref. 64.

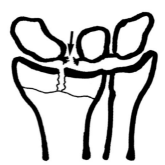

FIG. 23. Diagram shows intra-articular fracture to the junction of the lunate and radial facets of the distal radius with secondary shear forces through the scapholunate ligament *(arrow)*.

distal radius or the radial shaft (Galeazzi fracture). Pronation results in disruption of the dorsal radioulnar ligament, whereas supination results in disruption of the volar radioulnar ligament.

Although subluxation may be evident on conventional radiographs, positional instability may be detected using MRI by reviewing axial images acquired in pronation, neutral position, and supination and by reviewing the relationship of the distal ulna to the sigmoid notch (73).

Scaphoid Fractures

The scaphoid bone is the second most commonly fractured bone of the wrist, typically complicating a fall on a dorsiflexed hand. Undisplaced fractures heal without complication in up to 95% of cases. Displaced fractures occur in up to 30% of cases, and when displacement is greater than 1

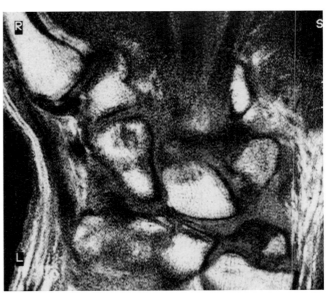

FIG. 25. Coronal TSE T1-weighted image shows a displaced ulnar styloid fracture with an intact triangular fibrocartilage.

mm, approximately 50% of cases develop either nonunion, avascular necrosis, or both (74,75).

Fractures are classified by site and orientation into those affecting the proximal pole, the waist, and the distal pole (Fig. 28). Fractures of the distal pole rarely develop either nonunion or avascular necrosis. In contrast, fractures of the proximal pole develop nonunion in almost all cases. Healing of fractures through the midzone or waist is variable. Complications are more common in fractures with displacement or humpback angulation at the fracture margin (75).

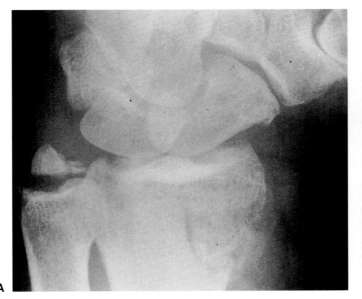

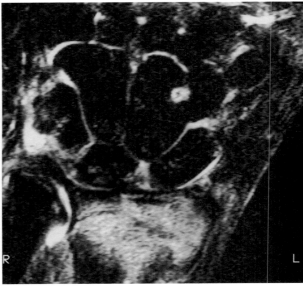

FIG. 24. (A) Radiograph shows a distal radial fracture with associated displaced fracture of the ulnar styloid process. **(B)** Coronal IR TSE image in the same patient shows an intact triangular fibrocartilage. With permission from ref. 64.

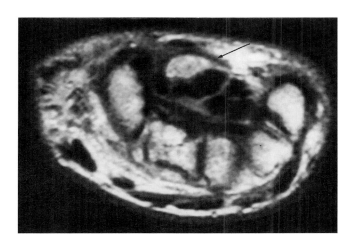

FIG. 26. Axial TSE T2-weighted image shows diffuse swelling and edema within the median nerve (pseudoneuroma, *arrow*) in a professional oarsman with chronic carpal tunnel syndrome. Additional images showed encroachment of the carpal tunnel by the body of a dorsally tilted lunate, complicating scapholunate ligament disruption.

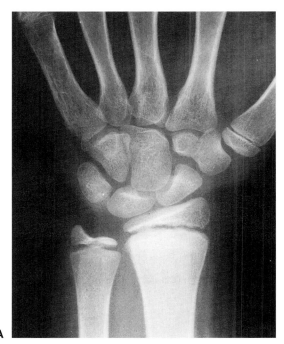

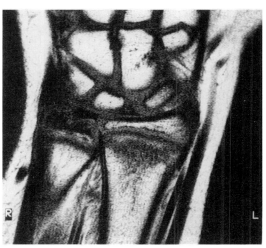

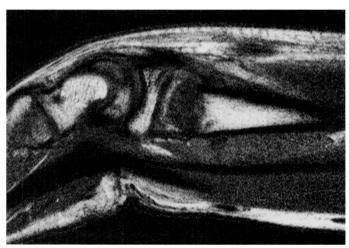

FIG. 27. (A) Radiograph shows increased density of the distal radial metaphysis in a gymnast thought to have presented with chronic epiphysiolysis. The TSE T1-weighted coronal **(B)** and sagittal **(C)** images show a fracture with subtle dorsal tilt and displacement of the distal fragment.

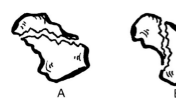 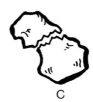

FIG. 28. Diagram shows (A) an oblique, (B) a vertical, and (C) a transverse fracture through the waist of the scaphoid.

Untreated, nonunion results in altered carpal equilibrium and the development of a DISI configuration. As a result, radiocarpal arthritis is commonly identified within 5 years in affected patients, midcarpal arthritis is commonly identified at 5 to 10 years, and generalized arthritis is identified at 20 years (76).

Magnetic Resonance Imaging in Scaphoid Fractures

Magnetic resonance imaging has two specific roles in the evaluation of scaphoid fractures: in the detection of radiographically occult fractures and in the evaluation of vascular integrity.

Occult Fracture Detection

Although many still refer patients with suspected scaphoid fractures for technetium-99m MDP scintigraphy (74), MR imaging presents several advantages. On scintigraphy, fractures are detected only if there is an attempt at bone healing or reactive marginal osteoblastic activity with secretion of hydroxyapatite. In health, healing response is often delayed to 48 hr, and in the elderly, the response may be delayed as long as a week. In effect, by scintigraphy, a result may not be obtained at the time of injury. Similarly, on scintigraphy, uptake by overlying inflamed soft tissues may be misleading and generate inaccuracy (75).

In contrast, MR imaging using a single turboSTIR sequence may be performed in 1 min 30 sec and allow definitive immediate diagnosis (77,78). Absent marrow edema confirms normality. In patients in whom edema is identified, anatomic information is obtained by performing a single coronal turbo spin-echo T1-weighted sequence (Fig. 29). Of interest, using MRI, it is apparent that despite clinical anxiety based on snuff-box tenderness, an occult fracture will be identified in only a minority.

Because cost of MRI is a function of scan time, dedicated MR scaphoid studies are considerably cheaper than scintigraphy, allow immediate diagnosis, and therefore reduce patient morbidity (75,77,79). With echo-planar-based inversion recovery, both single and multishot technique, diagnosis may now be made in less than 10 sec.

Vascular Integrity of Fracture Fragments

There are three patterns of blood supply to the carpal bones. Single vessels supply the scaphoid, capitate, and lu-

nate in 20%. The trapezium, triquetrum, and pisiform and 80% of the lunate receive nutrient arteries through two nonarticular surfaces with a consistent intraosseous anastomosis. The trapezoid and hamate lack an intraosseous anastomosis and after fracture are at risk of ischemic necrosis (80,81).

The proximal 70% to 80% of the scaphoid is supplied by the dorsal branch of the radial artery. Disruption of this vessel invariably occurs in fracture through the proximal pole and occasionally in fracture through the waist, resulting in ischemic necrosis (atraumatic interruption of vascular supply to the proximal pole is termed Preiser's disease). The tuberosity and distal pole are supplied by the volar branches, rarely interrupted by fracture (82).

Following fracture, a relative increase in density is identified in the ischemic portion between 4 and 8 weeks. Such a change is readily manifest at MR, with loss of normal marrow signal and replacement by signal hypointensity on both T1- and T2-weighted sequences (Fig. 30) (82). Dynamic imaging with gadolinium bolus tracking may be used in patients in whom loss of vascular integrity is suspected before loss of normal marrow signal. For this purpose we use a dynamic gradient or fast field-echo fat-saturated T1-weighted keyhole sequence. With this sequence, vascular enhancement may be both visually and graphically mapped through both fracture fragments (Fig. 31). Although acute fragment ischemia is common, evaluation of vascular integrity at 6 weeks is a useful marker of ultimate patient outcome. A similar protocol is employed in patients with chronic nonunion in an attempt to triage them into groups in whom graft and Herbert screw fixation is attempted and those in whom resection of the proximal vascular fragment is undertaken (83).

Lunate Fractures and Kienbock's Disease

Acute trauma to the lunate may manifest as dislocation or rarely fracture. When they occur, fractures may involve the palmar or dorsal surfaces or extend through the body (84). Although often clearly identified on both frontal and lateral radiographs, fractures are often best evaluated by tomographic sections; in this regard, both coronal and sagittal turbo spin-echo T1-weighted images are of considerable value.

Because the lunate is poorly vascularized, ischemic necrosis may complicate fractures, particularly those extending through body and proximal pole (85). Ischemia may also follow repetitive minor trauma, enhanced by increased lunate axial loading induced by a short ulnar (negative ulnar variance), termed Kienbock's disease. This entity most frequently occurs in young male manual laborers, affects the dominant hand, and is most frequently unilateral (86).

At MR imaging, Kienbock's disease is staged according to pattern and extent of signal changes. In stage 1 disease, focal signal changes are observed, hypointense on T1- and hyperintense on T2-weighted images. In stage 2 disease, signal changes progress to involve the entire lunate. In stage 3

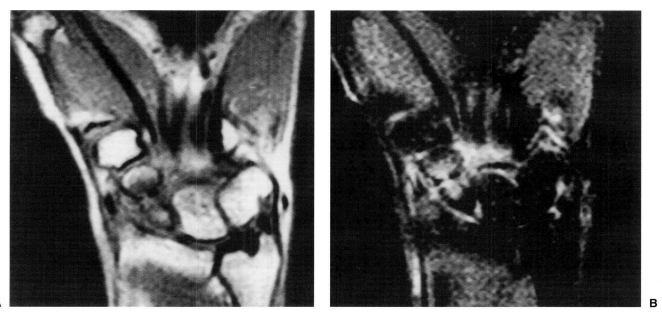

FIG. 29. Coronal T1 **(A)** and inversion recovery **(B)** images show a transverse fracture through the waist of the scaphoid. (Courtesy of Lunar Artoscan, Madison WI.)

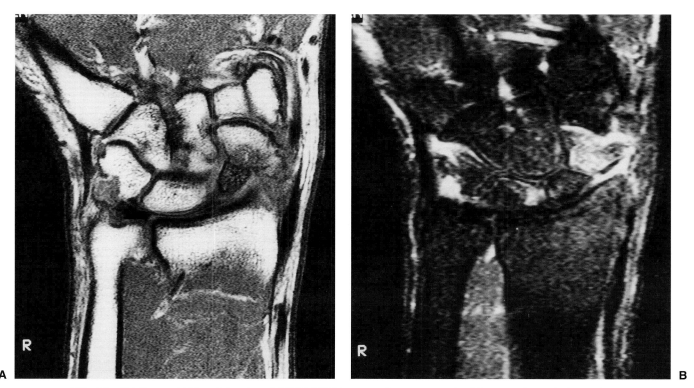

FIG. 30. (A) Coronal T1-weighted and **(B)** IR TSE images show an ununited fracture through the waist of the scaphoid with avascular necrosis of the proximal fragment, with characteristic signal hypointensity secondary to infarction. Note extensive edema within the distal fragment on fat-suppressed image secondary to abnormal motion and impaction.

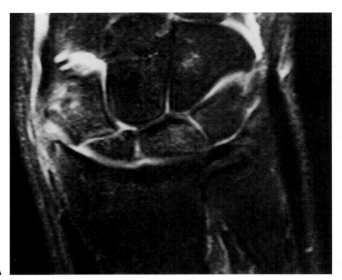
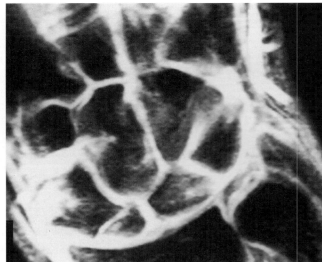

FIG. 31. (A) Coronal IR TSE image shows an ununited scaphoid fracture. **(B)** T1-weighted fast field-echo, keyhole acquisition shows gadolinium enhancement in the proximal and distal fragments, confirming the presence of vascular integrity.

disease, there is collapse of fragments, and in stage 4 disease, there is complicating osteoarthritis (87–89).

Kienbock's Disease		
Stage 1	Focal T1 Hypointensity, T2 Hyperintensity	Immobilize
Stage 2	Diffuse T1 Hypointensity, T2 Hyperintensity	Ulnar Lengthening
Stage 3	Articular Collapse	Ulnar Lengthening
Stage 4	Osteoarthritis	Excise or Fuse

Triquetral Fractures

Dorsal avulsions of the triquetrum are the second most common fracture of the carpal bones. They arise from an avulsion of the dorsal radiotriquetral ligament in hyperflexion or rarely from an avulsion of the ulnotriquetral ligament with hyperextension. With MRI in the sagittal plane, both inversion recovery and turbo TSE T1-weighted images allow clear identification of dorsal radiotriquetral ligament avulsions (90,91).

Pisiform Fractures

Fractures of the pisiform are rare and most commonly follow a direct blow to the volar ulnar aspect of the wrist. Although they are often identified on the carpal tunnel radiographic projection, injuries are also readily identified in coronal, axial, and sagittal planes at MRI.

Capitate Fractures

Capitate fractures are usually transverse in orientation and extend through the carpal waist and are therefore readily identified on conventional radiographs. Complex intra-articular fractures occasionally accompany fractures through the bases of the third and fourth metacarpals. Occasionally, radiographically occult capitate fractures are identified accompanying impaction fractures of the distal radius at MRI, particularly on fat-suppressed inversion recovery sequences (92).

Hamate Fractures

Hamate fractures are uncommon, but are occasionally identified following motorcycle accidents and in professional cyclists.

Three types of hamate fracture are recognized: sagittal split, fracture of the dorsal articular surface accompanying carpometacarpal fracture dislocation, and fracture of the hook. Hook fractures are best visualized using oblique and carpal tunnel projections. Improved detection is yielded by tomographic imaging using either computed tomography or magnetic resonance. When ulnar neuropathy complicates the injury, MRI allows simultaneous evaluation of structures of Guyon's canal and determination of fragment position to ulnar nerve (Figs. 32 and 33) (93,94).

Guyon's Canal

Guyon's canal is a fibro-osseous canal superficial to the flexor retinaculum, intimately related to both the pisiform and the hook of the hamate. The canal contains the ulnar nerve, artery, and vein. At the level of the hook of hamate, the nerve divides to a superficial palmar branch and a deep motor unit, such that fracture may disrupt either or both branches by direct contusion or persistent compression (95).

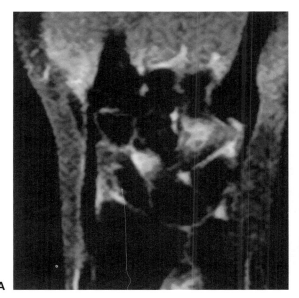

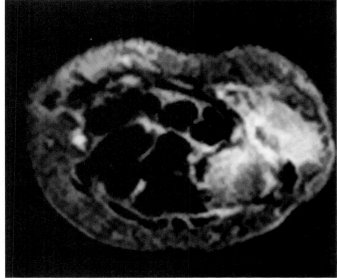

A

B

FIG. 32. Coronal **(A)** and axial **(B)** inversion recovery images show extensive marrow edema in the body and hook of the hamate and edema in the muscles of the hypothenar eminence. (Courtesy of Lunar Artoscan, Madison WI.)

MAGNETIC RESONANCE IMAGING OF ACUTE TRAUMA TO THE HAND

Injury to the Base of the Thumb: Gamekeeper's Thumb

Gamekeeper's thumb derives its name from an injury to the metacarpophalangeal articulation acquired by Scottish gamekeepers attempting to kill rabbits by strangulation. A contemporary term, skier's thumb is now more frequently employed, as it is in this group that the injury is now more frequently recognized.

The injury is characterized by disruption of the ulnar collateral ligament at the base of the thumb, integrity of which

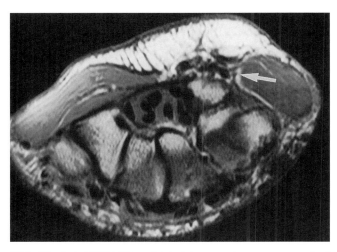

FIG. 33. Axial TSE T1-weighted image shows an ununited fracture of the hook of the hamate with proximity to Guyon's canal and the ulnar nerve *(arrow).*

dictates the ability to successfully appose the thumb and digits. Two forms of injury are recognized: in one, a small ossific fragment is avulsed at the insertion of the ligament (type 1) and is readily identified on radiographs; the second type, which is radiographically occult, is characterized by intrasubstance rupture without avulsion of bone (type 2) (Fig. 34).

Both forms of the injury result in instability; complete rupture is indicated by more than 35° of abduction on stress (96).

In practice, most injuries are now treated conservatively by immobilization within a splint. Surgery is undertaken in a minority. In type 1 injuries, surgery is undertaken when the avulsed fragment is displaced. In this setting, healing can be achieved only by surgically restoring apposition at the site of the avulsion with fragment fixation using hooked K wire. In type 2 injuries, surgery is undertaken when the margins of the torn ulnar collateral ligament are retracted (Stener lesion). Classically, the term Stener lesion is employed only when the proximal portion of the torn ligament is retracted sufficiently to allow the adductor aponeurosis to lie between the torn edges of the collateral ligament. Surgical repair must be undertaken within 3 weeks of injury if successful reconstruction is to be achieved (97).

Successful MR imaging of gamekeeper's thumb requires a dedicated wrist or digital coil allowing a small field of view less than 8 cm, with imaging prescribed off an axial localizer. In such a way, coronal images are prescribed parallel to the volar aspect of the flattened base of the thumb and allow visualization of the ulnar collateral ligament in its entirety. We prefer to image in the coronal plane with T1-weighted turbo spin-echo and turbo inversion recovery sequences; other authors have emphasized the value of T2-

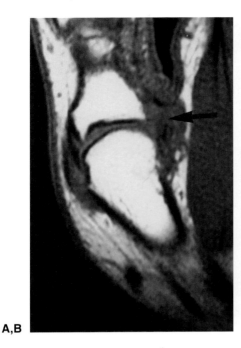 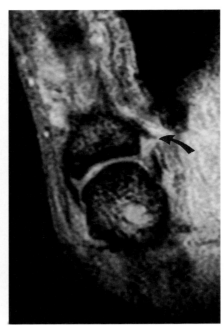

A,B

FIG. 34. Coronal TSE T1 **(A)** and FFE (gradient-echo) **(B)** images show rupture of the ulnar collateral ligament at the first metacarpophalangeal articulation without significant retraction *(arrows).*

weighted images. In the coronal plane, the normal ulnar collateral ligament is band-like and is uniformly hypointense, lying deep to the adductor aponeurosis. Following injury, fluid is noted to bridge the site of the tear. In patients with a Stener lesion, the proximal ligament is noted to be retracted with interposition of lax adductor aponeurosis at the site of tear (98).

Radial collateral ligament injury is considerably less common than injury to the ulnar collateral, and diagnosis is usually late. Affected patients often complain of local tenderness immediately following attempts at opening of a large jar lid or car door.

In suspected cases, radiographs, arthrography, ultrasound, or MR imaging may be employed to confirm diagnosis (96).

Similar collateral ligaments are responsible for radial and volar stability in all the interphalangeal joints and may be imaged using MRI following suspected trauma.

Thumb Dislocation and Proximal Interphalangeal Dislocation

Dorsal dislocation at the proximal interphalangeal (PIP) joint is the most common articular injury in the hand. Dislocation at the base of the thumb is less common, occurring either in isolation or accompanying intra-articular fractures (Bennet, simple intra-articular; Rolando, comminuted intra-articular).

The thumb and phalanges dislocate dorsally more often than volarly. Following dislocation, reduction is often difficult, and when this occurs, interposition of the volar plate or flexor pollicis longus or digitorum tendons should be suspected. Volar dislocation is invariably associated with collat-

eral ligament disruption and interposition of the dorsal capsule to the joint space, impairing reduction (Fig. 35) (99).

Volar Plate Injuries

The volar plate represents the ligamentous thickening of the volar capsule bridging and stabilizing the volar aspect of the interphalangeal and metacarpophalangeal joints. The volar plate is primarily responsible for passive resistance to hyperextension at these articulations, active resistance being provided by contraction of flexor muscle groups.

Volar pain on induced hyperextension with local tenderness suggests the injury, which can be clearly visualized in both passive and stressed sagittal views of the digits using MRI (see Fig. 35).

In symptomatic cases, volar capsulodesis, ligamentous reconstruction, and arthrodesis are occasionally undertaken (99,100).

Sesamoid Injuries

Two sesamoids are identified adjacent to the volar aspect of the metacarpophalangeal joint of the thumb in almost all patients, where they reside within the volar plate. The tendon of the adductor pollicis inserts into the ulnar sesamoid, and the tendon of the flexor pollicis brevis into the radial sesamoid, accounting for loss of tendon function and distraction of fragments following sesamoid injury (101).

Extensor Tendon Injury: Mallet Finger

The term mallet finger is used to describe the flexion deformity of the DIP joint resulting from loss of extensor ten-

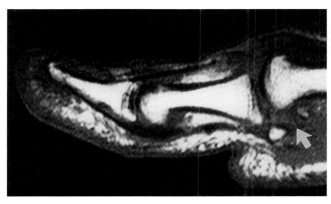

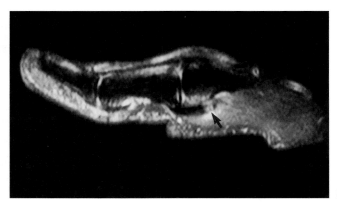

A   B

FIG. 35. Sagittal TSE T1 **(A)** and IR TSE **(B)** images show a volar plate injury at the base of the thumb *(arrows)* complicating a dislocation.

don continuity to the distal phalanx. The term mallet finger of bony origin is used to describe the same deformity occurring secondary to intra-articular fracture of the dorsal lip of the distal phalanx (Fig. 36).

Three patterns of tendon-related mallet finger are recognized and include type 1 injury, resulting from stretching of the ligament, type 2 injury, characterized by rupture of the tendon at its insertion, and type 3 injury, characterized by a subtle avulsion at the site of tendon insertion (102).

When uncertainty exists and surgical repair is contemplated, MR imaging is occasionally used to differentiate between tendon stretching and complete tear. In a cadaver model, authors (103) have previously demonstrated the ability of high-resolution MR to differentiate between different degrees of tendon injury. In practice, conservative management is undertaken if lacerations involve less than 60% of tendon cross-sectional area.

Extensor Tendon Injury: Boutonniere Deformity

Boutonierre deformity or buttonhole deformity is caused by disruption of the central slip of the extensor tendon combined with tearing of the triangular ligament on the dorsum of the middle phalanx, allowing the lateral bands of the extensor tendon to slip below the axis of the PIP articulation.

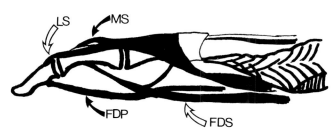

FIG. 36. Diagram of tendon insertions in the phalanges: LS, lateral slip of the extensor digitorum (avulsion results in a mallet finger); MS, middle slip of the extensor digitorum (avulsion results in a boutonniere deformity); FDP, flexor digitorum profundus (avulsion results in jersey finger); FDS, flexor digitorum superficialis.

Although the deformity is clinically apparent, MR imaging allows detailed evaluation of tendon position and integrity, triaging patients into surgical and nonsurgical groups (104).

Flexor Digitorum Profundus Tendon Injury: Jersey Finger

Avulsion of the flexor digitorum profundus tendon from its insertion into the base of the distal phalanx is a relatively uncommon injury, usually occurring during active sports, typically when a football or rugby player attempts to tackle the opposition but ends up grabbing at a handful of jersey, hence the term jersey finger.

Affected patients complain of an inability to flex at the DIP articulation; however, the injury is often overlooked unless specifically sought. Leddy and Packer have identified three patterns of injury. Type 1 injury is characterized by retraction of tendon to the palm, severing all blood supply and necessitating repair within 7 days. In type 2 injury, the tendon retracts to the PIP articulation, where it becomes entangled with the flexor digitorum superficialis. In type 3 injury, a large bony fragment is avulsed and becomes entrapped at the site of the distal pulley. Because of the importance of localizing the position of the avulsed tendon stump before surgical exploration, MR imaging in the sagittal plane is frequently employed in preoperative evaluation of these patients (105).

Soft Tissue Foreign Body Detection

Soft tissue foreign bodies—glass, wood, or plastic—may remain hidden within soft tissues following trauma and account for significant posttraumatic morbidity. Although ultrasound affords rapid and cheap screening, it is a subjective technique, and therefore sensitivity of the technique is extremely variable.

When MR imaging is employed for this purpose, gradient-echo or echo planar sequences should be employed. Lack of

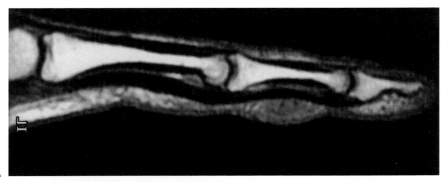

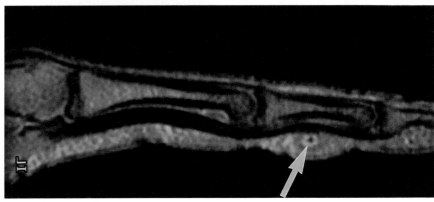

FIG. 37. (A) Sagittal T1-weighted image shows normal flexor digitorum profundus tendon without obvious soft tissue foreign body. **(B)** Sagittal fast field (gradient)-echo image shows susceptibility artifact *(arrow)* at the site of a wood fragment.

a refocusing pulse in both techniques enhances susceptibility differences at the site of the foreign body, dramatically improving visibility (Fig. 37).

REFERENCES

1. Kneeland JB. Technical considerations for MR imaging of the hand and wrist. *Magn Reson Clin North Am* 1995;3:193.
2. Schweitzer ME, Brahme SK, Hodler J, et al. Chronic wrist pain. spin echo and short tau inversion recovery MR imaging and conventional and MR arthrography. *Radiology* 1992;182:205.
3. Gilula LA, Carpal injuries: Analytical approach and case exercises. *Am J Roentgenol* 1979;133:503.
4. Andrews JG, Youm Y. A biomechanical investigation of wrist kinematics. *J Biomech* 1979;12:83.
5. Brumbaugh RB, Crowninshield RD, Blair WF, Andrews JG. An *in vivo* study of normal wrist kinematics. *J Biomech* 1982;104:176.
6. Erdman AG, Mayfield JK, Dorman F, Wallrich M, Dahlof W. Kinematic and kinetic analysis of the human wrist by stereoscopic instrumentation. *J Biomech Eng* 1979;101:124.
7. Linscheid RL. Kinematic considerations of the wrist. *Clin Orthop* 1986;202:27.
8. MacConaill MA. The mechanical anatomy of the carpus and its bearings on some surgical problems. *J Anat* 1941;75:166.
9. Sarrafian SK, Melamed JL, Goshgarian GM. Study of wrist motion in flexion and extension. *Clin Orthop* 1977;126:153.
10. Mayfield JK. Patterns of injury to carpal ligaments. A spectrum. *Clin Orthop Rel Res* 1984;187:36–42.
11. Stoller DW, Brody GA. The wrist and hand. In: Stoller D, ed. *Magnetic Resonance Imaging in Orthopaedics and Sports Medicine, 2nd ed.* Philadelphia: Lippincott–Raven, 1997;901–915.
12. Bogumill GP. *Anatomy of the Wrist.* Philadelphia: WB Saunders, 1988;14.
13. Taleisnik J. The ligaments of the wrist. *J Hand Surg* 1976;1:110.
14. Mayfield JK, Johnson RP, Kilcoyne RK. The ligaments of the human wrist and their functional significance. *Anat Rec* 1976;186:417.
15. Green DP. Dislocations and ligamentous injuries of the wrist. In: *Surgery of the Musculoskeletal System, 2nd ed, vol 1.* New York: Churchill Livingstone, 1990;449.
16. Johnson RP. The acutely injured wrist and its residuals. *Clin Orthop* 1980;149:33.
17. Linscheid RL, Dobyns JH, Beckenbaugh RD, Cooney WP, Wood MB. Instability patterns of the wrist. *J Hand Surg* 1983;8:682.
18. Sennwald G. *The Wrist, Anatomical and Pathophysiological Approach to Diagnosis and Treatment.* Berlin: Springer Verlag, 1987.
19. Smith DK. Scapholunate interosseous ligament of the wrist: MR appearances in asymptomatic volunteers and arthrographically normal wrists. *Radiology* 1994;192:217–221.
20. Berger RA, Blair WF, Crowninshield RD, Flatt AE. The scapholunate ligament. *J Hand Surg* 1982;7:87.
21. Linscheid RL, Dobyns JH, Beabout JW, Bryan RS. Traumatic instability of the wrist: diagnosis, classification and pathomechanics. *J Bone Joint Surg [Am]* 1972;54:1612–1632.
22. Ruby LK. Carpal instability. *J Bone Joint Surg [Am]* 1995;77:476.
23. Romginer MB, Bernreuter WK, Kenney PJ, Lee DH. MR imaging of anatomy and tears of wrist ligaments. *Radiographics* 1993;13:1233–1246.
24. Timins ME, Jahnke JP, Krah SF, et al. MR imaging of the major carpal stabilizing ligaments: normal anatomy and clinical examples. *Radiographics* 1995;15:575–587.
25. Herbert TJ, Faithfull RG, McCann DJ, Ireland J. Bilateral arthrography of the wrist. *J Hand Surg* 1990;15B:233–235.
26. Lavernia CJ, Cohen MS, Taleisnik J. Treatment of scapholunate dissociation by ligamentous repair and capsulodesis. *J Hand Surg* 1992;17:354–359.
27. Blatt G. Capsulodesis in reconstructive hand surgery: Dorsal capsulodesis for the unstable scaphoid and volar capsulodesis following excision of the distal ulna. *Hand Clin* 1987;3:81.
28. Augsburger S, Necking L, Horton J, Bach AW, Tencer AF. A comparison of scaphoid–trapezium–trapezoid fusion and four bone tendon weave for scapholunate dissociation. *J Hand Surg* 1992;17:360–369.
29. Smith DK. Lunatotriquetral interosseous ligament of the wrist: MR appearances in asymptomatic volunteers and arthrographically normal wrists. *Radiology* 1994;191:199–202.
30. Viegas SF, Patterson RM, Hokanson JA, Davis J. Wrist anatomy: Incidence, distribution, and correlation of anatomic variations, tears, and arthrosis. *J Hand Surg* 1993;18:463–475.

31. Tirman RM, Weber ER, Snyder LL, Koonce TW. Midcarpal wrist arthrography for detection of tears of the scapholunate and lunatotriquetral ligaments. *Am J Roentgenol* 1985;144:107–108.

32. Zlatkin MB, Chao PC, Osterman AL, Schnall MD, Dalinka MK, Kressel HY. Chronic wrist pain: evaluation with high resolution MR imaging. *Radiology* 1989;173:723–729.

33. Binkovitz lA, Ehman RL, Cahill DR, Berquist TH: Magnetic resonance imaging of the wrist. *Radiographics* 1988;8:1171.

34. Palmer AK, Werner FW. The triangular fibrocartilage complex of the wrist: anatomy and function. *J Hand Surg* 1981;6A:153.

35. Totterman SM, Miller RJ. MR imaging of triangular fibrocartilage complex. *Magn Reson Clin North Am* 1995;3:213.

36. Totterman SM, Miller RJ. Triangular fibrocartilage complex: Normal appearances on coronal three dimensional gradient recalled echo MR images. *Radiology* 1995;195:521–527.

37. Kang HS, Kindynis P, Brahme SK, et al. Triangular fibrocartilage in asymptomatic subjects: Investigation of abnormal signal. *Radiology* 1991;181:401.

38. Berger RA, Blair WF, el-Khoury GY. Arthrotomography of the wrist: The triangular fibrocartilage complex. *Clin Orthop* 1983;172:257.

39. Metz VM, Schratter M, Dock WI, et al. Age associated changes of the triangular fibrocartilage of the wrist: Evaluation of the diagnostic performance of MR imaging. *Radiology* 1992;184:217.

40. Oneson SR, Scales LM, Timins ME, et al. MR imaging interpretation of the Palmer classification of triangular fibrocartilage complex lesions. *Radiographics* 1996;16:97.

41. Palmer AK. Triangular fibrocartilage complex lesions: A classification. *J Hand Surg* 1989;14A:594.

42. Palmer AK, Glisson RR, Werner FW, Mech ME. Relationship between ulnar variance and triangular fibrocartilage complex thickness. *J Hand Surg* 1984;9A:681.

43. Palmer AK. The distal radioulnar joint. In: Lichtman DM, ed. *The Wrist and Its Disorders*. Philadelphia: WB Saunders, 1988;220–231.

44. Stern PJ. Tendinitis, overuse syndromes and tendon injuries. *Hand Clin* 1990;6:467–476.

45. Klug JD. MR diagnosis of tenosynovitis about the wrist. *Magn Reson Clin North Am* 1995;3:305–312.

46. Glajchen N, Schweitzer ME. MRI features in De Quervain's tenosynovitis of the wrist. *Skeletal Radiol* 1996;25:63.

47. Thorson E, Szabo RM. Common tendinitis problems in the hand and forearm. *Orthop Clin North Am* 1992;23:65.

48. Knirk JL, Jupiter JB. Intraarticular fractures of the distal end of the radius in young adults. *J Bone Joint Surg [Am]* 1986;68:647–659.

49. Johnston GHF, Freidman L, Kriegler JC. Computerized tomographic evaluation of acute distal radial fractures. *J Hand Surg* 1992;17A:738–744.

50. Pruitt DL, Gilula LA, Manske PR, Vannier MW. CT scanning with image reconstruction in the evaluation of distal radius fractures. *J Hand Surg* 1994;19A:720–727.

51. Cooney WP, Dobyns JH, Linscheid RL. Complications of Colles fractures. *J Bone Joint Surg* 1980;62A:613–619.

52. McMurtry RY, Jupiter JB. Fractures of the distal radius. In: Browner B, Jupiter J, Levine A, Trafton P, eds. *Skeletal Trauma*. Philadelphia: WB Saunders, 1991;1063.

53. Trumble TE, Schmitt SR, Vedder NB. Factors affecting functional putcome of displaced intra-articular distal radius fractures. *J Hand Surg* 1994;19A:325.

54. Fontes D, Lenoble E, De Somer B, et al. Lesions ligamentaires associees aux fractures distales du radius. A propos de cinquante-huit arthrographies peroperatoires. *Ann Chir Main* 1992;11:119–125.

55. Mohanti RC, Kar N. Study of triangular fibrocartilage of the wrist joint in Colles fracture. *Injury* 1980;11:321.

56. Geissler WB, Freeland AE, Savoie FH, et al. Intracarpal soft-tissue lesions associated with an intra-articular fracture of the distal end of the radius. *J Bone Joint Surg* 1996;78A(3):357.

57. Colles A. On the fracture of the carpal extremity of the radius. *Edinb Med Surg J* 1814;10:182.

58. Barton JR. Views and treatment of an important injury to the wrist. *Med Examiner* 1838;1:365.

59. Smith RW. *A Treatise on Fractures in the Vicinity of Joints and on Certain Forms of Accidental and Congenital Dislocations*. Dublin: Hodges & Smith, 1854.

60. Frykman G. Fracture of the distal radius including sequelae—shoulder hand syndrome, disturbance in the distal radioulnar joint, and impairmant of nerve function: A clinical and experimental study. *Acta Orthop Scand* 1967;108:1.

61. Melone CP Jr. Open treatment for displaced articular fractures of the distal radius. *Clin Orthop* 1986;202:103.

62. Cooney WP, Linscheid RL, Dobyns JH. Fractures and dislocations of the wrist. In: Rockwood CA, Green DP, Bucholz RW, Heckman JD, eds. *Fractures in Adults*. Philadelphia: Lippincott–Raven, 1996; 745.

63. Doczi J, Renner A. Epidemiology of distal radial fractures in Budapest. A retrospective study of 2,241 cases in 1989. *Acta Orthop Scand* 1994;65:432.

64. Spence L, Savenor A, Eustace S. MR imaging of fractures of the distal radius. *Skeletal Radiol* 1998;27:244–249.

65. Mudgal CS, Jones WA. Scapho-lunate diastasis. A component of fractures of the distal radius. *J Hand Surg* 1990;15B:503.

66. Golimbu CN, Firooznia H, Melone CP, et al. Tears of the triangular fibrocartilage of the wrist: MR imaging. *Radiology* 1989;173:731.

67. Wright TW, Del Charco M, Wheller D. Incidence of ligament lesions and associated degenerative changes in the elderly wrist. *J Hand Surg* 1994;19A:313.

68. Broder H. Rupture of flexor tendons associated with a malunited Colles fracture. *J Bone Joint Surg [Am]* 1954;36:404.

69. Burkhart SS, Wood MB, Linscheid RL. Posttraumatic recurrent subluxation of the extensor carpi ulnaris tendon. *J Hand Surg* 1982;7:1.

70. Atkins RM, Duckworth T, Kanis JA. Algodystrophy following Colles fracture. *J Hand Surg* 1989;14B:161.

71. Mesgarzadeh M, Schneck CD, Bonakdarpour A, et al. Carpal tunnel: MR Imaging. Part 11. Carpal tunnel syndrome. *Radiology* 1989;171: 749.

72. Shih C, Chang CY, Penn IW, Tiu CM, Chang T, Wu JJ. Chronically stressed wrists in adolescent gymnasts: MR imaging appearances. *Radiology* 1995;197:319.

73. Taleisnik J. Clinical and technologic evaluation of ulnar wrist pain. *J Hand Surg* 1988;13A:801.

74. Tiel van Buul MMC, Broekhuizen TH, Van Beek EJR, et al. Choosing a strategy for the diagnostic management of suspected scaphoid fracture: cost effectiveness analysis. *J Nucl Med* 1995;36:45.

75. Munk PL, Lee MJ, Logan PM, et al. Scaphoid bone waist fractures, acute and chronic: imaging with different techniques. *Am J Roentgenol* 1997;168:779.

76. Verdan C. Fractures of the scaphoid. *Surg Clin North Am* 1960;40: 461.

77. Hunter JC, Escobedo EM, Wilson AJ, et al. MR imaging of clinically suspected scaphoid fractures. *Am J Roentgenol* 1997;168:1287.

78. Breitenseher MJ, Metz VM, Gilula LA, et al. Radiographically occult scaphoid fractures: value of MR imaging in detection. *Radiology* 1997;203:245.

79. Thorpe AP, Murray AD, Smith FW, et al. Clinically suspected scaphoid fracture: comparison of magnetic resonance imaging and bone scintigraphy. *Br J Radiol* 1996;51:285.

80. Golimbu CN, Firooznia H, Rafii M. Avascular necrosis of carpal bones. *Magn Reson Imag Clin North Am* 1995;3:281–303.

81. Gelberman RH, Menon J. The vascularity of the scaphoid bone. *J Hand Surg* 1980;5:508–513.

82. Trumble TE. Avascular necrosis after scaphoid fracture: A correlation of magnetic resonance imaging and histology. *J Hand Surg* 1990; 15A:556–564.

83. Eustace S. MR Imaging of acute orthopedic trauma to the extremities. *Radiol Clin North Am* 1997;35:615.

84. Gelberman RH, Bauman TD, Menon J, Akeson WH. The vascularity of the lunate bone and Kienbock's disease. *J Hand Surg* 1980;5A: 272–278.

85. Almquist EE. Kienbock's disease. *Orthop Clin North Am* 1986;17: 461–472.

86. Almquist EE. Kienbock's disease. *Clin Orthop* 1986;202:68–78.

87. Imaeda T, Nakamura R, Miura T, Makino N. Magnetic resonance imaging in Kienbock's disease. *J Hand Surg* 1992;17B:12.

88. Agerholm JC, Goodfellow JW. Avascular necrosis of the lunate bone treated by excision and prosthetic replacement. *J Bone Joint Surg [Br]* 1963;45:110–116.

89. Sowa DT, Holder LE, Patt PG, Weiland AJ. Application of MRI to ischemic necrosis of the lunate. *J Hand Surg* 1989;14A:1008–1016.

90. Bartone NF, Grieco RV. Fractures of the triquetrum. *J Bone Joint Surg [Am]* 1956;38:353.

91. Smith DK, Murray PM. Avulsion fractures of the volar aspect of

triquetral bone of the wrist. A subtle sign of carpal ligament injury. *Am J Roentgenol* 1995;166:609.

92. Adler JM, Shaftan GW. Fractures of the capitate. *J Bone Joint Surg [Am]* 1962;44:1537.

93. Andress MR, Peckar VG. Fracture of the hook of Hamate. *Br J Radiol* 1970;43:141.

94. Boulas HJ, Miler MA. Hook of Hamate fractures: Diagnosis, treatment and complications. *Orthop Rev* 1990;19:518.

95. Zeiss J, Jakab E, Khimji T, Imbriglia J. The ulnar tunnel at the wrist (Guyon's canal): Normal MR anatomy and variants. *Am J Roentgenol* 1992;158:1081.

96. Louis DS, Buckwalter KA. Magnetic resonance imaging of the collateral ligaments of the thumb. *J Hand Surg* 1984;14:739.

97. Stener B. Displacement of the ruptured ulnar collateral ligament of the metacarpo-phalangeal joint of the thumb. *J Bone Joint Surg [Br]* 1962;44:869.

98. Spaeth HJ, Abrams RA, Bock GW, et al. Gamekeeper thumb: differentiation of nondisplaced and displaced tears of the ulnar collateral ligament with MR imaging. *Radiology* 1993;188:553.

99. Kaplan EB. Dorsal dislocation of the metacarpophalangeal joint of the index finger. *J Bone Joint Surg [Am]* 1957;39:1081.

100. Moberg E, Stener B. Injuries to the ligaments of the thumb and fingers. Diagnosis, treatment and prognosis. *Acta Chir Scand* 1953;106:166.

101. Hansen CA, Peterson TH. Fracture of the thumb sesamoid bones. *J Hand Surg* 1987;12A:269.

102. Stark HH, Boyes JH, Wilson JN. Mallet finger. *J Bone Joint Surg [Am]* 1962;44:1061.

103. Rubin DA, Kneeland JB, Kitay GS, Naranja RJ Jr. Flexor tendon tears in the hand: use of MR imaging to diagnose degree of injury in a cadaver model. *Am J Roentgenol* 1996;166:615.

104. Calandruccio JH, Steichen JB. Magnetic resonance imaging for diagnosis of digital flexor tendon rupture after primary repair. *J Hand Surg* 1995;20B:289.

105. Parellada JA, Balkissoon ARA, Hayes CW, Conway WF. Bowstring injury of the flexor tendon pulley system. MR imaging. *Am J Roentgenol* 1996;167:347.

Subject Index